Clinical Haematology

SECOND EDITION

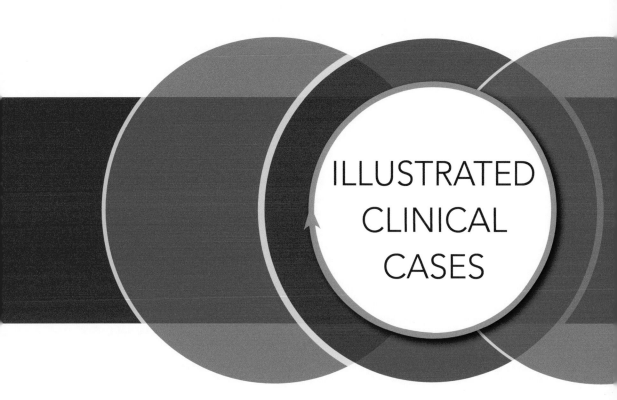

ILLUSTRATED CLINICAL CASES

Clinical Haematology

SECOND EDITION

ATUL B. MEHTA
MA, MD, FRCP, FRCPath
Haemophilia Centre and Thrombosis Unit
Royal Free London NHS Foundation Trust
London, UK

KEITH GOMEZ
MBBS, PhD, MRCP, FRCPath
Haemophilia Centre and Thrombosis Unit
Royal Free London NHS Foundation Trust
London, UK

CRC Press
Taylor & Francis Group
Boca Raton London New York

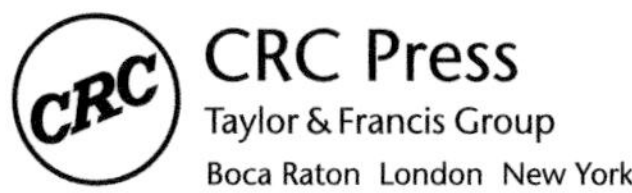

CRC Press is an imprint of the
Taylor & Francis Group, an **informa** business

CRC Press
Taylor & Francis Group
6000 Broken Sound Parkway NW, Suite 300
Boca Raton, FL 33487-2742

Printed on acid-free paper

International Standard Book Number-13: 978-1-4822-4379-6 (Paperback); 978-1-138-63591-3 (Hardback)

Library of Congress Cataloging-in-Publication Data

Names: Mehta, Atul B., author. | Gomez, Keith, author.
Title: Clinical haematology / Atul B. Mehta and Keith Gomez.
Other titles: Self-assessment colour review of clinical haematology | Illustrated clinical cases.
Description: Second edition. | Boca Raton : CRC Press, [2018] | Series:
Illustrated clinical cases | Preceded by Self-assessment colour review of
clinical haematology / Atul B. Mehta. London : Manson Pub., "1995.
Identifiers: LCCN 2016051832| ISBN 9781482243796 (pbk. : alk. paper) | ISBN
9781138635913 (hardback : alk. paper)
Subjects: | MESH: Hematologic Diseases–diagnosis | Hematologic
Diseases–therapy | Case Reports
Classification: LCC RC636 | NLM WH 120 | DDC 616.1/5–dc23
LC record available at https://lccn.loc.gov/2016051832

Visit the Taylor & Francis Web site at
http://www.taylorandfrancis.com

and the CRC Press Web site at
http://www.crcpress.com

Printed and bound in Great Britain by
TJ Books Limited, Padstow, Cornwall

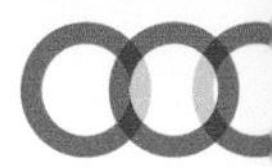

CONTENTS

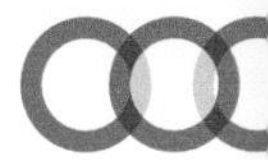

FOREWORD

In his foreword to the first edition of *Clinical Haematology*, Professor Luccio Luzzatto identified the interest in a combined laboratory and clinical specialty as one of the key features that attract young clinicians to haematology. This continues to be the case and it is this interest in interpreting laboratory data relevant to a clinical presentation that haematologists find compelling. This attraction is also evident in clinical laboratory scientists who are likewise drawn to the clinical interface in their roles in data interpretation and quality assurance.

Atul Mehta and Keith Gomez have produced a book which absolutely captures the essence of clinical haematology, using a range of clinical histories illustrated with numerous different forms of diagnostic material, from clinical photographs to photomicrographs of blood and bone marrow, CT, MRI, and PET scans, haemoglobin electrophoresis and HPLC, FACS plots, and platelet aggregation, to mention a few. The book takes us through general and malignant haematology to haemostasis and thrombosis, and finishes with several scenarios related to quality control and quality assurance.

What I really like about this book is the way the cases are presented, such that the reader ends up working through them in a way that replicates the process in real life. I think this book will appeal to trainees in medicine and especially trainees in haematology. There is little doubt that those preparing for exit exams in haematology such as the membership of the Royal College of Pathologists UK, and similar, will find this book helpful. In addition, the book will appeal to clinical scientists, established consultants and specialty grade doctors practising haematology.

I would like to congratulate both authors on their book and hope that their readers enjoy working through the cases as much as I did.

Henry Watson
Chief Examiner for Haematology, Royal College of Pathologists
London, UK
Consultant Haematologist, NHS Grampian
Aberdeen, UK

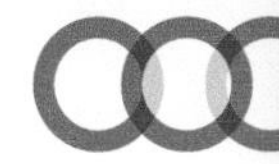

ACKNOWLEDGEMENTS

We wish to acknowledge the help and support of medical and scientific colleagues in the Department of Haematology, Royal Free Hospital and School of Medicine, and in our Medical Illustration Department.

With a Foreword by Dr. Henry Watson
Royal College of Pathologists
London, UK

Atul B. Mehta, MA, MD, FRCP, FRCPath
Keith Gomez, MBBS, PhD, MRCP, FRCPath

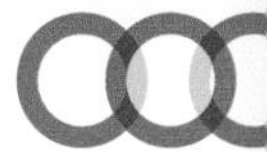

LIST OF ABBREVIATIONS

ABC activated B cell
ACD anaemia of chronic disease
AIHA autoimmune haemolytic anaemia
ALL acute lymphoblastic leukaemia
AML acute myeloid leukemia
ANF anti-nuclear factor
APML acute promyelocytic leukemia
APTT activated partial thromboplastin time
AST aspartate aminotransferase
ATRA all-trans retinoic acid
CALR calreticulin
CBF core binding factor
CLL chronic lymphocytic leukaemia
CMV cytomegalovirus
CNS central nervous system
CT computed tomography
DAT direct anti-globulin
DVT deep vein thrombosis
EBV Epstein–Barr virus
EPO erythropoietin
ERCP endoscopic retrograde cholangiopancreatography
ERT enzyme replacement therapy
ESR erythrocyte sedimentation rate
FAB French–American–British
FDP fibrin degradation product
FFP fresh-frozen plasma
FISH fluorescent in situ hybridization
FLAER fluorescently labeled aerolysin
G6PD glucose-6-phosphate dehydrogenase
GGL chronic granulocytic leukaemia
GGT Gamma-glutamyl transferase
GI gastrointestinal
GP general practitioner
GVHD graft versus host disease
Hb Haemoglobin
HL Hodgkin's lymphoma
HLA human leukocyte antigen
HLH haemophagocytic lymphohistiocytosis
HMWM high-molecular weight multimers
HPA human platelet antigen
HPLC high-performance liquid chromatography
INR international normalised ratio
IPS International Prognostic System
ITP immune thrombocytopenia
IV intravenous
IVIG intravenous immunoglobulin
IVU intravenous urogram
LDH lactate dehydrogenase
MCHC mean corpuscular haemoglobin concentration
MCV mean corpuscular volume
MRI magnetic resonance imaging
NADPH nicotinamide adenine dinucleotide phosphate
NAP neutrophil alkaline phosphatase
NHL non-Hodgkin's lymphoma
PA Pernicious anaemia
PA posteroanterior
PCV packed cell volume
PET positron emission tomography
PNH paroxysmal nocturnal haemoglobinuria
PT prothrombin time
RBC red blood cells
RE reticuloendothelial
RIPA ristocetin-induced platelet aggregation
SRT substrate reduction therapy
TK tyrosine kinase
TNF tumour necrosis factor
TSH thyroid-stimulating hormone
TTP thrombotic thrombocytopenic purpura
VWF von Willebrand factor
WBC white blood cells
WHO World Health Organization

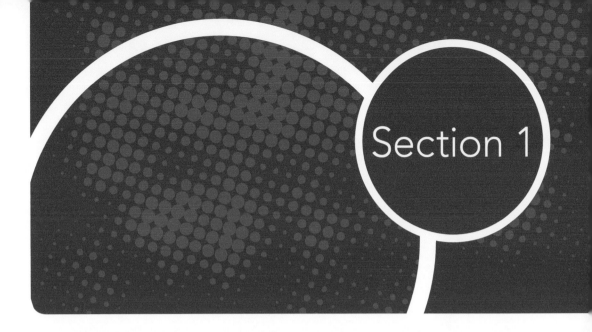

GENERAL AND MALIGNANT HAEMATOLOGY

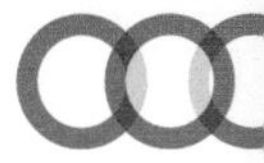

CASE 1

QUESTIONS

A 76-year-old man has a 2-week history of abdominal pain, polyuria and nocturia. He has also noticed a skin nodule which is increasing in size. Investigations show

Haemoglobin (Hb)	71 g/L
White blood cells (WBC)	4.6 × 10^9/L
Platelets	112 × 10^9/L
Urea	46 mmol/L
Creatinine	905 mmol/L
Ca^{2+}	3.60 mmol/L (N 2.1–2.6 mmol/L)
Albumin	26 g/L (N 35–42 g/L)
Total protein	120 g/L (N 65–80 g/L)
Alkaline phosphatase	143 U/L (N 30–130 U/L)
Uric acid	0.48 mmol/L (N 0.3–0.4 mmol/L)

Q1.i Comment on the above results.

Q1.ii Comment on the bone marrow aspirate.

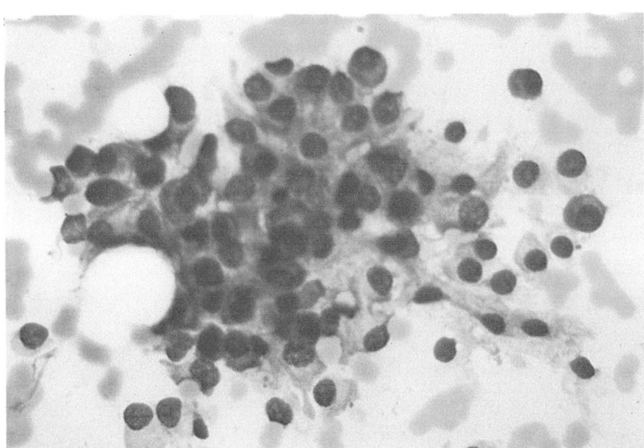

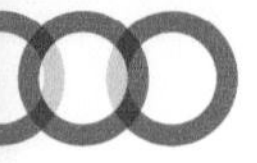

Case 1: ANSWERS

A1.i The results indicate anaemia and thrombocytopenia with marked renal failure. Hypercalcaemia with normal alkaline phosphatase suggests primary bone marrow malignancy. The raised total protein suggests myeloma.

A1.ii The bone marrow is infiltrated by plasma cells, confirming myeloma. Plasma cell leukaemia is an aggressive form of myeloma characterised by large numbers of circulating plasma cells.

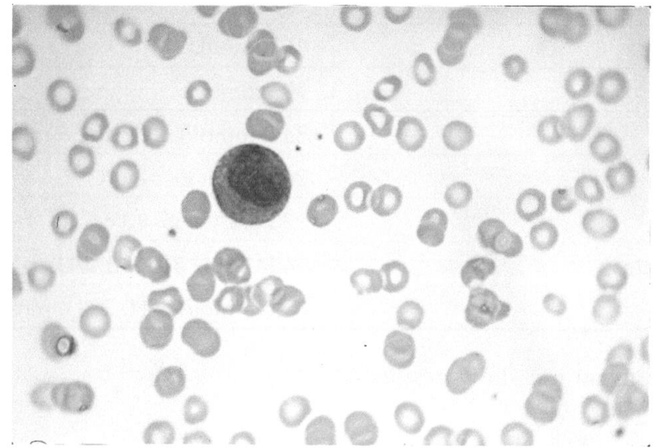

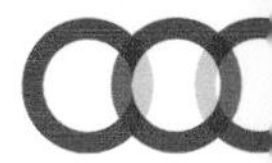

Case 1: QUESTIONS (Continued)

Q1.iii Comment on the aspirate of this patient's skin nodule.

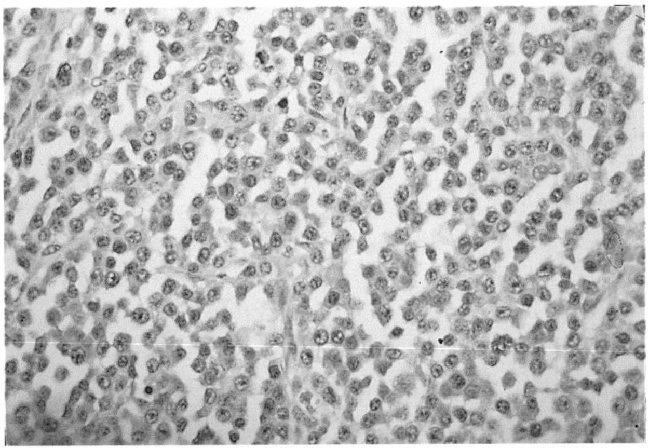

Q1.iv Comment on the skull x-ray.

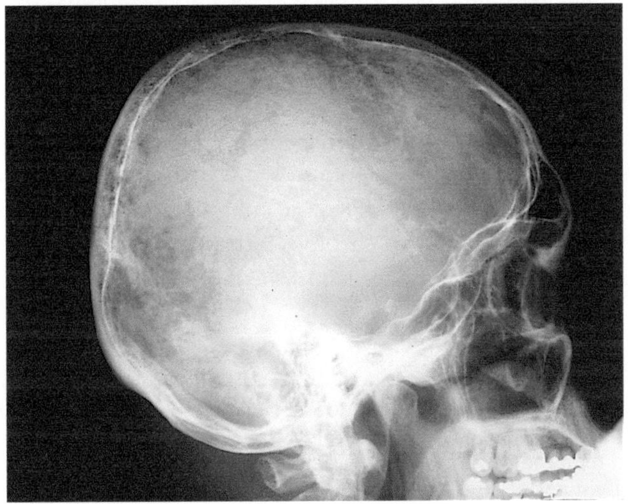

Q1.v What is the diagnosis?

Q1.vi How should he be treated?

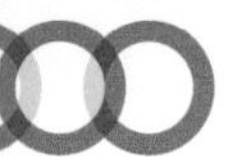

Case 1: ANSWERS (Continued)

A1.iii The skin deposit is also due to myeloma infiltration.

A1.iv The skull x-ray shows multiple lytic lesions, a characteristic finding in myeloma.

A1.v Myeloma.

A1.vi The hypercalcaemia and renal failure require urgent therapy with rehydration to promote diuresis. An intravenous urogram (IVU) should not be done as the patient should not be dehydrated. However, abdominal ultrasound scan to exclude renal obstruction is valuable in acute renal failure.

Baseline tests should include paraprotein quantification in serum and urine (Bence Jones protein), skeletal survey, beta-2 microglobulin and C-reactive protein. Other baseline tests should include a coagulation profile, culture of mid-stream urine and assessment of antibodies to hepatitis A, B and C. Serum-free light chains should be estimated as they are elaborated by the tumour cells and are often the principal cause of the renal toxicity. A renal biopsy should be considered, and the nephrologist will wish to undertake a range of tests to exclude other causes of acute renal impairment. A complete cardiac assessment including echocardiography is important, and the presence of amyloid deposition, for example, in heart and kidneys should be considered. Baseline assessment should also include genetic analysis of the cells by fluorescent in situ hybridization (FISH) and/or chromosome analysis. The International Staging System (ISS) for myeloma is given in the table.

Molecular changes in myeloma

1. Translocations involving immunoglobulin heavy chain (Igh) locus, e.g. t(11;14) (translocation of *CCNDI*), t(4;14) (dysregulation of fibroblast growth Factor III and multiple myeloma SET [*MMSET*] domain)
2. Copy number alterations, e.g. hyperdiploidy, deletion 13, gains of 1q, trisomies, 17p deletion
3. Mutation – e.g. in ERK pathway
4. Methylation modification
5. Late events as markers of clonal progression, e.g. *RAS* activation, *MYC* dysregulation

ERK, extracellular signal-related kinases.

International Staging System

Stage I	Beta-2 microglobulin <5.3 mg/dL, albumin >35 mg/dL
Stage II	Remainder
Stage III	Beta-2 microglobulin >5.5 mg/dL

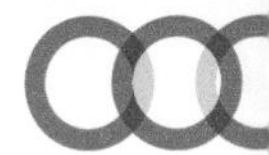

Case 1: ANSWERS (Continued)

Imaging techniques are important for detection of skeletal and neurologic involvement. There is increasing interest in the use of fluorodeoxyglucose (FDG)–positron emission tomography (PET) scans for detection of active myeloma deposits (as opposed to old and possibly healed skeletal deposits) and treatment can be targeted towards resolution of observed abnormalities. Thus, a set of pre- and post-treatment images are recorded as shown in the figure.

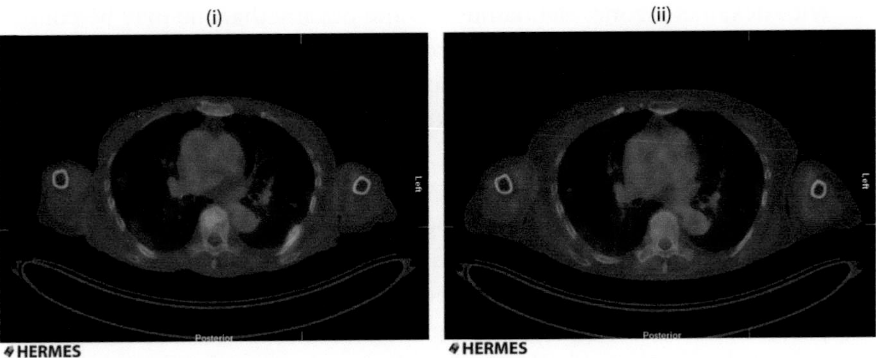

Fluorodeoxyglucose (FDG)–positron emission tomography (PET) scan in myeloma to show active bone disease. (i) Pre-treatment. (ii) Post-treatment.

The patient should receive allopurinol (at a reduced dose of 100 mg/day because of his renal failure) followed by steroid therapy for hypercalcaemia. If the calcium remains elevated, consider bisphosphonates, for example, zoledronic acid or pamidronate, given by intravenous (IV) infusion, dose adjusted for renal impairment. The renal failure may warrant institution of dialysis.

Chemotherapy should be commenced once he is stabilised. Bortezomib is a proteosome inhibitor which is administered subcutaneously alongside dexamethazone. Addition of an anthracycline drug, for example, Adriamycin should be considered; it can be given as an infusional regime with the bortezomib and dexamethazone. There is evidence that intensive early treatment aimed at reducing the tumour burden and the serum level of free light chains may help to restore renal function. Cyclophosphamide may be added as a weekly bolus; it is preferred in renal failure, as it is metabolised by the liver. Thalidomide is an immunomodulatory agent which also has direct anti-myeloma effects; side effects include drowsiness, constipation, neuropathy and a critical need to avoid pregnancy (self or partner). A stable ('plateau') phase of the disease is typically achieved after four to six cycles of chemotherapy. Long-term bisphosphonate therapy (e.g. sodium clodronate) may slow progress of skeletal disease in myeloma. The typical course of myeloma is that patients relapse but will respond to reinstitution of chemotherapy. Thalidomide derivatives include lenalidomide, which has an

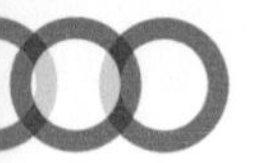

increasing role as a first-line agent as it has greater activity than thalidomide and less neurotoxicity and it is also less likely to provoke thrombosis. Pomalidomide is a derivative that has activity in subjects who are resistant to lenalidomide. Other options include melphalan and (intermittent oral) prednisolone (+/− thalidomide); further courses of bortezomib or its newer derivatives (e.g. carfilzomib, a newly licensed proteosome inhibitor with less neurotoxicity than bortezomib; or ixazomib, which can be given orally) with dexamethazone. Bendamustine and dexamethazone may be considered. Older regimes which may have a role in relapsed patients include vincristine, adriamycin, both by IV infusion, and dexamethasone (VAD), and the combination of idarubicin and dexamethazone.

Younger patients (those under 65) with myeloma may benefit from intensive therapy, including autologous transplant of peripheral blood stem cells. Patients under 50 who have a human leukocyte antigen (HLA)-matching sibling may be considered for allogeneic haemopoietic stem cell transplantation, though this has a greater toxicity and lesser efficacy than in acute leukaemia and relapsed lymphoma. A monoclonal antibody with specificity against CD38 has been recently licensed and has activity both as a single agent and in combination with pomalidomide.

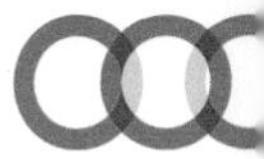

CASE 2

QUESTIONS

A 42-year-old woman gives a 2–3 month history of abdominal pain, diarrhoea and rectal bleeding. She passes blood-stained motions four to six times each day. She has also developed progressive tiredness and loss of appetite. On examination she is pale. There is no lymphadenopathy. She has mild generalised abdominal tenderness, but there is no organomegaly. Her blood count shows

Haemoglobin (Hb)	84 g/L
Mean corpuscular volume (MCV)	110 fL
White blood cells (WBC)	3.1×10^9/L
Platelets	80×10^9/L

Biochemistry is normal, but the erythrocyte sedimentation rate (ESR) is raised at 86 mm/h.

Q2.i What diagnosis is suggested by the barium meal and follow-through (Figure 2a)?

Q2.ii What abnormalities are seen in her bone marrow aspirate (Figures 2b through 2d)? What is the diagnosis?

Q2.iii What further investigations would you perform?

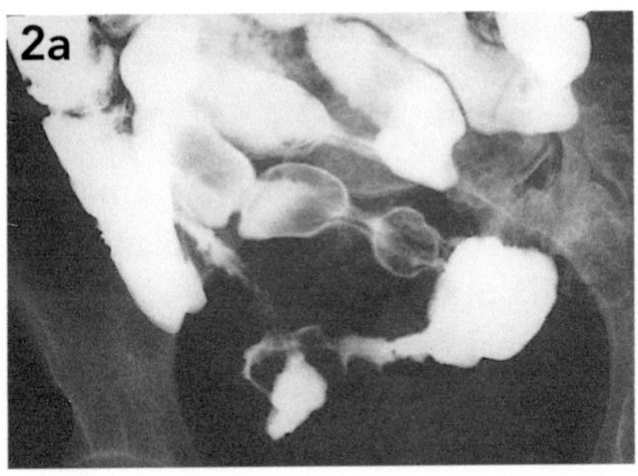
2a

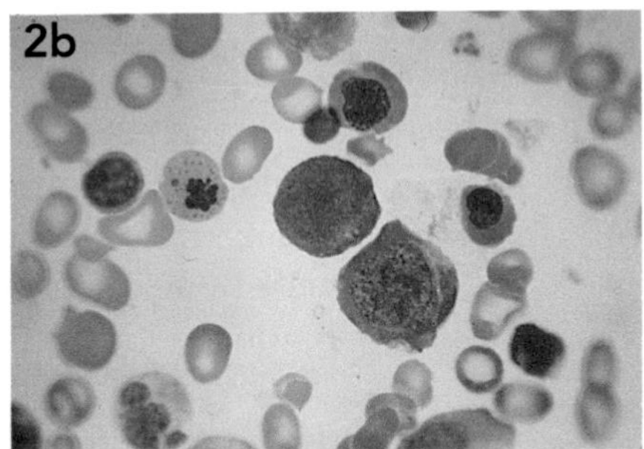
2b

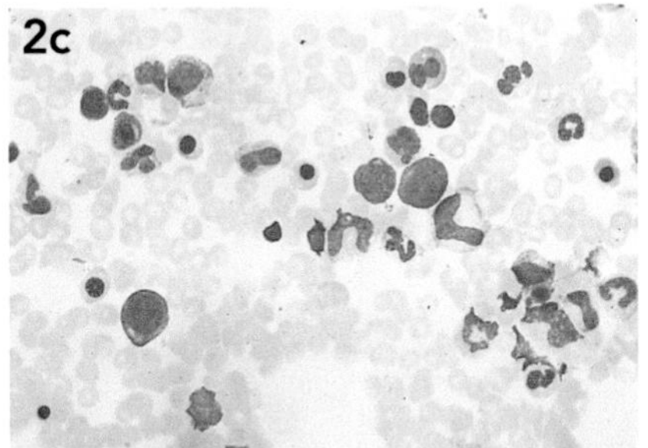
2c

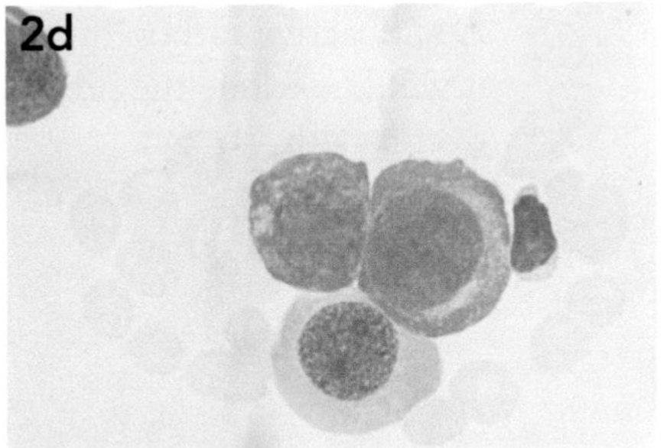
2d

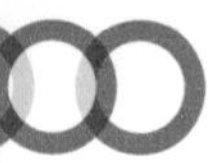

Case 2: ANSWERS

A2.i The barium meal and follow-through show classical changes of Crohn's disease. There is evidence of mucosal thickening and oedema with flocculation of barium.

A2.ii The bone marrow appearances are those of megaloblastic anaemia. The nucleated red cells show an open nuclear chromatin pattern (most clearly seen on the high-power view of erythroblasts, Figure 2d). There are giant metamyelocytes in the white cell series (Figures 2c and 2e).

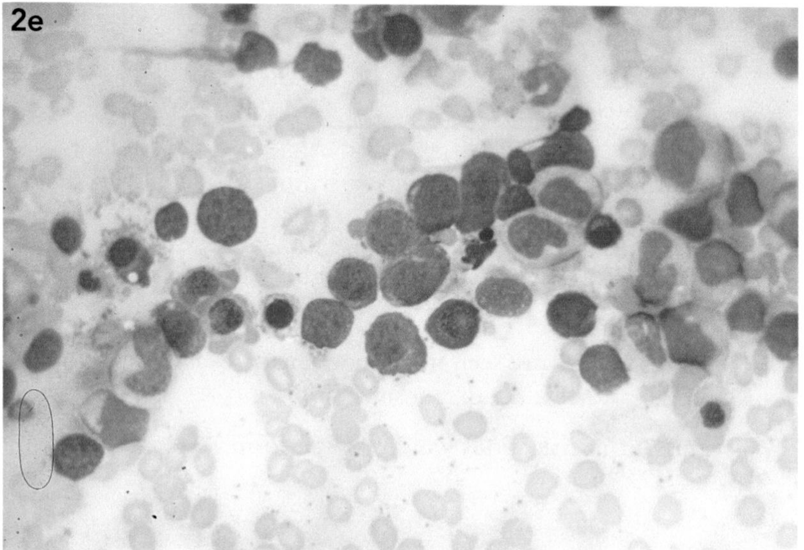

A2.iii Important additional investigations include assessment of haematinics – iron studies, serum ferritin, serum B_{12} and serum and red cell folate levels. The likeliest cause of megaloblastic anaemia in Crohn's disease is malabsorption of vitamin B_{12} due to disease of the terminal ileum.

Vitamin B_{12} absorption studies are no longer performed.

A radioactive carbon breath test would be a helpful further investigation, as it would exclude the presence of an intestinal stagnant loop with bacterial overgrowth.

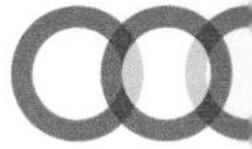

CASE 3

QUESTIONS

A 36-year-old female presented with a short history of increasing tiredness and bruising. Her blood count shows as follows:

Haemoglobin (Hb)	79 g/L
White blood cells (WBC)	34.8×10^9/L
Platelets	21×10^9/L

A bone marrow aspirate was taken (Figure 3a). Six weeks later, she developed a febrile illness with facial swelling and orbital oedema (Figure 3b). She also became short of breath and hypotensive, and had a single episode of haemoptysis. A chest x-ray (Figure 3c) and thoracic computed tomography (CT) scan (Figure 3d) were performed.

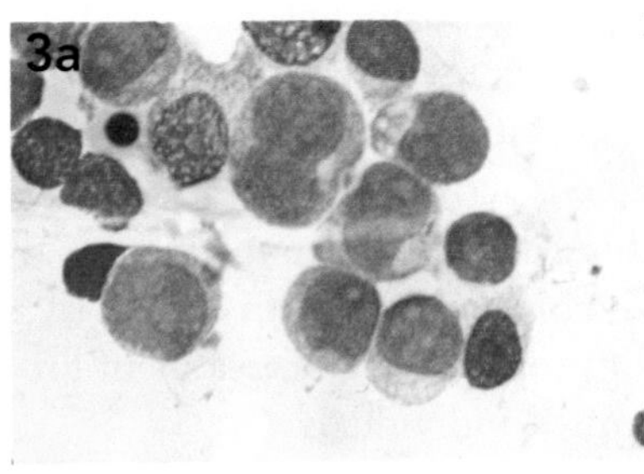

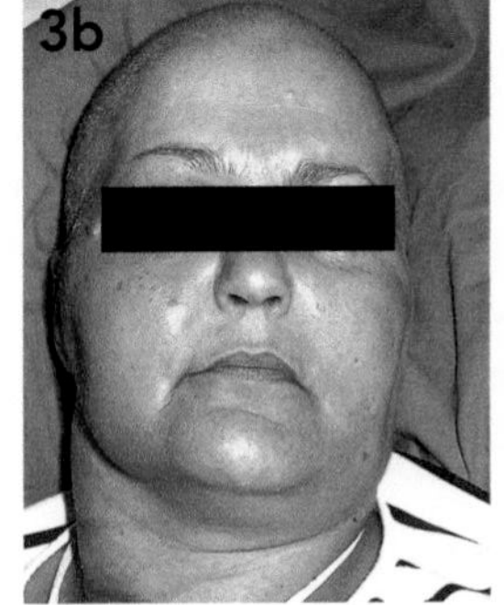

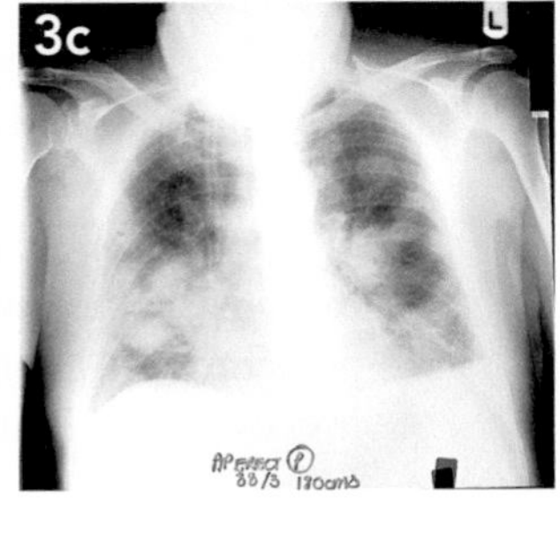

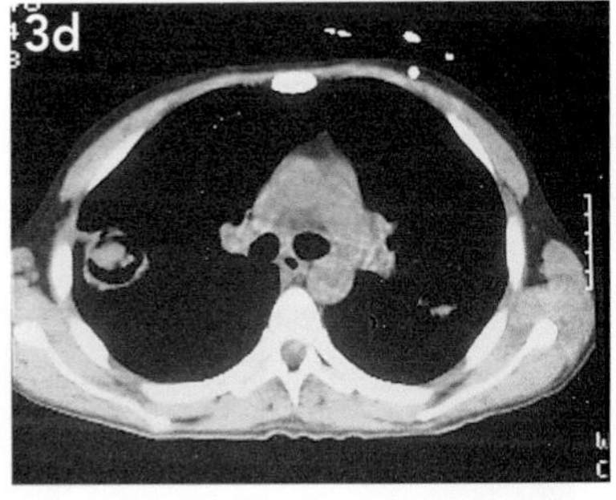

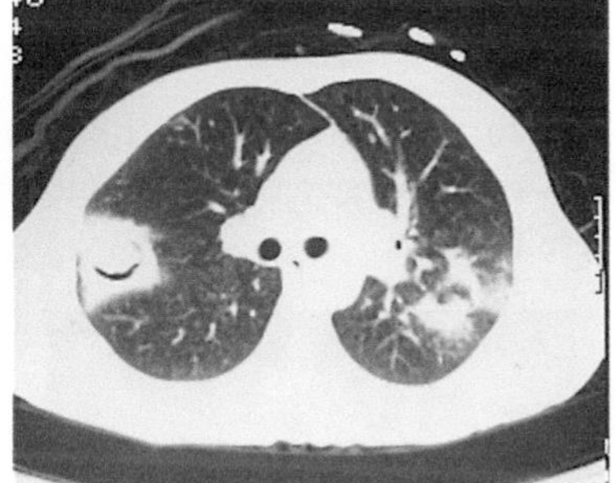

Q3.i What is the presentation diagnosis?

Q3.ii What is the likeliest cause of her febrile illness?

Q3.iii How should she be treated?

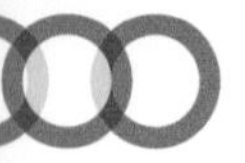

Case 3: ANSWERS

A3.i The bone marrow aspirate is infiltrated by primitive leukaemic cells which have Auer rods. The diagnosis is therefore acute myeloid leukaemia.

A3.ii Infection is clearly the likeliest cause in this setting. The marked facial cellulitis would be compatible with a Gram-positive skin infection but an x-ray of her sinuses should also be carried out. The chest x-ray shows widespread consolidation with ring shadows. Cavitation should be carefully looked for, and, if present, would support a diagnosis of staphylococcal pneumonia. The CT scan confirms cavitation, but the nature of these peripheral, triangular and enhancing lesions is highly suggestive of a fungal pneumonia.

A3.iii Every attempt must be made to make a microbiological diagnosis (blood cultures, culture of aspirate from skin, sputum culture, possibly bronchoalveolar lavage). She should receive broad-spectrum antibiotic and anti-fungal therapy, and this should include systemic liposomal amphotericin or some other lipid formulation of amphotericin B. Oral itraconazole is used as prophylaxis and intravenous itraconazole is active in the treatment of aspergillosis. Caspofungin is a newer anti-fungal agent active in both candidiasis and aspergillosis. Voriconozole has a broader spectrum of activity; posaconazole has recently become available for prophylaxis and treatment for invasive fungal infections in immunocompromised individuals.

The development of haemoptysis is disturbing, as there is a high risk of massive pulmonary haemorrhage in thrombocytopenic patients with invasive pulmonary fungal infections, and surgical resection should be considered for solitary lesions – this is probably inappropriate in this patient, who has multiple lesions.

The images below show thoracic CT scans in a leukaemic patient before and after therapy with liposomal amphotericin, demonstrating substantial resolution.

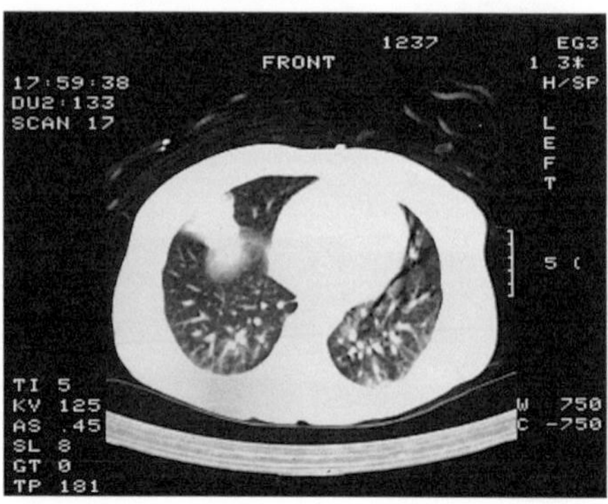

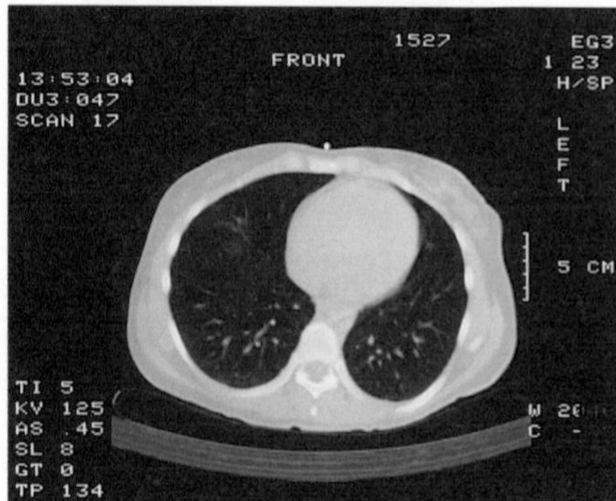

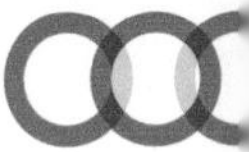

CASE 4

QUESTIONS

A 52-year-old woman with a history of carcinoma of the breast and progressive bone pain is admitted to hospital.

Q4.i Comment on the blood film appearances (Figure 4a).

Q4.ii Comment on the bone marrow aspirate (Figure 4b).

Q4.iii Comment on the bone marrow trephine (Figure 4c).

Q4.iv What further tests are indicated?

Q4.v What is the diagnosis?

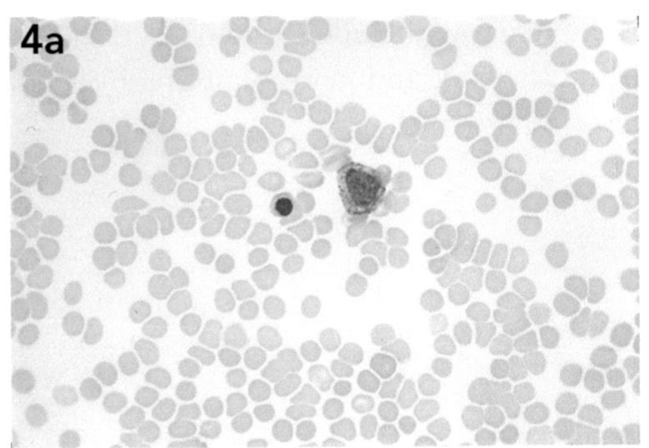

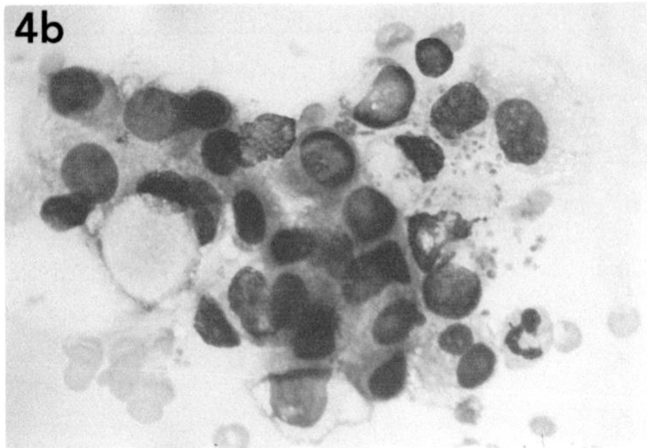

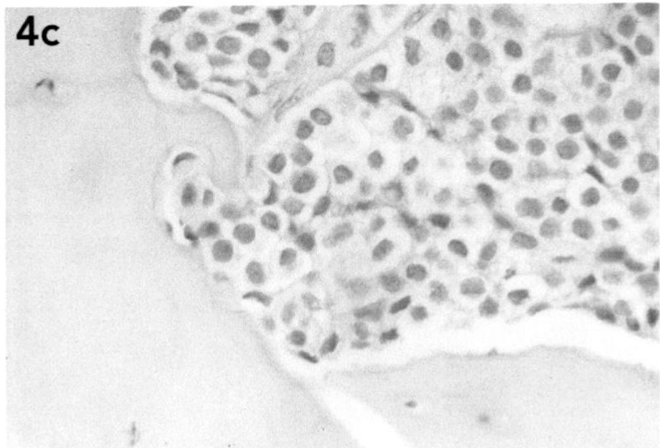

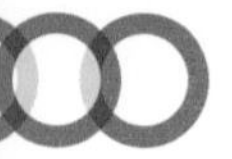

Case 4: ANSWERS

A4.i The blood film shows immature red and white blood cell forms, and is thus leukoerythroblastic. Possible causes are bone marrow infiltration, acute haemolysis and overwhelming sepsis or bleeding – that is, situations in which the marrow is either replaced by abnormal cells (including fibrous tissue) or responding to an acute and overwhelming systemic illness.

A4.ii The marrow is infiltrated by abnormal, non-myeloid cells.

A4.iii Trephine biopsy confirms marrow infiltration.

A4.iv A bone scan will confirm secondary deposits. This patient may have hypercalcaemia (which can lead to renal failure) and the alkaline phosphatase (bone isoenzyme) may be raised. Immunocytochemistry and flow cytometry may be used to confirm the origin of the infiltrating cells, for example, epithelial cells are usually positive for cytokeratin.

A4.v Carcinoma of the breast with bone marrow secondaries.

Other tumours that frequently affect the marrow include tumours of the bronchus (Figure 4d), prostate, renal and thyroid, and neuroblastoma in childhood (Figure 4e).

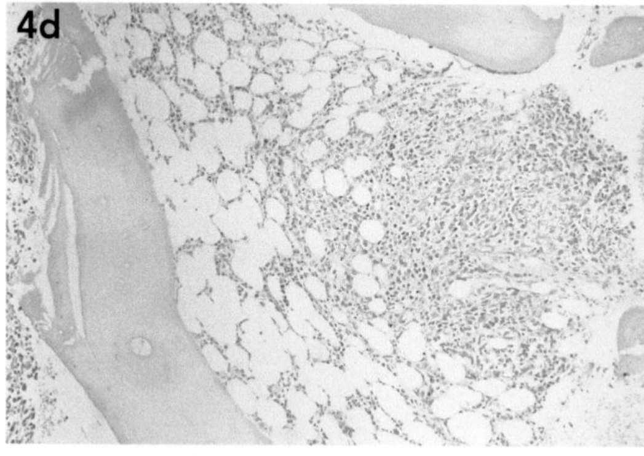

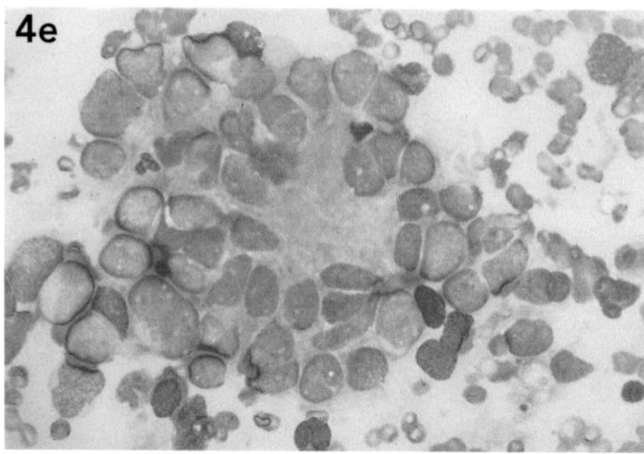

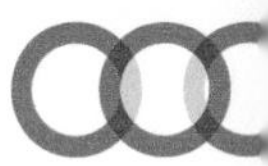

CASE 5

QUESTIONS

A 4-year-old child has a 3- to 4-day history of bruising over her face, neck and lower limbs. She has just recovered from a viral infection. Examination shows purpura over the legs and over her face (Figures 5a and 5b). The spleen is not palpable. Her blood count shows

Haemoglobin (Hb)	119 g/L
White blood cells (WBC)	9.3 × 10^9/L (neutrophils 37%, lymphocytes 61%)
Platelets	9 × 10^9/L
Prothrombin time	12 seconds (control 10–12 seconds)
Activated partial thromboplastin time (APTT)	35 seconds (control 30–40 seconds)
Fibrinogen	2.3 g/L (NR 2–4 g/L)
Creatinine	72 mmol/L

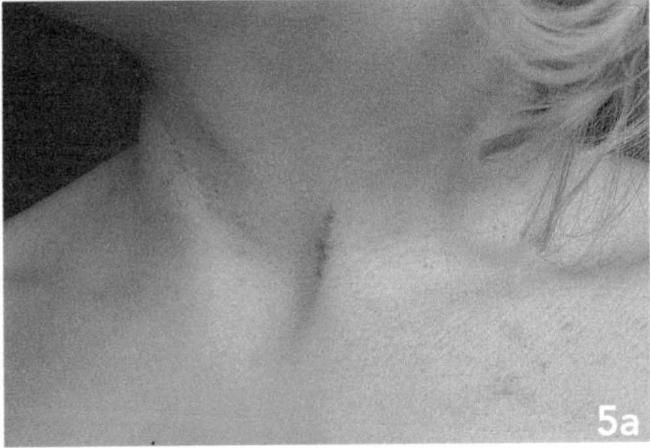
5a

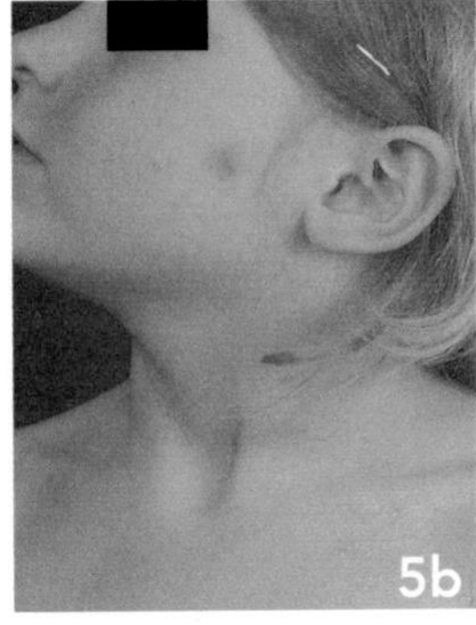
5b

The blood film is shown (Figure 5c).

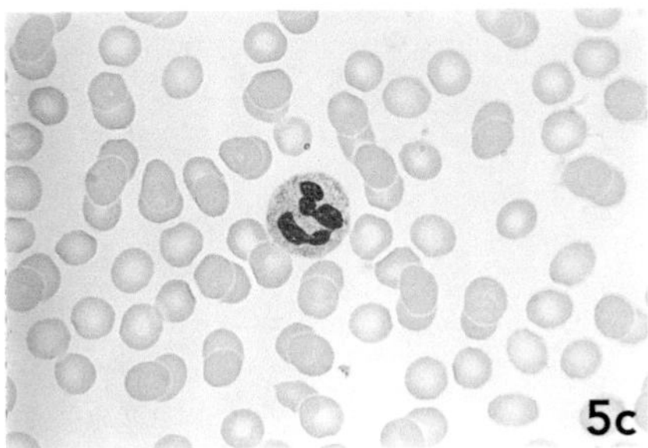
5c

Q5.i What is the likeliest diagnosis?

Q5.ii What further tests are required?

Q5.iii What treatment would you recommend?

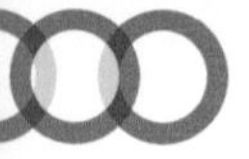

Case 5: ANSWERS

A5.i The blood film confirms thrombocytopenia, but there is no polychromasia, no red cell fragmentation and there is a normal neutrophil. The coagulation tests are normal, effectively excluding disseminated intravascular coagulation, and the creatinine is normal, excluding haemolytic uraemic syndrome. Immune thrombocytopenia (ITP) is the likeliest diagnosis.

A5.ii ITP in childhood is a self-limiting condition. Invasive investigations should be avoided if the child is well and the parents should be alerted to the importance of observing signs of mucosal bleeding – for example, from the nose and mouth. If mucosal bleeding occurs, treatment should be considered and it is reasonable to exclude other causes of thrombocytopenia (drugs, infection including rubella, infectious mononucleosis, hepatitis C, bacterial infections). Haematological malignancy can present as thrombocytopenia and should be excluded if the platelet count does not improve spontaneously over the course of a few days and prior to treatment of the ITP. A bone marrow aspirate (Figure 5d) confirms the presence of megakaryocytes (large, multinuclear cells), thus suggesting platelet destruction. Platelet antibody testing is of much less value than the corresponding tests for red cells. An anti-nuclear factor assay should be performed. The preceding history of viral infection is consistent with ITP, though this is by no means seen universally.

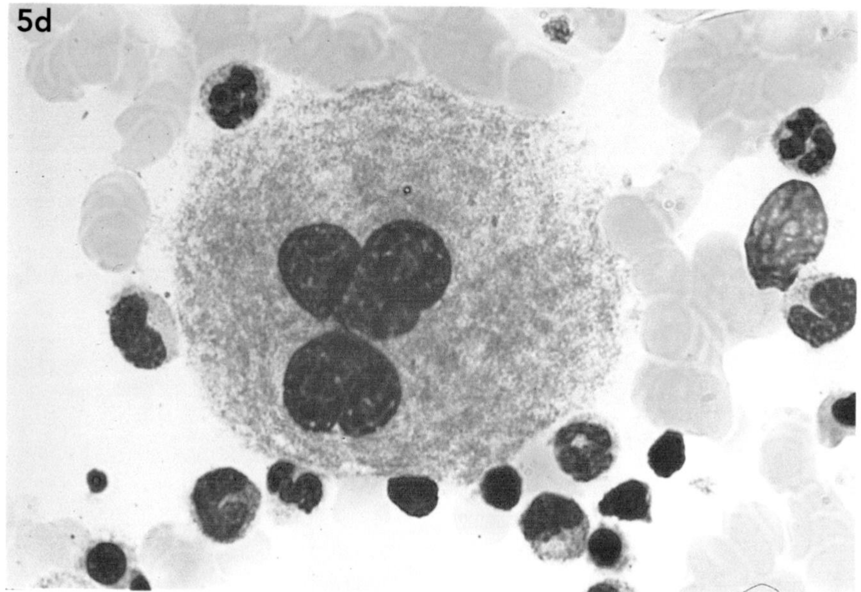

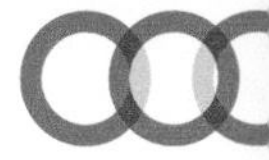

A5.iii Avoidance of injury and anti-platelet drugs, for example, aspirin. The majority of children will recover spontaneously and need no therapy.

If the count does not recover spontaneously (e.g. within 2 weeks) or if there is symptomatic bruising, particularly affecting mucous membranes such as the nose and mouth, then treatment is indicated. Prednisolone, starting at 0.5 mg/kg/day and reducing according to response, is the first-line therapy. Intravenous immunoglobulin (0.4 mg/kg/day) for 3–5 days is equally effective, but best reserved for non-responders. The thrombopoietin receptor analogues are a new class of drugs which are used if and when steroids or intravenous immunoglobulin (IVIG) are ineffective. Romiplostin has to be given by parenteral injection whereas eltrombopag can be given orally. Other immunosuppressive drugs (e.g. cyclophosphamide, azathioprine, mycophenolate and the anti-CD20 monoclonal antibody rituximab) are other possible approaches, but for adults with resistant or relapsed ITP but are generally contraindicated in children.

Splenectomy is best avoided in children under five and should, in any event, be preceded by vaccination against pneumococcus and *Haemophilus influenzae* B, and followed by long-term oral penicillin V as prophylactic therapy against infection.

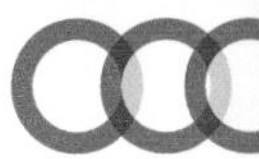

CASE 6

QUESTIONS

A 36-year-old woman gives a 1-week history of tiredness. Her menstrual period has been going on for 10 days, and she has also noticed blood loss when brushing her teeth. Over the past day, she has developed a fever. Investigations show

Haemoglobin (Hb)	79 g/L
White blood cells (WBC)	3.2×10^9/L
Platelets	11×10^9/L
Prothrombin time	19 seconds (control 11–13 seconds)
Activated partial thromboplastin time (APTT)	64 seconds (control 30–40 seconds)
Thrombin time	28 seconds (control 18–20 seconds)
Fibrinogen	0.03 g/L (NR 0.2–0.4 g/L)
Fibrin degradation product (FDP) titre	1:60 (NR 2–4 g/L)

Q6.i What abnormalities are seen on the blood film (Figure 6a) and bone marrow (Figure 6b)?

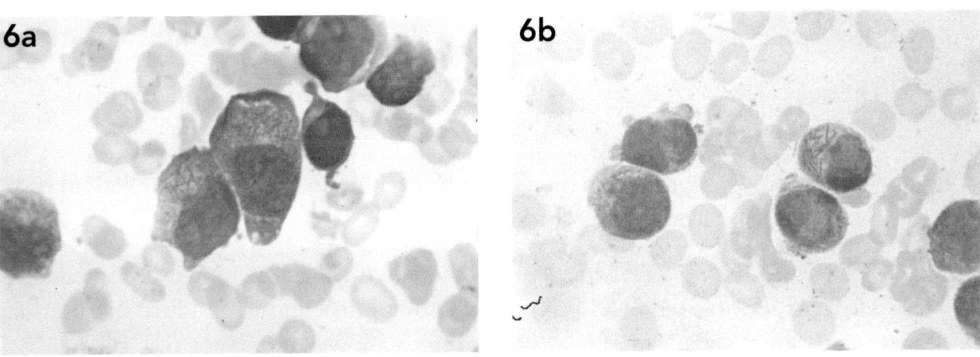

Q6.ii What is the cause of the abnormal coagulation?

Q6.iii What is the diagnosis?

Q6.iv How is this condition managed?

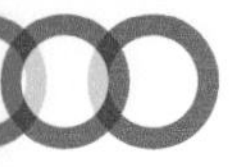

Case 6: ANSWERS

A6.i The blood and bone marrow film show leukaemic blast cells containing dense granules, many of which have condensed to form Auer rods. Some cells have multiple Auer rods. This appearance is typical of acute promyelocytic leukaemia (PML). This form of leukaemia is associated with a translocation of material from chromosome 15 (PML) to chromosome 17 (at the site of the retinoic acid alpha receptor, RARA) (t15–17). Figure 6c shows a variant form of M_3 (microgranular variant) where cytoplasmic granulation is less marked, but the 'dumbbell'-shaped nucleus is a characteristic. Molecular analysis shows a disease-specific fusion gene (*PML-RARA*). Cytogenetic and fluorescence in situ hybridization (FISH) changes of acute promyelocytic leukemia (APML) are illustrated in Figure 6d.

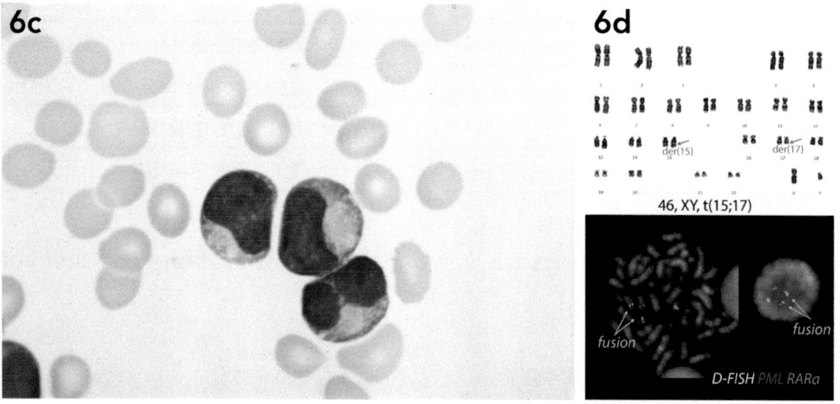

A6.ii The coagulation changes are consistent with disseminated intravascular coagulation (DIC).

A6.iii Acute promyelocytic leukaemia complicated by disseminated intravascular coagulation – a well-recognised association.

A6.iv The coagulopathy frequently gets worse when chemotherapy is commenced. All-trans retinoic acid (ATRA) is given by mouth and can induce maturation of leukaemic cells; its use is associated with a lower incidence of DIC, a higher rate of remission and improved long-term survival.

Modern chemotherapy regimes for APML focus on three to four courses of anthracycline-based chemotherapy (e.g. idarubicin plus cytosine arabinoside). Once the PML-RARA transcript becomes undetectable, the patient is in remission and ATRA can be stopped. Arsenic trioxide is used as the first-line therapy for patients who relapse. It can also be used as first-line treatment in patients who are unsuitable for intensive chemotherapy; however, it is cardiotoxic and must be carefully monitored. Other treatment approaches for relapsed disease include the anti-CD33 monclonal antibody (Myelotarg), or allogeneic stem cell transplant.

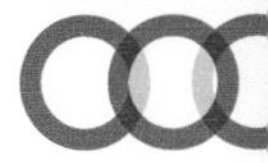

CASE 7

QUESTIONS

Q7.i What abnormality is seen on the blood film?

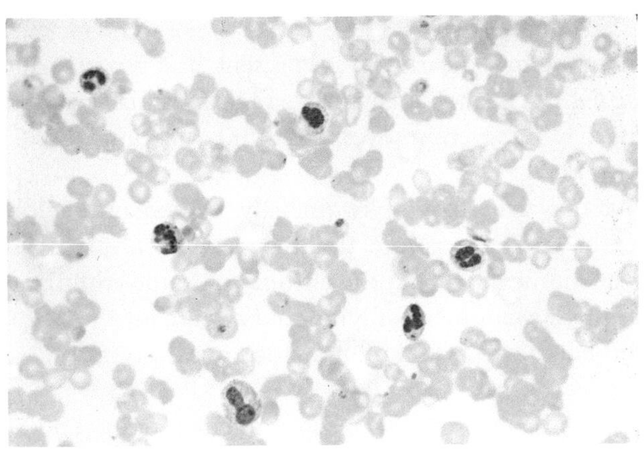

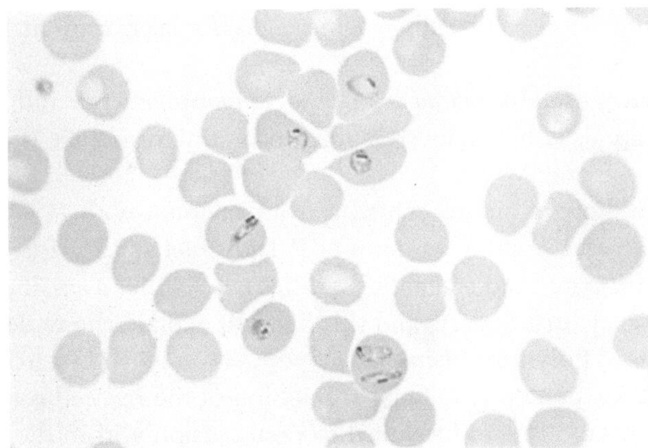

Q7.ii What are the important haematological complications of this condition?

Q7.iii What treatment should be offered?

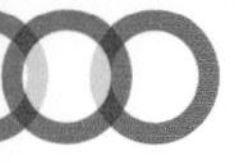

Case 7: ANSWERS

A7.i Malaria. The presence of more than one ring form per red cell strongly suggests *Plasmodium falciparum*.

A7.ii Anaemia, which is principally due to haemolysis of infected erythrocytes but is also due to immune haemolysis, splenomegaly and impaired marrow production.

Thrombocytopenia is nearly always present, and is partly due to splenomegaly. Low-grade disseminated intravascular coagulation can also occur; this may be severe in overwhelming infection.

Leukopenia may arise from splenomegaly. Hypergammaglobulinaemia is frequent. Chronic malaria infection may lead to substantial splenomegaly ('tropical splenomegaly'), and the chronic immune stimulation may be a factor in the development of lymphoid malignancy (e.g. lymphoma). Neutrophil leukocytosis and monocytosis may also occur.

A7.iii Falciparum malaria is commonly resistant to chloroquine, and is best treated with quinine (by intravenous infusion in severely ill patients). If quinine resistance is suspected, it should be followed by either fansidar or tetracycline. Mefloquine and halofantrine are also currently recommended for falciparum malaria.

Infections caused by *Plasmodium ovale*, *Plasmodium vivax* and *Plasmodium malariae* are usually less severe and chloroquine resistance is uncommon.

Figure 7a shows a mature schizont from a patient with *P. vivax* infection and Figures 7b and 7c show gametes of *P. falciparum* and *P. vivax*, respectively. Diverse inherited red cell abnormalities may confer a small degree of protection against malaria and this helps to explain the wide prevalence of 'balanced polymorphisms' at the population level. Heterozygosity for the sickle gene is beneficial as invasion of the red cell is followed by parasite metabolism and reduced oxygen tension within the cell. The resultant sickling leads to a deformed cell which can be cleared by the reticuloendothelial system. Homozygosity for the sickle cell gene is usually associated with hyposplenism and an underactive reticuloendothelial (RE) system; such subjects are not protected against malaria. Both alpha and beta thalassaemia and certain red cell membrane abnormalities, for example, ovalocytosis may offer a small degree of protection against malaria. There is excellent epidemiological evidence that glucose-6-phosphate dehydrogenase (G6PD) deficiency can also afford a small degree of protection.

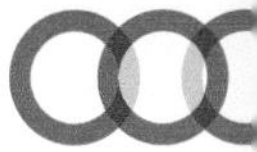

Case 7: ANSWERS (Continued)

7a

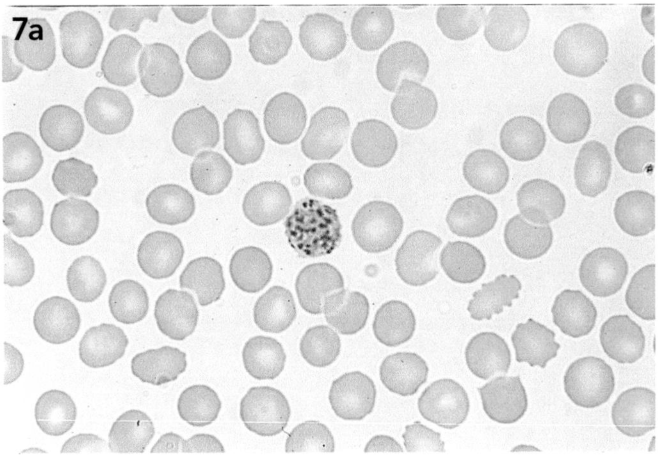

7b

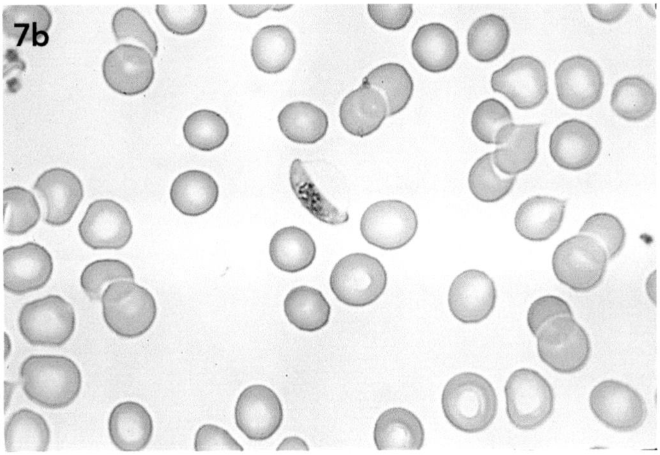

7c

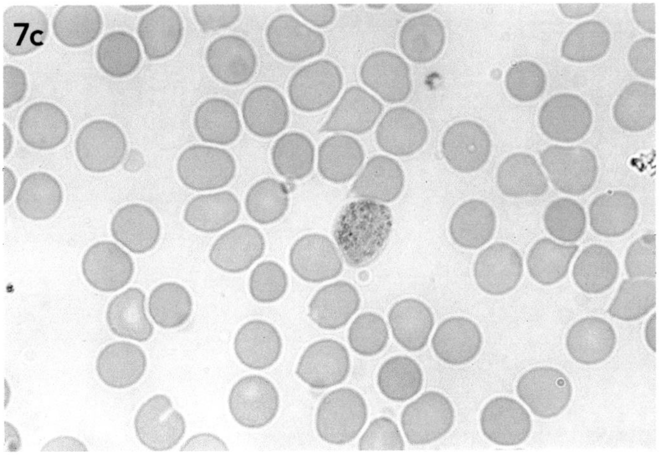

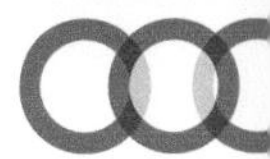

CASE 8

QUESTIONS

A 34-year-old man has a history of chronic anaemia that was improved by an operation at the age of 11. He develops tiredness and shortness of breath after moderate exertion but does not require blood transfusion and copes well with everyday activities. Drug therapy comprises folic acid 5 mg/day and penicillin V 250 mg twice daily. A full blood count shows

Haemoglobin (Hb)	85 g/L
Mean corpuscular volume (MCV)	107 f/L

Q8.i Comment on the blood film.

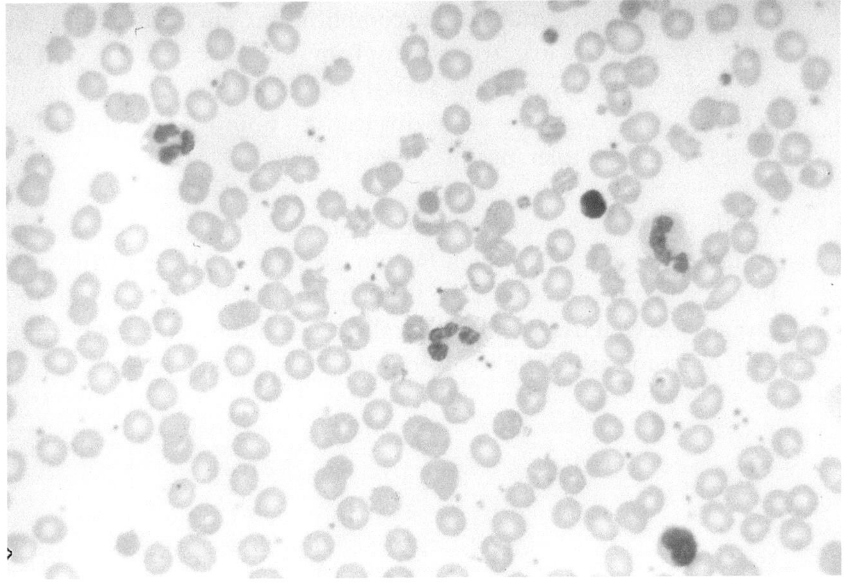

Q8.ii Suggest the likely diagnosis. How would you confirm it?

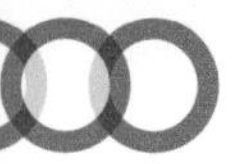

Case 8: ANSWERS

A8.i The blood film shows irregularly contracted cells (pyknocytes) with Howell–Jolly bodies and target cells. A splenectomy is suggested, though the red cell abnormalities exceed those usually seen, simply as a result of splenectomy.

A8.ii An important differential diagnosis is hereditary spherocytosis, but the blood film does not show spherocytes.

The commonest of the inherited glycolytic pathway enzymopathies, and the diagnosis in this case, is pyruvate kinase deficiency. The auto-haemolysis test is of historical and theoretical interest, and most laboratories would proceed directly to enzyme assay followed by DNA analysis to define the specific mutation. Even so, this is a rare disease, with less than 300 cases reported worldwide.

The red cell lacks a nucleus and is unable to undertake protein synthesis to renew its supply of deficient enzymes; other tissues are able to compensate, though neurological and cardiac complications can occur with inherited red cell enzymopathies (e.g. triose phosphate isomerase deficiency). The levels of 2,3-diphosphoglycerate (2,3-DGP) are usually elevated in patients with pyruvate kinase deficiency and this leads to improved oxygen delivery to tissues and better tolerance of anaemia.

Another cause of congenital haemolytic anaemia is the presence of an unstable haemoglobin variant (see image below). These usually involve amino acid substitutions in the beta chain, though alpha and gamma chain variants are well described. Clinically, these disorders range from severe, with onset in early childhood, to mild, compensated haemolysis.

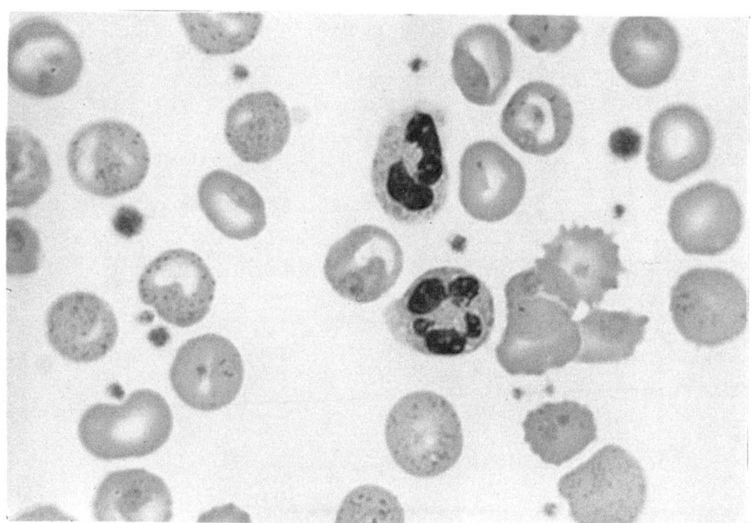

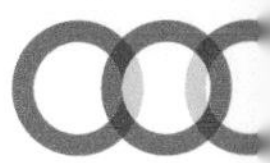

CASE 9

QUESTIONS

A 76-year-old woman gives a 2- to 3-month history of progressively cold and numb fingertips. The symptoms are persistent but episodic. She is a non-smoker. Her feet are normal, and physical examination is otherwise unremarkable. All pulses are present. Her blood count shows

Haemoglobin (Hb)	90 g/L
White blood cells (WBC)	14.6 × 10^9/L (neutrophils 67%)
Platelets	1246 × 10^9/L

Q9.i Comment on the appearance of the hands.

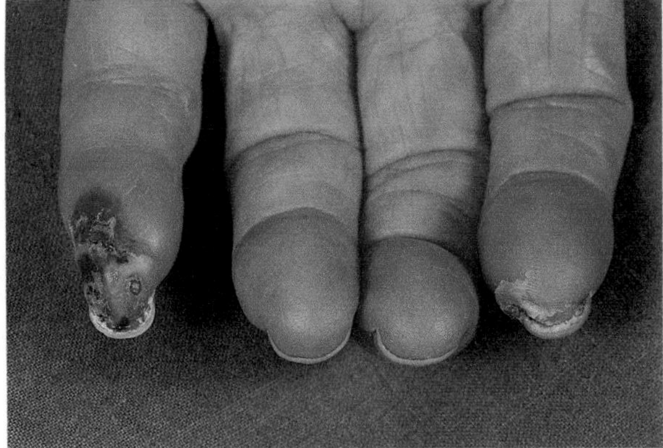

Q9.ii Comment on the blood film.

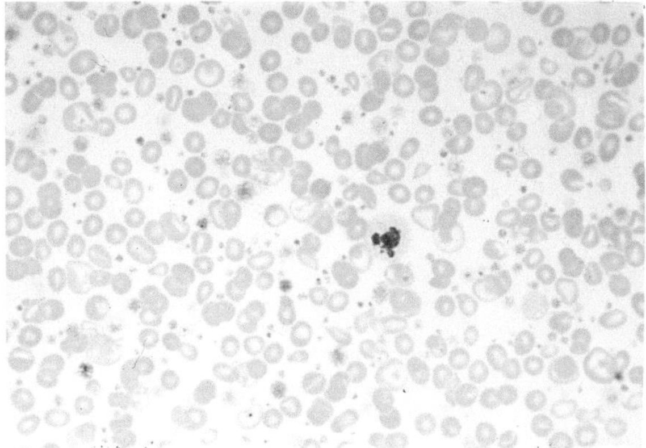

Q9.iii What are the possible causes of the abnormalities?

Q9.iv What further investigations would you undertake?

Q9.v What are the possible treatments?

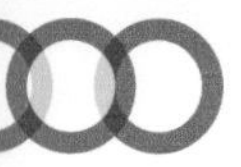

Case 9: ANSWERS

A9.i There are severe ischaemic changes affecting both hands (Figure 9a).

A9.ii The blood film shows increased numbers of circulating platelets, with marked platelet anisocytosis and many giant platelets (Figure 9b).

A9.iii Increased platelets may be primary or secondary. Primary thrombocythaemia turned out to be the diagnosis in this case, and this is a myeloproliferative disorder; a raised platelet count is also encountered as part of other myeloproliferative disorders, for example, chronic granulocytic leukaemia, polycythaemia vera. Secondary thrombocytosis occurs in response to infection, bleeding, iron deficiency and malignancy, and is seen after splenectomy.

A9.iv A full history and physical examination is needed to exclude causes of secondary thrombocytosis. A bone marrow aspirate with chromosome analysis and trephine biopsy may confirm primary thrombocythaemia. Approximately 50% of patients with essential thrombocythemia (ET) have a mutation at the janus kinase 2 (JAK2) locus (V617F), and a high proportion of JAK2 negative patients have a mutation at the CALR locus. A serum ferritin is required to exclude iron deficiency, and abdominal ultrasound scan may detect splenomegaly. Platelet function tests are typically abnormal in primary thrombocythaemia and normal in secondary or reactive states.

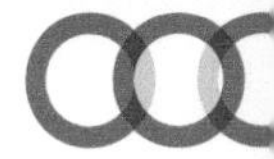

Case 9: ANSWERS (Continued)

A9.v Primary thrombocythaemia is treated with chemotherapy (e.g. oral hydroxyurea) to lower the platelet count and maintain it below 400×10^9/L, and anti-platelet therapy (e.g. aspirin 150 mg on alternate days) to inhibit platelet function.

Figure 9a shows increased platelet numbers in association with abnormal, hypogranular neutrophils. This patient had myelodysplasia; cytogenetic analysis showed the presence of 5q$^-$, which is associated with a slowly progressive form of myelodysplasia with macrocytosis and thrombocythaemia. Figure 9b illustrates the JAK2 assay and Figure 9c the calreticulin (CALR) assay.

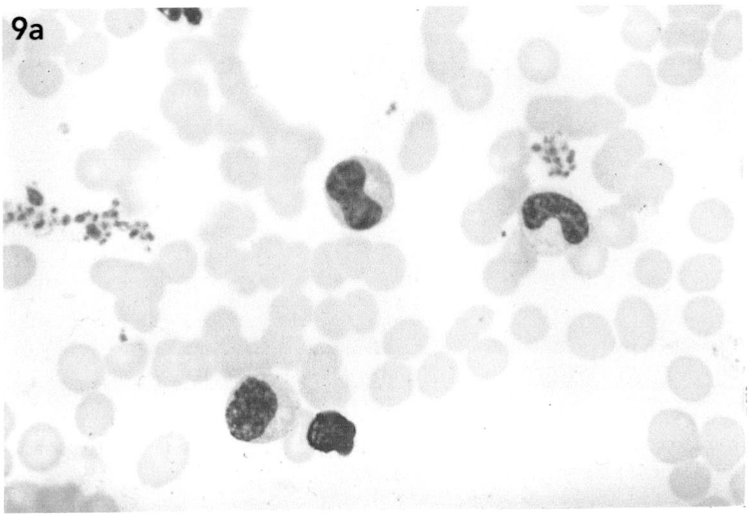

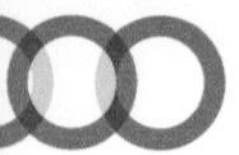

Case 9: ANSWERS (Continued)

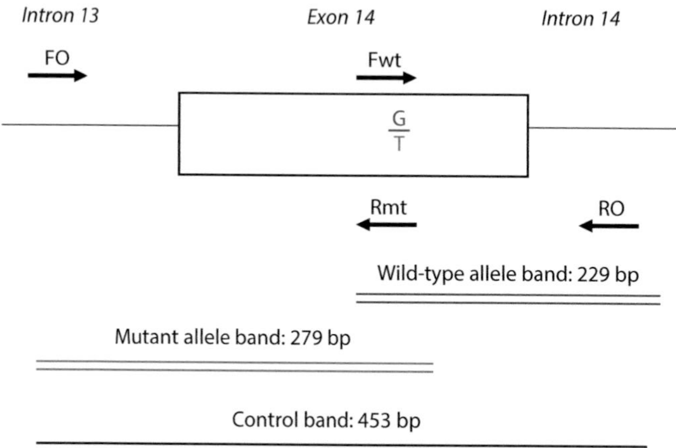

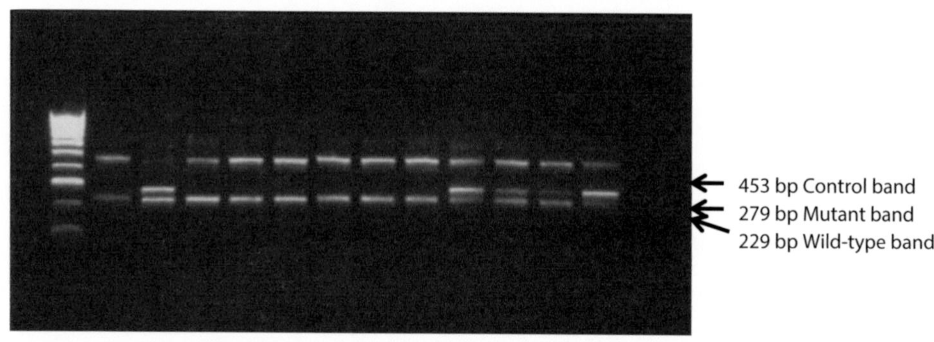

Figure 9b Janus kinase 2 (JAK2) assay is an amplification refractory mutation system polymerase chain reaction (PCR). The wild-type (WT) allele yields two bands, but the mutant (MT) allele yields three bands.

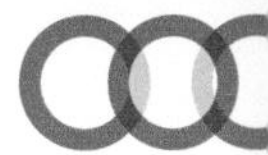

Case 9: ANSWERS (Continued)

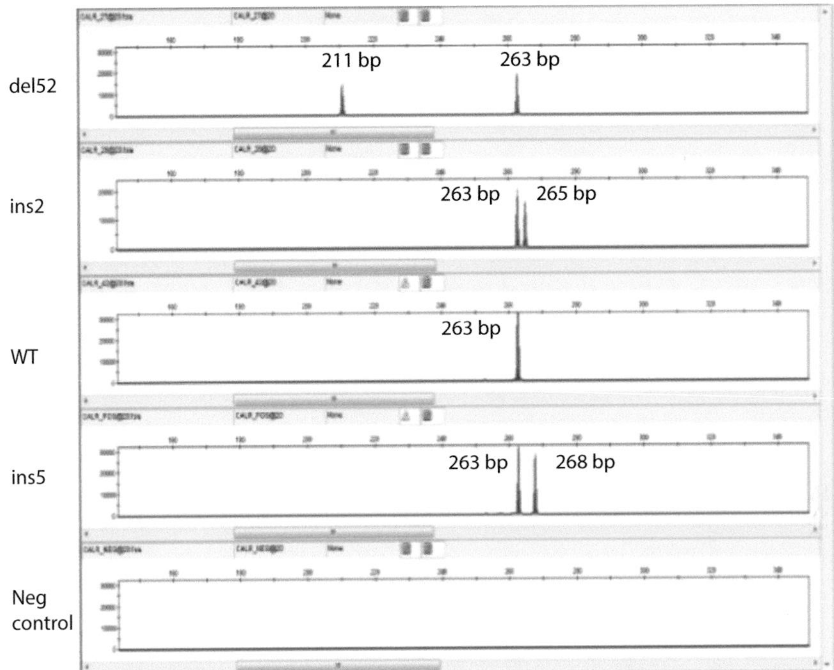

Figure 9c Calreticulin (CALR) assay. Over 30 different mutations are situated in exon 9 of the gene, and all give rise to an identical frame-shift and abnormal 3′ protein. The PCR products are analysed by capillary gel electrophoresis. The wild-type allele band is 263 bp.

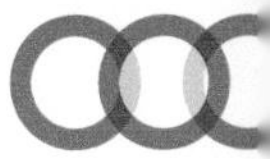

CASE 10

QUESTIONS

A 76-year-old female was diagnosed 3 years ago as suffering from chronic lymphocytic leukaemia (CLL). She has not required any therapy and was in good health until 4 weeks ago. She now complains of tiredness, polyuria and lethargy, and has also noticed increasing abdominal distension. On examination she is pale. She is not jaundiced, but she does have lymphadenopathy in both axillae. A marked swelling of the left elbow is noted. The spleen is easily palpable, and ascites is present. Neurological examination is normal.

Q10.i Comment on the peripheral blood film findings.

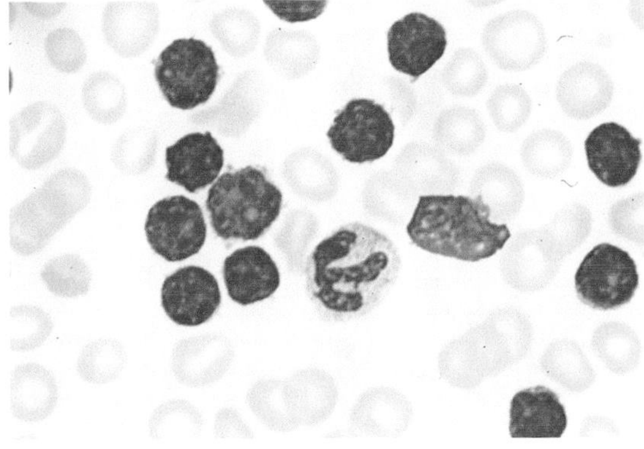

Q10.ii Comment on the abdominal computed tomography (CT) scan.

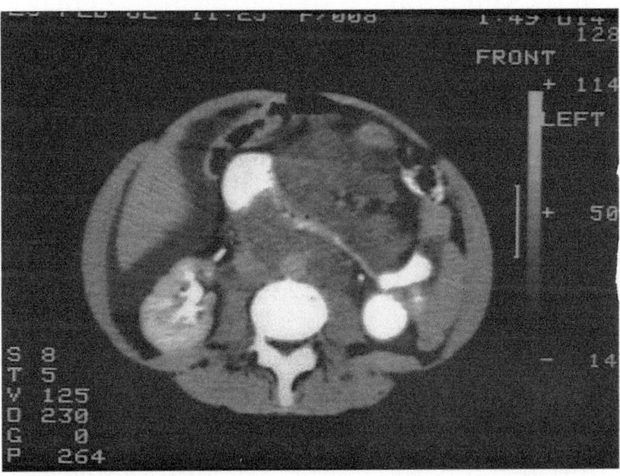

Q10.iii What is the likeliest diagnosis?

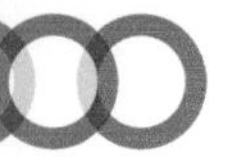

Case 10: ANSWERS

A10.i The film shows abnormal lymphoid cells which do not look like the mature B lymphocytes of CLL. These are larger cells with plentiful basophilic cytoplasm. These appearances are in keeping with an immunoblastic transformation of CLL. The bone marrow trephine biopsy is shown below; it is hypercellular and heavily infiltrated by pleomorphic lymphocytes.

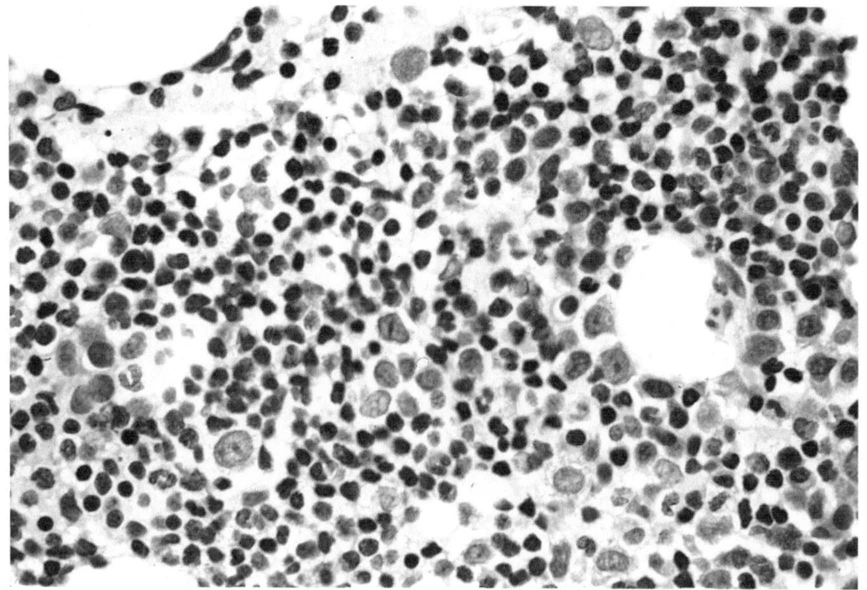

Flow cytometry will demonstrate that the cells in classic CLL are positive for the T-cell marker cluster of differentiation 5 (CD5) and the mature B-cell markers CD19, 20 and 23. FMC7 is negative on classic CLL but typically positive when the condition has transformed; CD5 may also become negative. In classic CLL, expression of the protein kinase ZAP-70 and of CD38 are both more common in cases which are germ line (unmutated) at the immunoglobulin heavy chain (IgH) locus and all these features are associated with a worse prognosis. Chromosome and fluorescence in situ hybridization (FISH) analysis will give useful prognostic information – for example, deletion of p53 is often seen in advanced CLL whereas 13q deletions are associated with a good prognosis.

A10.ii The CT scan shows enlarged retroperitoneal lymph nodes. These are affecting the ureters, possibly causing ureteric obstruction, and they are perhaps also affecting the bowel. The history suggests she may be developing renal failure.

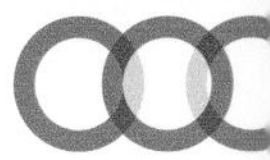

Case 10: ANSWERS (Continued)

A10.iii Richter's syndrome denotes a transformation of CLL into a more aggressive tumour, often with enlargement of lymph node tissue in unusual sites (e.g. retroperitoneally). This patient also had massive axillary and epitrochlear nodes.

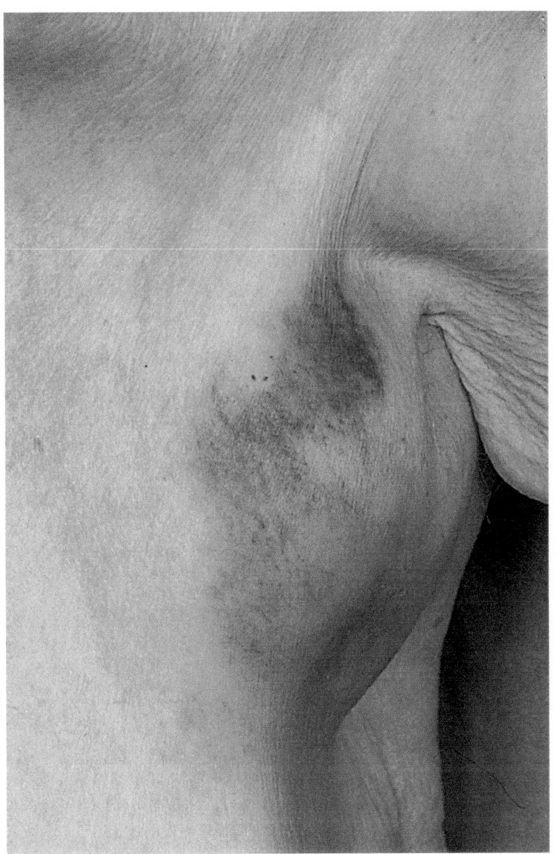

This condition responds poorly to therapy and is usually rapidly progressive. Treatment approaches in CLL have evolved rapidly. Advanced disease may respond to treatment with the anti-CD20 monoclonal antibody rituximab in combination with intensive chemotherapy – for example, R plus fludarabine and cyclophosphamide. Other monoclonals, for example, ofatumumab may also have a role. Ibrutinib is an orally administered, highly potent, selective and irreversible small-molecule inhibitor of Bruton's tyrosine kinase (Btk), an important component of the B-cell receptor signalling pathway. It has recently been licensed for patients with CLL who have relapsed. It has activity both as a single agent and in combination with monoclonals and chemotherapy. Venetoclax is a new agent that targets the BCL2 protein and has activity in refractory CLL. Venetoclax targets the BCL2 protein and has demonstrated activity in relapsed and refractory CLL.

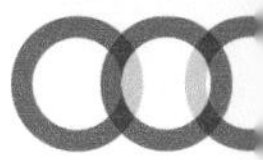

CASE 11

QUESTIONS

A 72-year-old woman presents with a 4- to 6-week history of gradually increasing tiredness and shortness of breath. A blood count shows

Haemoglobin (Hb)	86 g/L
Mean corpuscular volume (MCV)	65 fL
Mean corpuscular haemoglobin (MCH)	26.4 pg
Mean corpuscular haemoglobin concentration (MCHC)	29 g/dL
Red blood cells (RBC)	3.8 × 10^{12}/L
White blood cells (WBC)	6.7 × 10^{9}/L (differential normal)
Platelets	456 × 10^{9}/L

Q11.i What abnormalities are shown in the blood film?

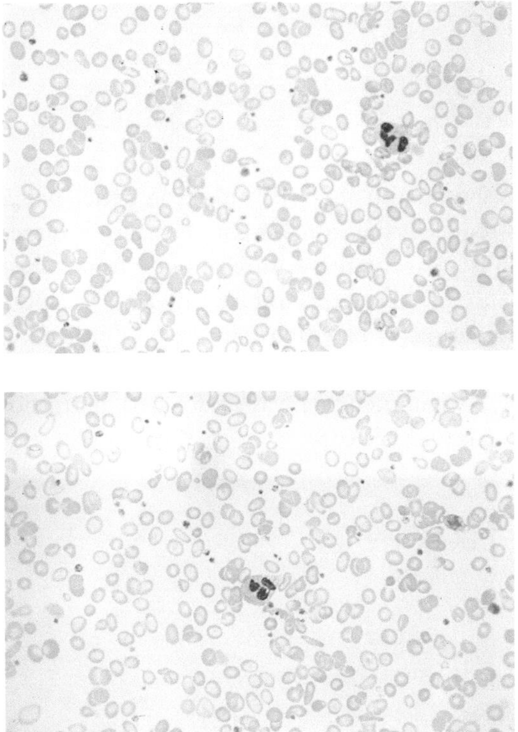

Q11.ii What is the diagnosis?

Q11.iii What further investigations should be performed?

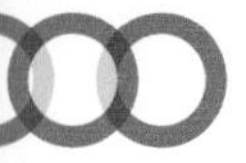

Case 11: ANSWERS

A11.i The blood count shows anaemia with microcytic, hypochromic red cell indices.

A11.ii The platelet count is raised, in keeping with iron deficiency anaemia. The blood film shows hypochromic, microcytic cells, with target cells, and increased platelet numbers. The differential diagnosis of hypochromasia and microcytosis is thalassaemia. The carrier states for both alpha thalassaemia and beta thalassaemia are rarely associated with anaemia. Other causes of target cells include liver disease, post-splenectomy and other haemoglobinopathies, for example, haemoglobin C.

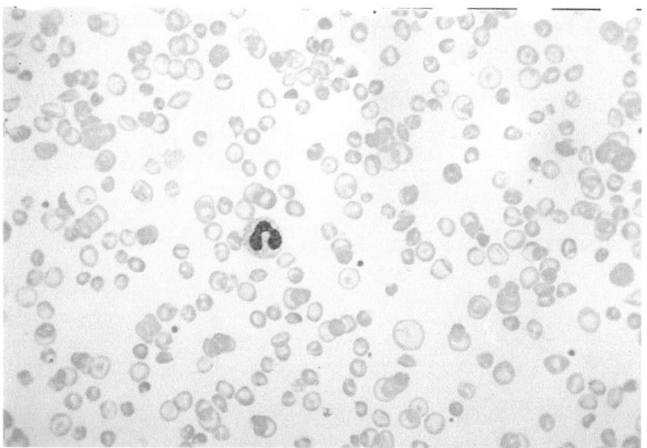

A11.iii Investigations should aim at confirming iron deficiency and defining a cause. Serum iron is reduced, the iron-binding capacity is increased and the serum ferritin (which is an accurate measure of body iron stores) is reduced. The commonest cause of this picture is bleeding and, in a post-menopausal female or in a male, the cause of bleeding must be established.

In this patient, a barium enema was performed. This showed a carcinoma of the colon at the splenic flexure.

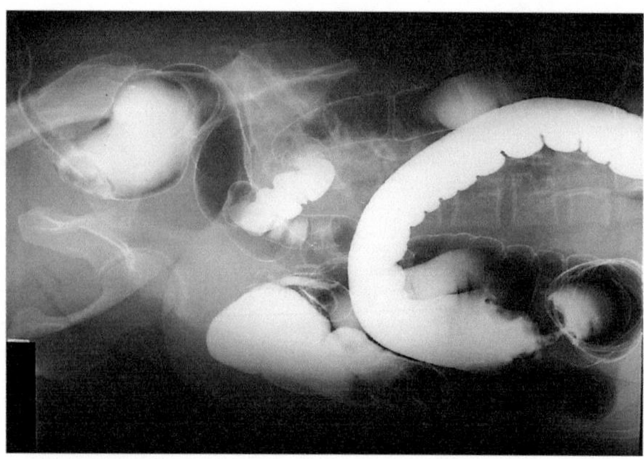

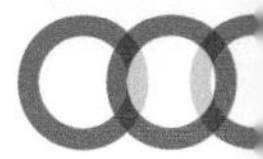

CASE 12

QUESTIONS

A 6-year-old girl presents with a 4-week history of gradually increasing tiredness and lack of energy. She has also become jaundiced. There is no relevant past medical history. Examination reveals a pale, jaundiced child with no lymphadenopathy but with a spleen palpable 6 cm below the left costal margin. There are no signs of chronic liver disease. Cardiovascular examination reveals a soft apical systolic murmur. Investigations show

Haemoglobin (Hb)	61 g/L
Mean corpuscular volume (MCV)	110 fL
Reticulocytes	22%
White blood cells (WBC)	15.1×10^9/L (neutrophils 12.3×10^9/L)
Platelets	103×10^9/L

Q12.i What abnormalities are seen on the blood film?

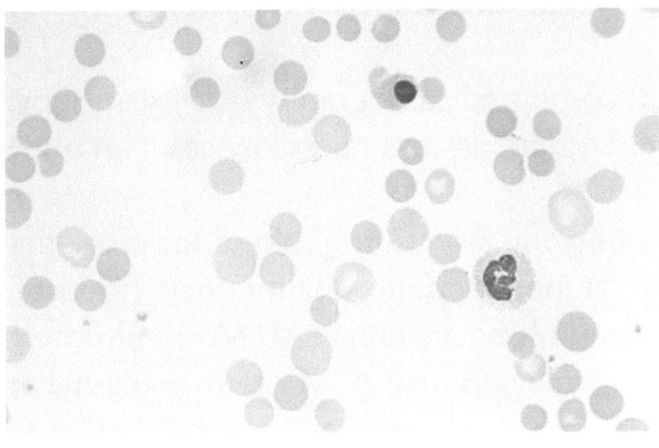

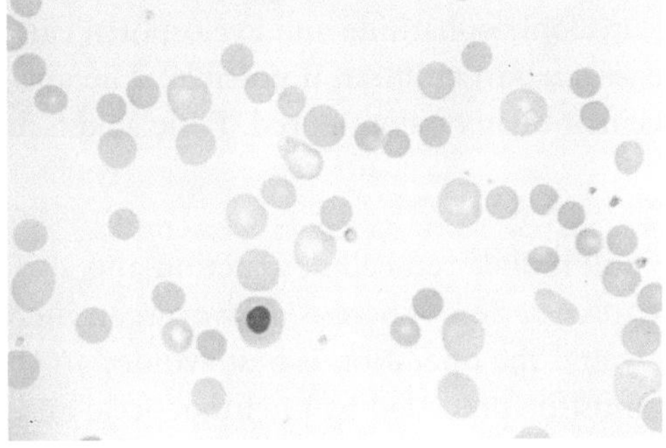

Q12.ii What is the likely diagnosis?

Q12.iii What further investigations are indicated?

Q12.iv How would you treat this patient?

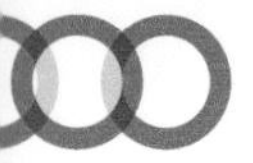

Case 12: ANSWERS

A12.i The blood film shows polychromasia, anisocytosis, poikilocytosis and spherocytes, with circulating nucleated red blood cells.

A12.ii Autoimmune haemolytic anaemia.

A12.iii The direct anti-globulin test (DAT, Coombs test) is strongly positive, with complement and IgG detectable on the red cell surface.

Liver function tests show an elevated bilirubin (320 mmol/L) which is largely unconjugated. Her serum contains a pan-reacting red cell antibody that has no clear specificity and there is no evidence of an additional red cell alloantibody. The antibody reacts most strongly at 37°C.

Serum haptoglobin is often reduced and urine haemosiderin is present in the presence of intravascular haemolysis.

An auto-antibody screen reveals a positive anti-nuclear factor (ANF) at a titre of >1:100, suggesting underlying systemic lupus erythematosus (SLE).

An abdominal computed tomography (CT) scan shows splenomegaly but no lymph node enlargement, and no evidence of an underlying lymphoma.

Red cell grouping and selection of blood for cross-matching should be done with care at an experienced laboratory. Important infectious causes of autoimmune haemolytic anaemia (AIHA) in children include Epstein–Barr virus (EBV), cytomegalovirus (CMV), mycoplasma and parvo virus.

A12.iv Prednisolone 1.0 mg/kg of body weight is first-line immunosuppression. Azathioprine, cyclophosphamide and cyclosporin can all be considered but should be avoided in children if possible. The anti-CD20 monoclonal antibody rituximab may be considered. Folic acid 5 mg should be given daily.

Splenectomy will reduce red cell destruction and also remove a site of auto-antibody production. There is, however, an increased risk of infection postoperatively and the operation is best avoided in children under 5. Splenectomy must be preceded by pneumococcal and *Haemophilus influenzae* B vaccination and followed by long-term prophylactic penicillin.

Evans syndrome is the association of AIHA with immune thrombocytopenic purpura (ITP) and is seen in over one-third of children with AIHA.

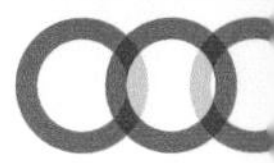

CASE 13

QUESTIONS

The blood film is from a 35-year-old male who has the following blood count:

Haemoglobin (Hb)	63 g/L
Mean corpuscular volume (MCV)	81 fL
White blood cells (WBC)	6.1×10^9/L
Platelets	137×10^9/L

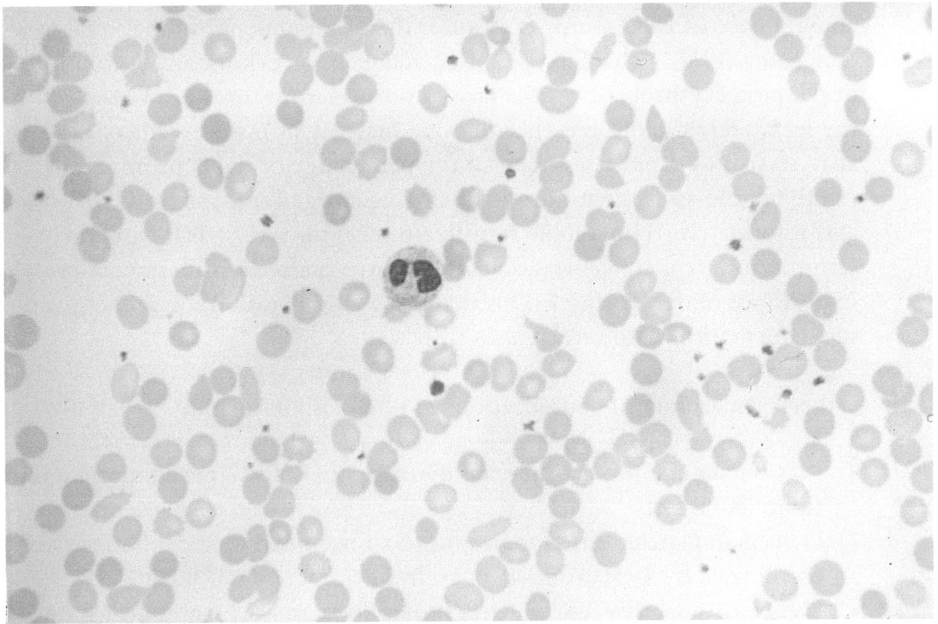

Q13.i What is the diagnosis?

Q13.ii What is the pathogenesis of the anaemia?

Q13.iii What other haematological complications may occur?

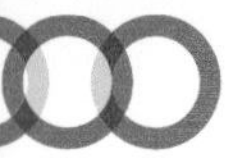

Case 13: ANSWERS

A13.i This patient is suffering from renal failure. The blood film shows characteristic echinocytes (Burr cells). The reticulocyte count is usually normal or slightly low, and bone marrow examination shows normoblastic erythropoiesis, often without the erythroid hyperplasia expected for the level of anaemia.

A13.ii The most important pathogenic mechanism is reduced production of erythropoietin by diseased kidneys. Treatment has been revolutionised by the availability of recombinant erythropoietin (EPO). Diminished red cell survival, iron deficiency through blood loss (e.g. at haemodialysis) and secondary hyperparathyroidism are contributory factors. Most patients with established renal failure will be on treatment with EPO. An important consequence of EPO administration is the development of functional iron deficiency (FID) – characterised by inadequate incorporation of iron into developing erythroblasts in the face of normal iron stores as assessed by the serum ferritin and presence of bone marrow iron stores. Many modern analysers allow rapid assessment of the percentage of hypochromic cells (%HRC); the assessment of reticulocyte haemoglobin content (CHr) is also informative. The soluble transferrin receptor assay (sTfR) and the serum transferrin concentration can also give useful information. The importance of diagnosing FID is that early consideration should be given to supplementation with intravenous iron.

A13.iii Other haematological complications of renal failure include

- Polycythaemia, for example, following ectopic EPO production by renal tumours or cysts
- Defects in platelet function, leading to a haemorrhagic diathesis partly correctable by 1-deamino-8-D-arginine vasopressin (DDAVP)
- Hypercoagulability, particularly in nephrotic syndrome, which is partly related to reduced fibrinolysis, reduced protein C and reduced anti-thrombin
- Changes due to the underlying pathology causing renal failure (e.g. autoimmune haemolytic anaemia and idiopathic thrombocytopenic purpura in systemic lupus erythematosus; low platelet count in disseminated intravascular coagulation)
- Treatment-induced changes (e.g. immunosuppression)

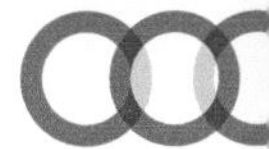

The image below shows Burr cells and basophilic stippling in the blood film of another patient with renal failure.

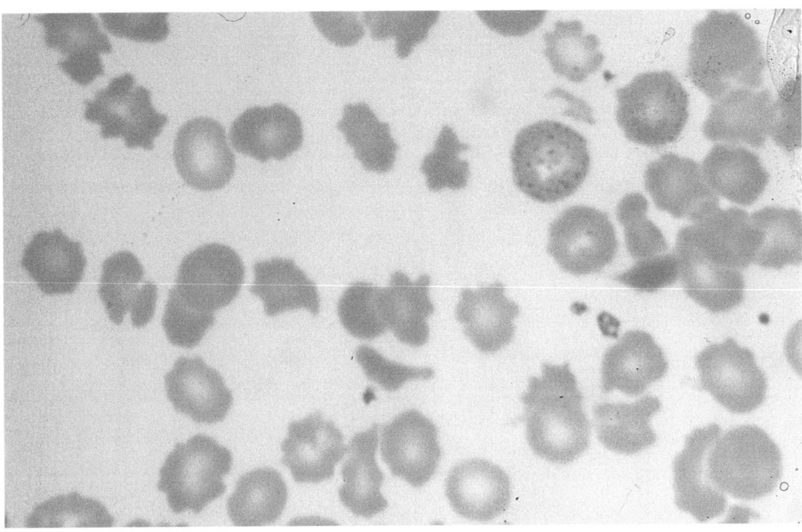

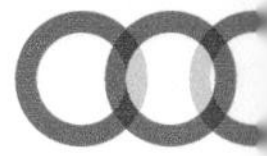

CASE 14

QUESTIONS

A 22-year-old male complains of acute onset of generalised pains in the back, abdomen and limbs. He has also had increased urinary frequency and pain in passing urine over the previous week. On examination, he has a painful swelling of his right upper arm. His blood count shows

Haemoglobin (Hb)	84 g/L
Mean corpuscular value (MCV)	81 fL
White blood cells (WBC)	33.4 × 10^9/L (neutrophils 86%)
Platelets	390 × 10^9/L

Q14.i What abnormalities are shown in the blood film (Figure 14a)?

Q14.ii Haemoglobin electrophoresis was performed on the patient, his family and controls (Figure 14b):

- Lane a is his mother.
- Lane b is his father.
- Lane c is his sister.
- Lane d is his brother.
- Lane e is the patient.
- Lane f is another brother.
- Lane g is a control sample of haemoglobin A/C blood.
- Lane h is a control of haemoglobin A/S blood.

What is the haematological diagnosis? Which of the siblings is likely to be symptomatic?

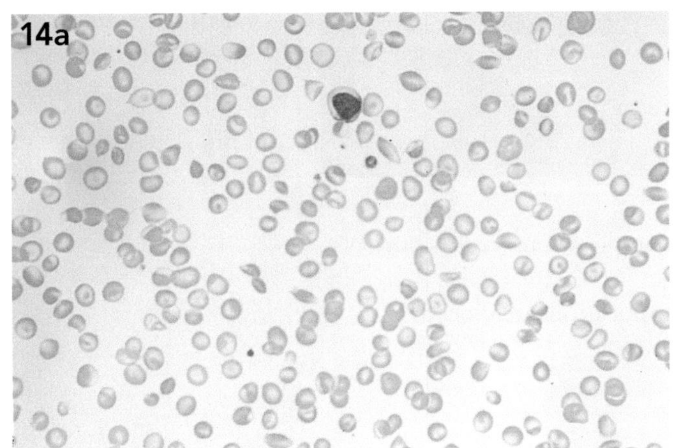

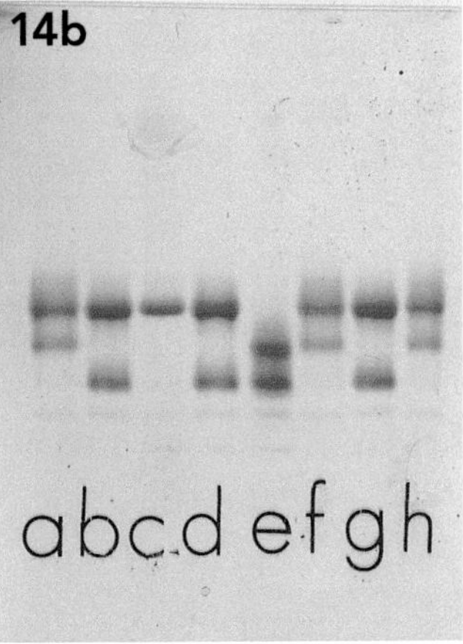

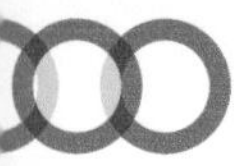

Case 14: QUESTIONS (Continued)

Q14.iii What abnormality is on the x-ray (Figure 14d), and what complication has occurred?

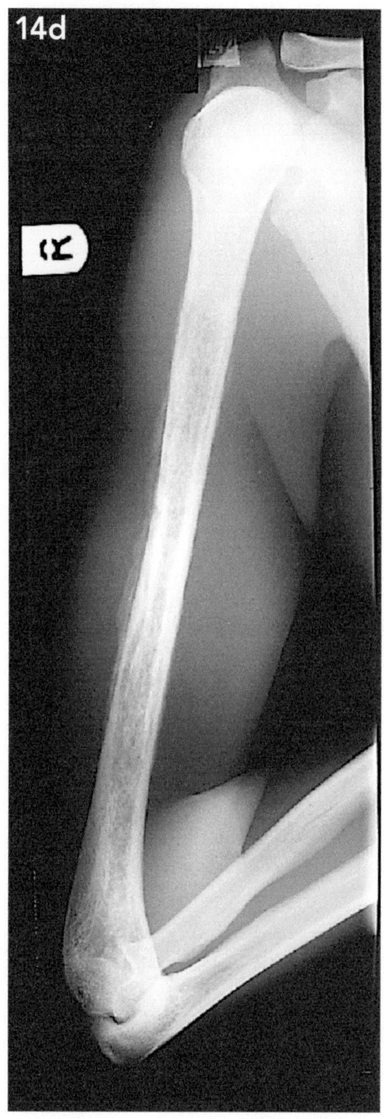

Q14.iv What other skeletal complications may occur?

Q14.v What other renal complications may occur?

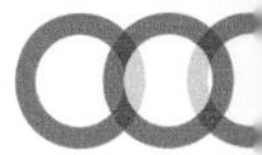

Case 14: ANSWERS

A14.i The blood film shows target cells and irregularly contracted red blood cells. Sickle cells are not prominent. Rectangular cells and cells in which the cytoplasm has shrunk away from the membrane are also seen.

A14.ii The findings in the blood film and the haemoglobin electrophoresis patterns suggest haemoglobin SC disease, the compound heterozygous state for the two important beta-chain mutants, haemoglobin S and C. None of the siblings has a significant haemoglobinopathy, and none of them is likely to be symptomatic. SC disease is a variant of homozygous sickle cell anaemia (SS disease) which is of almost equal severity and has a similar clinical presentation. This patient appears to have a sickle cell crisis which may have been preceded by a urinary tract infection. Figure 14c is an illustration of high-performance liquid chromatography (HPLC) in sickle cell; this is now the standard diagnostic technique.

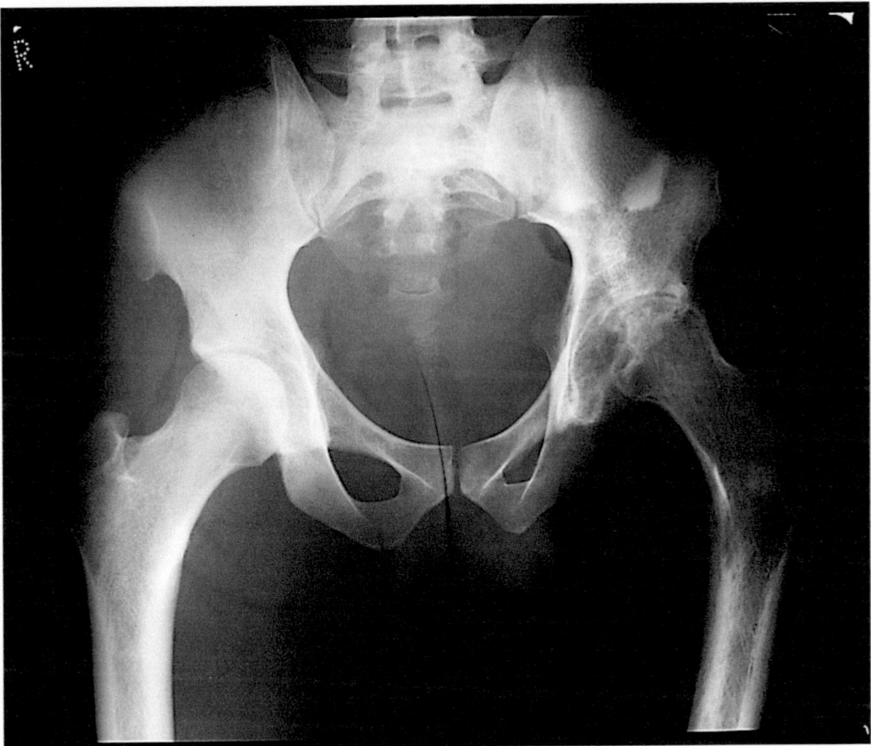

Figure 14c HPLC sickle cell disease – 91.3% of the Hb is sickle haemoglobin (Hbs).

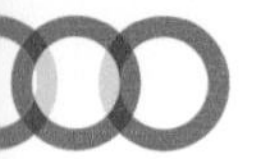

Case 14: ANSWERS (Continued)

A14.iii The x-ray (Figure 14c) shows sequestrum formation within the humerus. There is periosteal reaction. This suggests osteomyelitis. Blood culture revealed a bacteraemia with *Escherichia coli*, and the same organism was isolated from the right humerus. Patients with sickle cell anaemia have an increased risk of osteomyelitis, as organisms may enter the bloodstream from areas of mucosal damage (e.g. in the urinary and gastrointestinal tracts) subjects are hyposplenic, and areas of infarcted marrow can be readily colonised by organisms. Salmonella osteomyelitis is particularly common, as hyposplenism predisposes to this organism, and bile from haemolysis within the marrow provides an enriched culture medium.

A14.iv The most important additional skeletal abnormality is avascular necrosis of the femoral head (image on the left) or the humeral head.

A14.v Renal papillary necrosis (image on the right) may occur in haemoglobin SC disease.

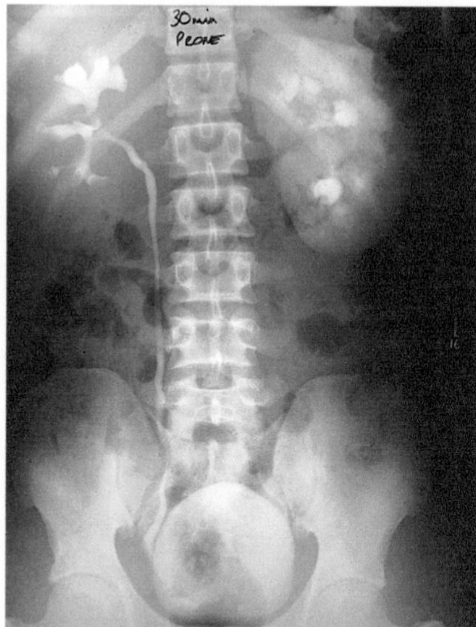

Peak name	Calibrated area %	Area %	Retention time (min)	Peak area
F	2.5*	---	1.08	30226
Unknown	---	0.1	1.23	1923
Unknown	---	0.8	2.12	10141
Ao	---	1.1	2.31	14589
A2	4.7*	---	3.65	59151
S-window	---	91.3	4.51	1215757

Total area: 1331787

F concentration = 2.5*%

A2 concentration = 4.7*%

*Values outside of expected ranges

Analysis comments:

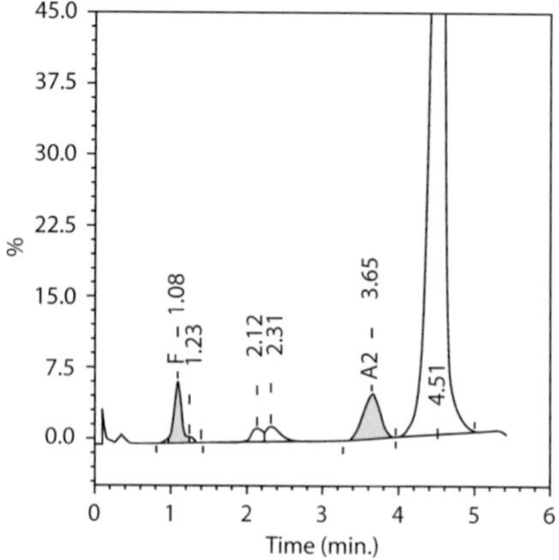

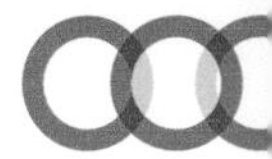

CASE 15

QUESTIONS

A 76-year-old woman presents with a 3- to 4-month history of gradually increasing tiredness and lethargy. She has also noticed numbness and tingling of the hands. On examination she is pale and slightly icteric. A skin rash is noted (Figure 15a). Sensory testing of the legs shows diminished sensation affecting both feet symmetrically. Both ankle jerks are absent and the knee jerks are brisk. Her blood count shows

Haemoglobin (Hb)	65 g/L
Mean corpuscular volume (MCV)	110 fL
White blood cells (WBC)	2.5 × 10^9/L
Platelets	103 × 10^9/L

Q15.i What is the dermatological diagnosis?

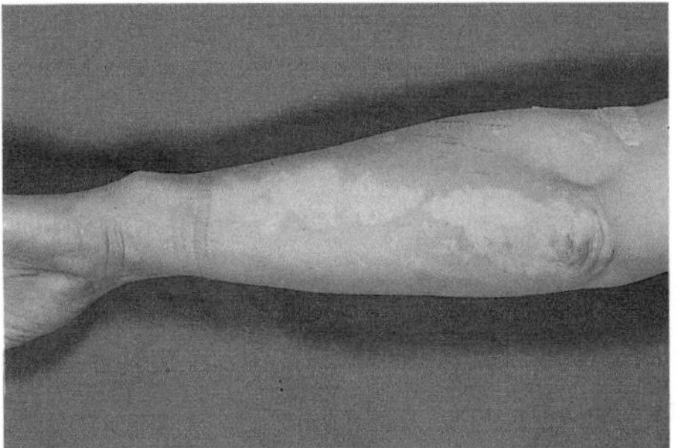

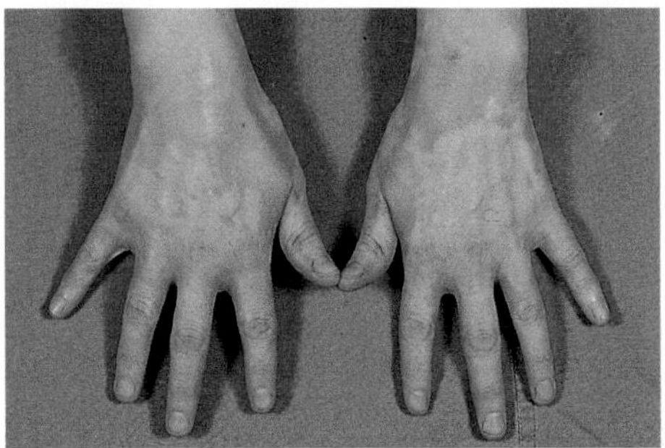

Q15.ii What is the haematological diagnosis? What abnormalities are shown on the blood film?

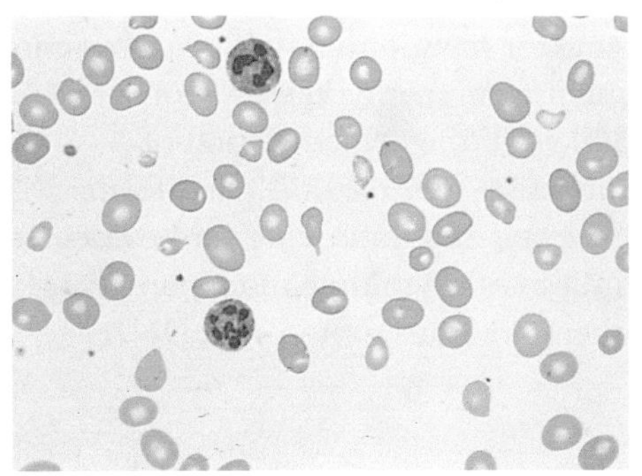

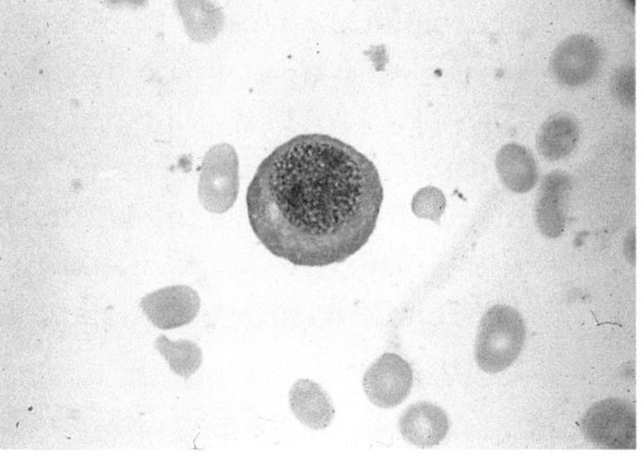

Q15.iii What is the neurological diagnosis?

Q15.iv What further investigations are warranted?

Q15.v How should the patient be treated?

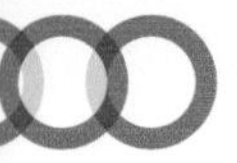

Case 15: ANSWERS

A15.i Vitiligo. This is associated with organ-specific autoimmune diseases, for example

- Pernicious anaemia
- Thyroid disease
- Addison's disease
- Hypoparathyroidism

A15.ii Pernicious anaemia (PA). The blood film shows macrocytosis, anisocytosis and hypersegmented polymorphonuclear leukocytes. There is also a circulating megaloblast. Deficiency of vitamin B_{12} is caused by failure of gastric absorption of the vitamin. Antibodies to gastric parietal cells are present in 95% of patients with pernicious anaemia but only 10% of normal individuals. Antibodies to intrinsic factor are found in 60% of people with pernicious anaemia.

A15.iii Subacute combined degeneration of the spinal cord, with a characteristic combination of upper and lower motor neuron signs in the legs.

A15.iv The following investigations should be carried out:

- Serum B_{12}
- Serum folate and ferritin, and red cell folate (a raised red cell folate with reduced serum folate is characteristically seen in B_{12} deficiency)
- Thyroid-stimulating hormone (TSH) level
- An upper gastrointestinal endoscopy is advised.

A15.v Administration of folic acid without B_{12} therapy can lead to worsening of the neurological changes. B_{12} is a coenzyme for methionine synthase, a reaction needed to activate folate by converting it from methyl tetrahydrofolate (me-THF) to THF. The reaction is linked to the demethylation of methionine to homocysteine, and emphasises the role of B_{12} and folate metabolism in reducing homocysteine levels and improving cardiovascular risk. Folate is a coenzyme for the synthesis of thymidine monophosphate (TMP); deficiency of B_{12} and folate therefore leads to impaired DNA synthesis.

Parenteral B_{12} – hydroxocobalamin 1000 mg intramuscularly weekly for 4 weeks followed by long-term injections every 3 months – is appropriate. Iron and folate supplements should be given orally for the first 2 months of treatment.

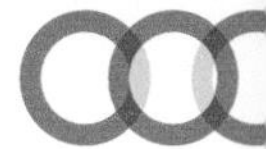

Case 15: ANSWERS (Continued)

Figure 15a shows facial pallor with mild jaundice ('lemon-yellow tinge') in a woman with PA who has dyed her hair (premature greying is characteristic). Figure 15b shows her fleshy tongue. These patients have an increased incidence of gastric carcinoma.

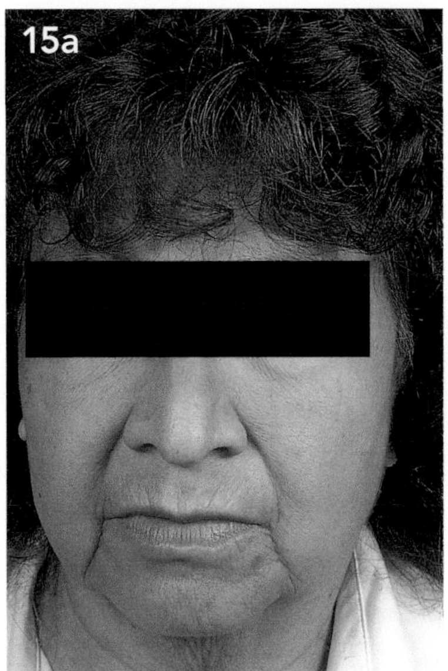

15a

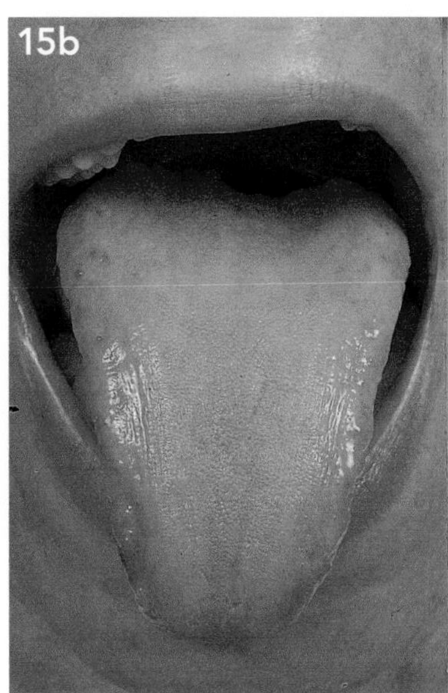

15b

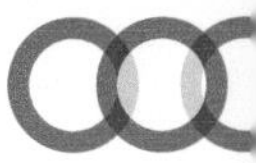

CASE 16

QUESTIONS

A 56-year-old woman has noticed increasing tiredness and malaise. She was intensively investigated for iron deficiency 1 year ago and no cause was found. She has subsequently noticed episodes of pain associated with passage of dark urine. Investigations show

Haemogloblin (Hb)	9.5 g/dL
Mean corpuscular volume (MCV)	72 fL
White blood cells (WBC)	4.1×10^9/L
Platelets	113×10^9/L

Q16.i Comment on the blood film and blood count.

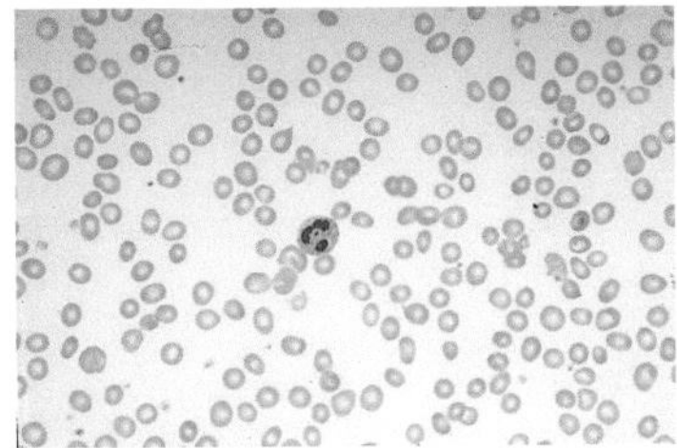

Q16.ii A specialised test is performed on her serum and cells. There are nine tubes, as follows:

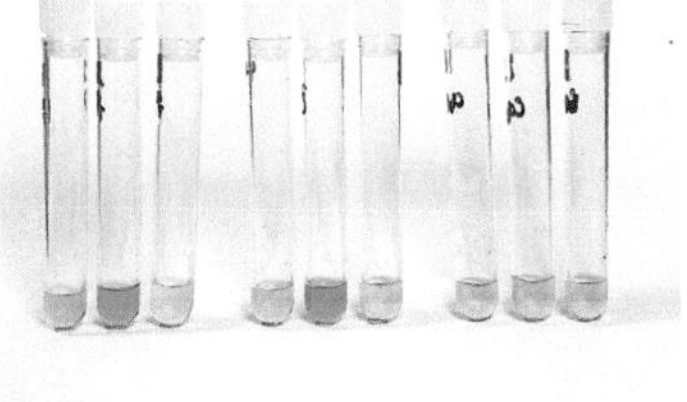

1. Patient cells with patient serum (unacidified).
2. Patient cells with patient serum (acidified).
3. Patient cells with patient serum (acidified and heated).
4. Patient cells with donor serum (unacidified).
5. Patient cells with donor serum (acidified).
6. Patient cells with donor serum (acidified and heated).
7. Donor cells with donor serum (unacidified).
8. Donor cells with donor serum (acidified).
9. Donor cells with donor serum (acidified and heated).

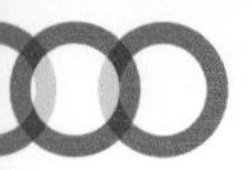

Case 16: QUESTIONS (Continued)

Q16.iii What is the diagnosis? How is the diagnosis confirmed?

Q16.iv What is the pathogenesis and natural history of this disease?

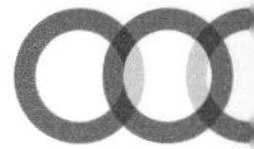

Case 16: ANSWERS

A16.i The blood film shows hypochromic microcytic red cells which are consistent with iron deficiency. There is a disproportionate degree of anisocytosis and polychromasia.

A16.ii This is an illustration of Ham's test, and demonstrates that her red cells have increased sensitivity to lysis by complement present in her own serum.

Heat inactivates complement, whereas low pH activates complement. Thus, lysis of her cells occurs to a small extent in the presence of her own serum and donor serum, is exaggerated by the presence of acidified serum and does not occur when complement is inactivated. Donor cells do not undergo lysis and would not do so even in the presence of the patient's serum. The intravascular haemolysis leads to the presence of haemosiderin, which can be stained by Perl's reaction (Figure 16a) on the urine deposit. The only other disorder that may give a positive Ham's test is a rare congenital dyserythropoietic anaemia (CDA type II, hereditary erythrocyte multinuclearity with positive acidified serum [HEMPAS] test, Figure 16b).

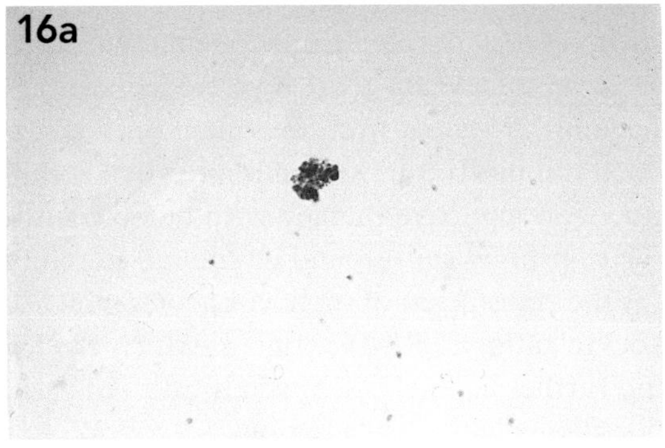

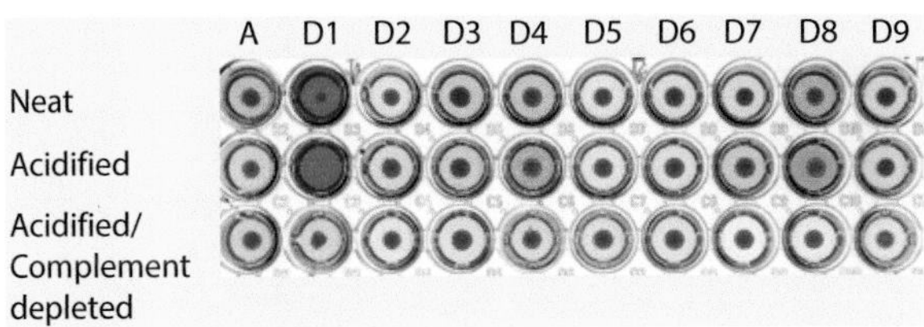

Figure 16b Hereditary erythrocyte multinuclearity with positive acidified serum (HEMPAS) screen.

HEMPAS cells carry an unusual antigen that reacts with a lytic antibody present in about 30% of normal sera; lysis would not occur in tube 2 but may occur in tubes 4 and 5.

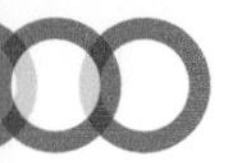

Case 16: ANSWERS (Continued)

A16.iii Paroxysmal nocturnal haemoglobinuria (PNH). Ham's test is no longer used for diagnosis but is included here as it illustrates the mechanism of haemolysis. The diagnosis is confirmed by flow cytometric analysis of blood cells to demonstrate reduced expression of CD55 and CD59 (see below).

A16.iv This is an acquired clonal disorder which arises due to acquired mutations of the PIG-A gene in haemopoietic stem cells. Affected cells are deficient in glucosyl-phosphatidylinositol-anchored proteins (GPI-APs) which leads to defects in the cell membrane which impair inactivation of complement, and thus to increased complement-mediated lysis. Many patients have defective platelet function and a thrombotic tendency, and presentation with hepatic vein thrombosis (Budd–Chiari syndrome) is well recognised. The fluorescently labelled aerolysin (FLAER) assay reveals haemopoietic cells deficient in GPI-APs and can be used to assess the size of the abnormal clone. The standard diagnostic test for PNH is by flow cytometry to demonstrate reduced expression of CD 55 and CD 59 on red cells. The illustration of the Ham's test is given to illustrate the pathological abnormality; the Ham's test is obsolete.

Patients with PNH may develop pancytopenia with aplastic anaemia, and a proportion go on to develop acute myeloid leukaemia. Patients with significant haemolysis benefit from treatment with ecluzimab, a monoclonal antibody which inhibits the activation of terminal complement components by binding to C5. Supportive therapy with blood transfusion may also be required. The transfused cells should be filtered to remove contaminating leukocytes, as the transfusion of such leukocytes may lead to sensitisation to human leukocyte antigen (HLA) antigens, which can lead to complement activation and further haemolysis. Severely affected patients should be considered for allogeneic transplantation.

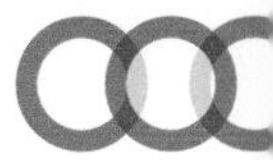

CASE 17

QUESTIONS

A 41-year-old male has a 6-week history of fever and night sweats. He has lost 2 kg in weight. He has had a recent cough with productive sputum, but his fever has failed to subside after a course of antibiotics. He smokes 10 cigarettes a day and drinks 16 units of alcohol a week. On examination, he is pale and looks unwell. There is no palpable lymphadenopathy or splenomegaly. Investigations show

Haemoglobin (Hb)	87 g/L
Mean corpuscular volume (MCV)	81 fL
Platelets	310×10^9/L
Erythrocyte sedimentation rate (ESR)	91 mm/h
Urea and electrolytes	Normal
Immunoglobulins	Normal
White blood cells (WBC)	9.1×10^9/L (differential normal)
Bilirubin	61 mmol/L (NR 5–17 mmol/L)
Aspartate aminotransferase (AST)	137 U/L (NR 5–40 U/L)
Alkaline phosphatase	250 U/L (NR 35–130 U/L)
Gamma-glutamyl transferase (GGT)	215 U/L (NR 10–48 U/L)
Albumin	34 g/L (NR 35–50 g/L)

Q17.i Comment on the chest x-ray and the thoracic computed tomography (CT) scan.

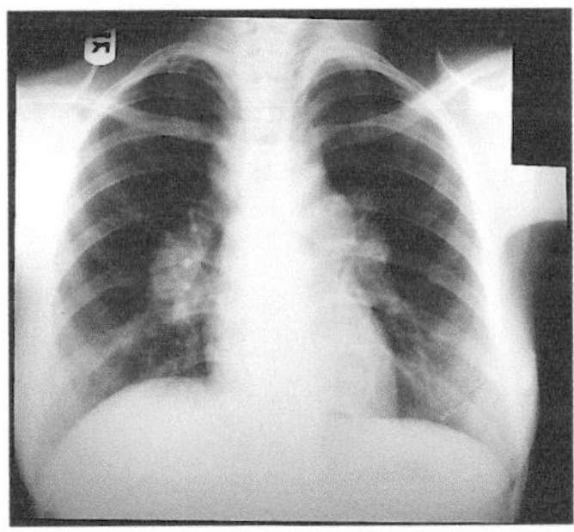

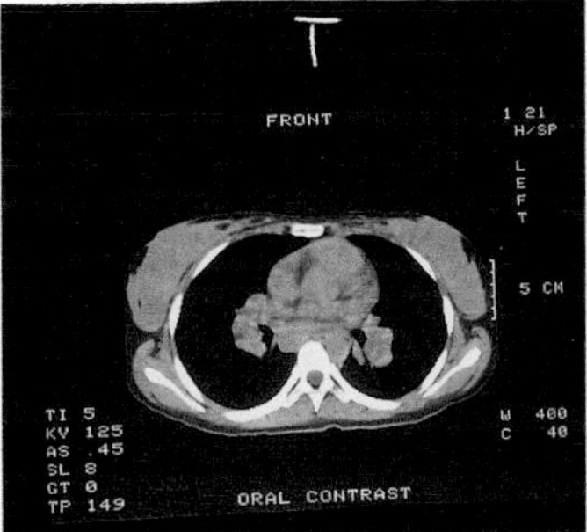

Q17.ii Comment on the abdominal CT scan.

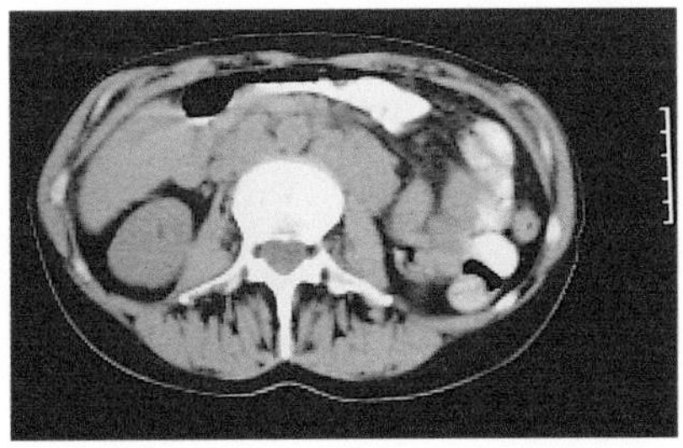

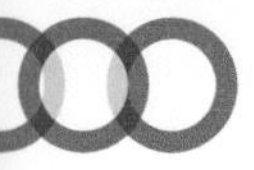

Case 17: ANSWERS

A17.i The chest x-ray shows a large mediastinal mass, compatible with lymph node enlargement.

A17.ii Abdominal CT scan shows enlargement of the retroperitoneal lymph nodes between the junction of the renal vessels and the bifurcation of the aorta.

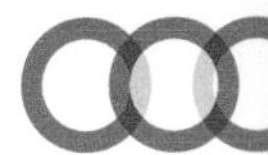

Q17.iii A liver biopsy (Figure 17a), and lymph node biopsy is performed. A bone marrow aspirate and trephine (Figure 17b) are also performed. Comment on the liver biopsy (Figure 17a). Comment on the bone marrow biopsy (Figure 17b).

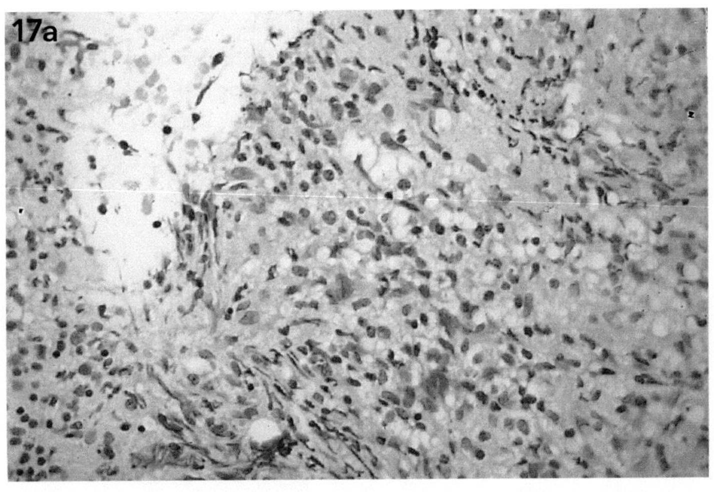

17a

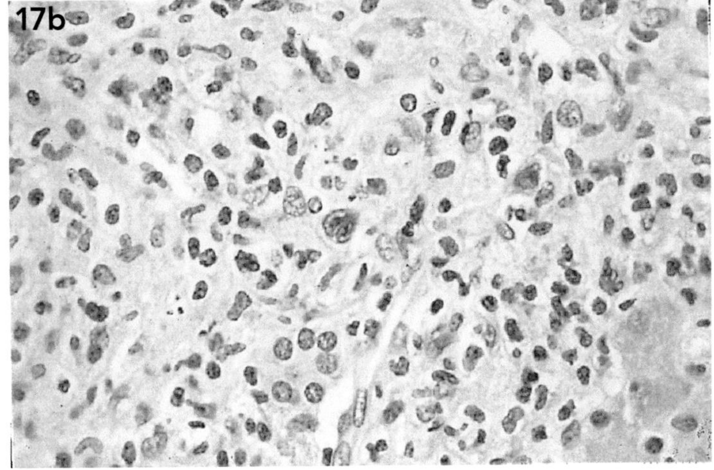

17b

Q17.iv What is the diagnosis? What further investigations should be performed?

Q17.v How should he be treated?

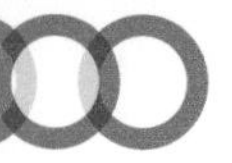

Case 17: ANSWERS (Continued)

A17.iii The liver biopsy shows infiltration of the liver by large multinucleated cells which have the appearance of Reed–Sternberg cells. Bone marrow trephine shows an abnormal area at one end of the core which, at high power, also reveals involvement by Hodgkin's disease. The cells were confirmed to be CD30 positive.

A17.iv Stage IV B mixed cellularity Hodgkin's lymphoma (HL). The advent of fluorodeoxyglucose–positron emission tomography (FDG–PET) scans has improved the management of HL as it allows accurate localisation of diseased tissue which resolves after successful treatment (Figure 17c, showing pre- and post-treatment scans).

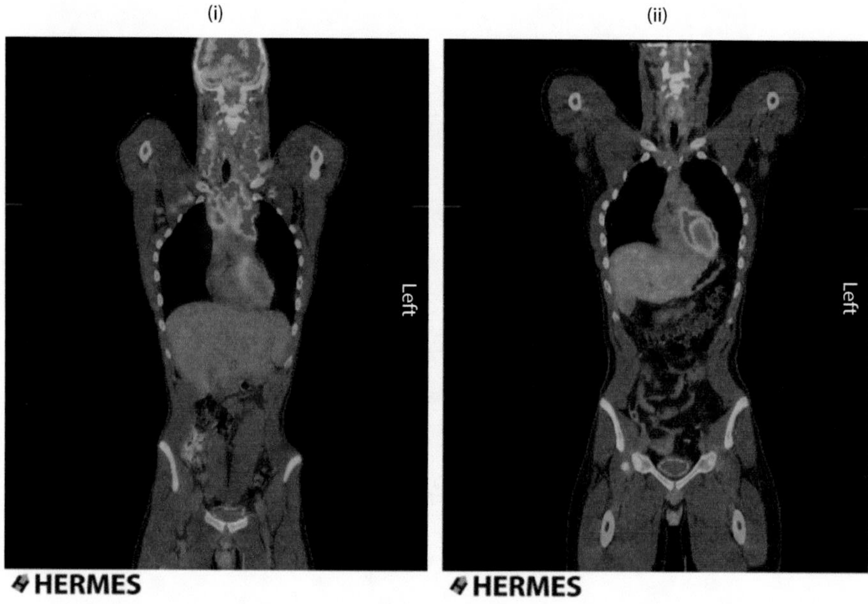

Figure 17c Hodgin lymphoma (HL) – fluorodeoxyglucose–positron emission tomography (FDG–PET) scans. (i) Pre-treatment. (ii) Post-treatment.

A17.v Localised Hodgkin's disease (e.g. Stages I and IA) responds well to radiotherapy. However, systemic symptoms, involvement of tissues both above and below the diaphragm (Stage III) and involvement extending outside the lymphoreticular system (e.g. into the liver, marrow, lung, central nervous system, skin – Stage IV) should be treated with combination chemotherapy. Suitable regimes are chlorambucil, vinblastine, procarbazine, prednisolone (ChlVPP) and adriamycin, BCNU, vinblastine, dacarbazine (ABVD). Failure to respond as assessed by PET scans is an indication to intensify chemotherapy.

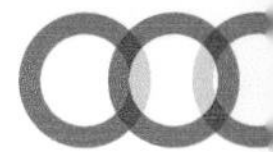

Side effects of combination chemotherapy include bone marrow suppression, hair loss, susceptibility to infection, and infertility. There is an increased risk of acute myeloid leukaemia in lymphoma patients who have received combination chemotherapy, particularly if they have also received radiotherapy.

Figure 17d shows gastric involvement and pyloric obstruction by high-grade non-Hodgkin's lymphoma; barium flow and symptoms were both improved by radiotherapy (Figure 17e). The following table shows the International Prognostic System (IPS) for HL (Hasenclever).

International Prognostic System for HL (Hasenclever)

The following are adverse prognostic features at diagnosis
Albumin <40 g/L
Haemoglobin concentration <105 g/L
Male sex
Age 45 or older
Stage IV disease according to Ann Arbor classification
Leukocytosis (WBC >15 × 10^9/L)
Lymphopenia (lymphocyte count <0.6 × 10^9/L)

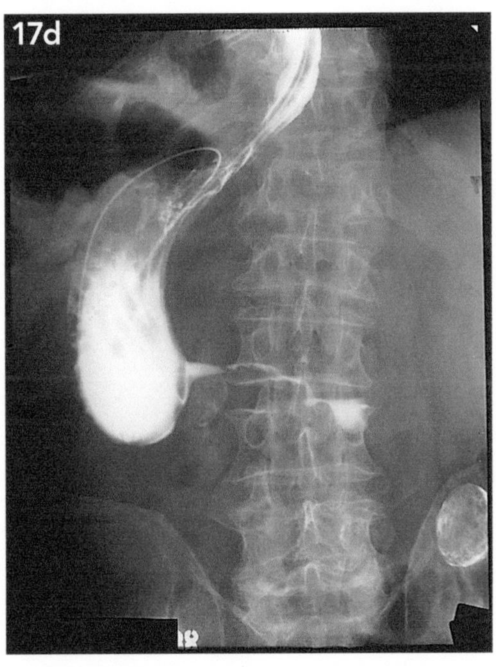

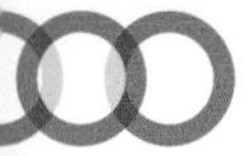

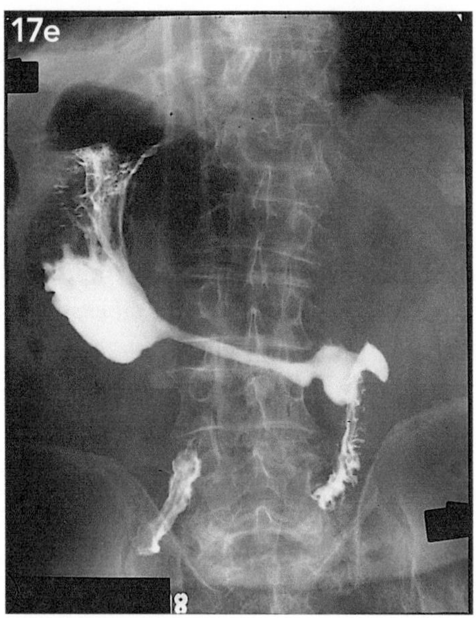
17e

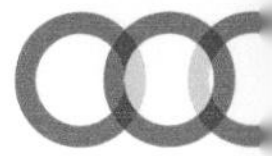

CASE 18

QUESTIONS

A 56-year-old woman, with a long history of arthritis, has an abnormal blood count:

Haemoglobin (Hb)	91 g/L
Mean corpuscular volume (MCV)	91 g/L
Mean corpuscular haemoglobin volume (MCHC)	32.1
White blood cells (WBC)	7.2×10^9/L
Platelets	195×10^9/L

Q18.i What diagnosis is suggested by the x-ray of her hands?

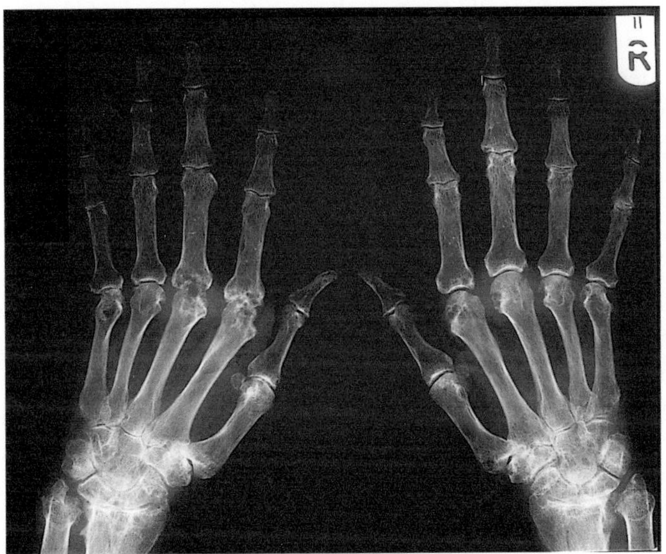

Q18.ii What is the likeliest cause of her anaemia?

Q18.iii What investigations would you perform on this patient?

Q18.iv What other haematological complications may occur in this condition?

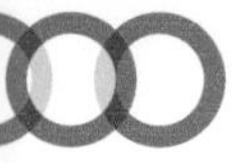

Case 18: ANSWERS

A18.i The x-ray confirms the diagnosis of rheumatoid arthritis – it shows an erosive arthritis affecting her hands.

A18.ii The anaemia of chronic disease (ACD). This normochromic normocytic (occasionally slightly microcytic) anaemia commonly complicates chronic inflammatory and infective conditions and neoplasia. The mechanism is poorly understood but it probably involves a suppressive effect that increased cytokine levels (e.g. tumour necrosis factor [TNF], interleukin 6) have on erythropoiesis, the release of iron from the reticuloendothelial system, and iron utilisation.

A18.iii The diagnosis of rheumatoid can be confirmed by demonstrating the presence of rheumatoid factor and anti-cyclic citrullinate peptide (anti-CCP) antibodies. Disease modifying treatments for rheumatoid include monoclonal antibodies to TNF, and these agents may improve the anaemia. The serum iron and the total iron-binding capacity are typically lowered in ACD.

The serum ferritin is usually normal, though it may be raised in the face of active inflammation. A lowered serum ferritin would suggest iron deficiency, which frequently complicates rheumatoid arthritis (e.g. due to gastric bleeding induced by ingestion of non-steroidal anti-inflammatory drugs). Vitamin B12 and folic acid levels, thyroid function, renal function, liver function and erythrocyte sedimentation rate (ESR) would be worth assessing.

A18.iv Other haematological complications of rheumatoid arthritis include

- Immunological disorders – autoimmune haemolytic anaemia, idiopathic thrombocytopenic purpura, leukopenia, Felty's syndrome (leukopenia and splenomegaly)
- Therapy-induced complications – gastrointestinal bleeding, cytopenias, aplastic anaemia (caused, e.g. by phenylbutazone); the blood film shows a fragment of a bone marrow aspirate taken from a patient with phenylbutazone-induced aplastic anaemia
- An increased incidence of lymphoma
- Amyloidosis

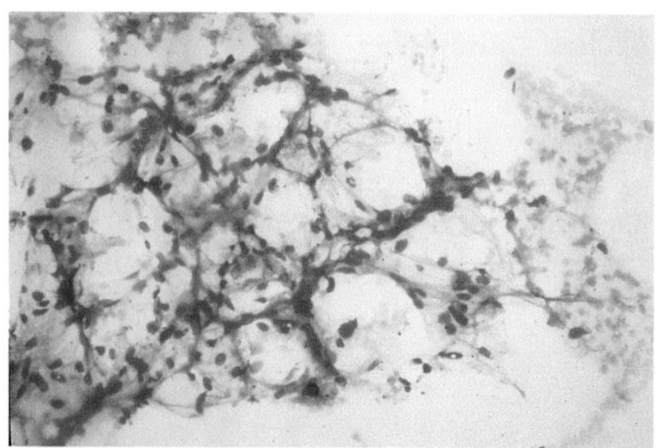

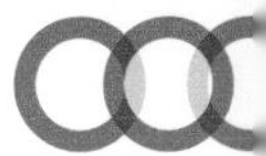

CASE 19

QUESTIONS

A 34-year-old patient, with a past history of intravenous drug abuse, presents with a 7-day history of progressive shortness of breath. On examination, he is pyrexial and has clear dyspnoea and tachycardia. His blood pressure is reduced at 90/60 mmHg. Oxygen saturation when breathing 40% oxygen is reduced at 86%, and he is sweating. His full blood count shows

Haemoglobin (Hb)	85 g/L
White blood cells (WBC)	17.5×10^9/L (neutrophils 79%)
Platelets	105×10^9/L

Q19.i What is the likeliest diagnosis from the history and chest x-ray?

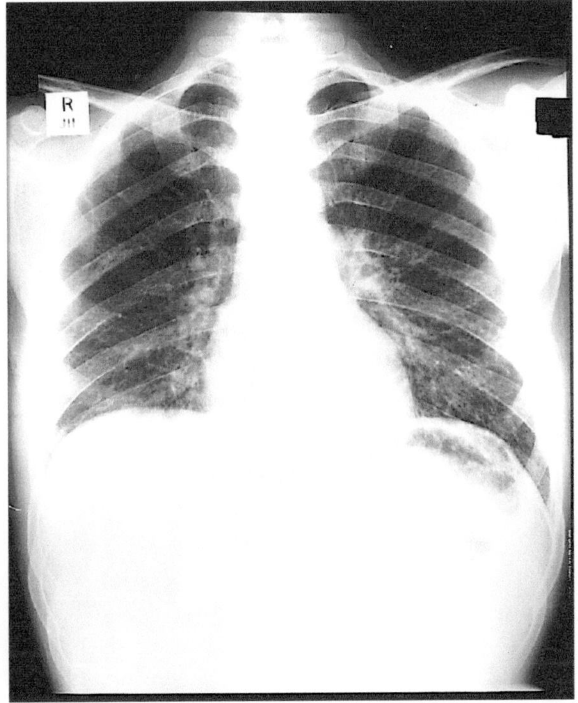

Q19.ii What further tests should be performed?

Q19.iii How should he be treated?

Q19.iv What other haematological complications may occur in this condition?

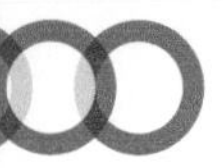

Case 19: ANSWERS

A19.i He probably has an infection with *Pneumocystis carinii*.

A19.ii HIV antibody. A bronchoalveolar lavage or bronchial secretions should be obtained so that a firm microbiological diagnosis can be made; this should be done after consultation with an anaesthetist. He needs to be assessed for admission to an intensive therapy unit. A full biochemical screen should be performed, and blood, urine and a throat swab should be sent for bacterial, viral, fungal and protozoan culture.

A19.iii He should be treated with high-dose intravenous co-trimoxazole for presumed Pneumocystis infection, but broad-spectrum antibiotics should be given until a bacteriological diagnosis is proven and in case of mixed infections. High-dose co-trimoxazole may cause myelosuppression, partly reversible with folinic acid.

A19.iv Immune thrombocytopenia, lymphopenia and anaemia of chronic disease are relatively common. The commonest haematological malignancy associated with HIV is non-Hodgkin's lymphoma; high-grade Burkitt-like B-cell lymphoma with central nervous system (CNS) involvement is characteristic (see Figure 19a). Paraproteins and myeloma may occur, and acute myeloid leukaemia (AML) is reported. Monocytosis, a haemophagocytic syndrome, immune haemolytic anaemia, myelodysplasia and aplastic anaemia are also reported.

The blood film (Figure 19b) is from an HIV-positive patient who is on zidovudine; it shows macrocytosis and thrombocytopenia. Figure 19c shows bone marrow aspirate from the same patient – he has developed acute myeloid leukaemia with erythroid differentiation.

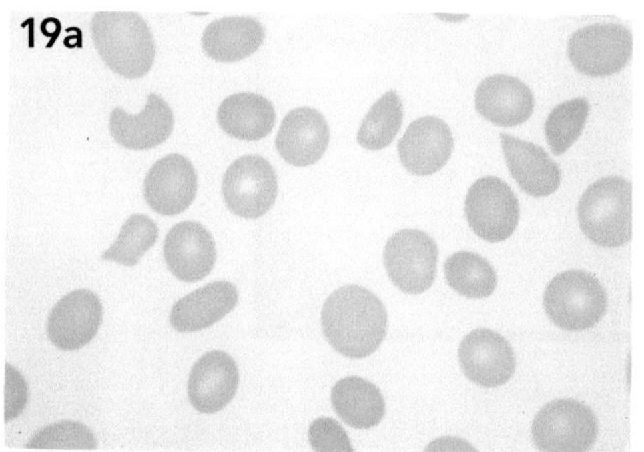

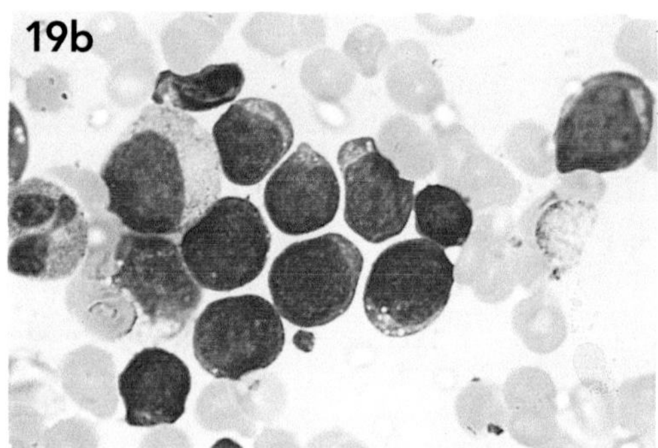

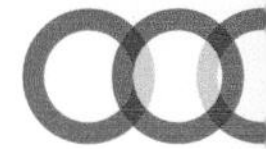

Case 19: ANSWERS (Continued)

Myelodysplasia and acute leukaemia are reported. A Ziehl–Nielson stain on a bone marrow trephine biopsy in an HIV-positive patient (Figure 19c) shows multiple organisms, which on culture were confirmed to be *Mycobacterium avium-intracellulare*. Bone marrow trephine biopsy in an HIV-positive patient (Figure 19d) shows an infection with *Cryptococcus neoformans*.

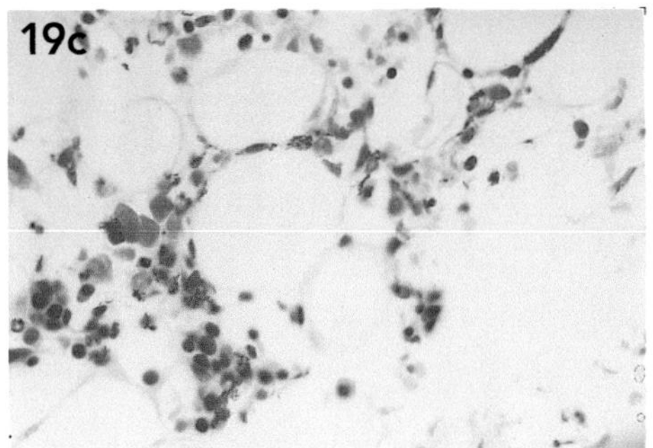

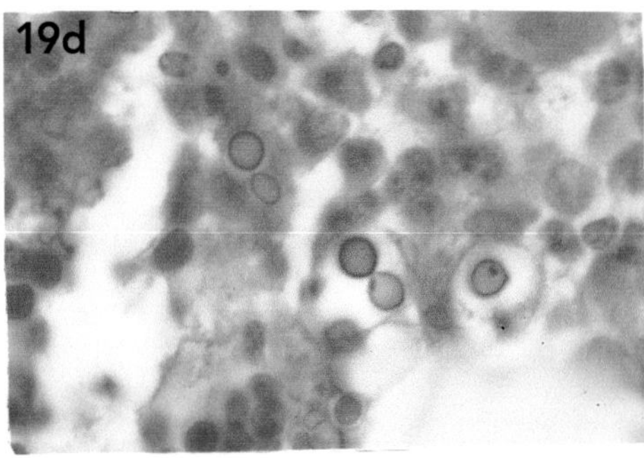

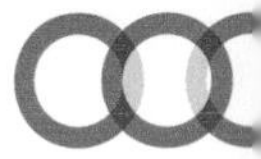

CASE 20

QUESTIONS

A 68-year-old man presents with a 12-hour history of headache, confusion and declining consciousness. His wife says that he has recently completed oral chemotherapy for an 'indolent form of leukaemia'. Examination reveals him to be responding to painful stimuli but not to verbal commands. He has bilateral axillary and inguinal lymphadenopathy. He is clinically jaundiced and anaemic. His spleen is palpably enlarged. He has neck stiffness, generalised hyper-reflexia and bilateral upgoing plantar reflexes. Fundal examination is normal, and there are no focal neurological signs. Full blood count shows

Haemoglobin (Hb)	7.5 g/dL
White blood cells (WBC)	37 × 109/L (lymphocytes 86%)
Platelets	26 × 109/L

Q20.i What abnormalities are seen on this patient's blood film?

Q20.ii Suggest a possible haematological diagnosis.

Q20.iii What abnormalities are seen on the enhanced computed tomography (CT) scan?

Q20.iv How should this patient be managed?

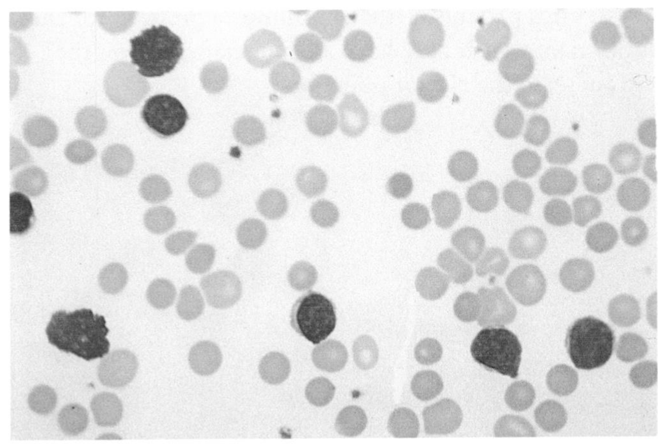

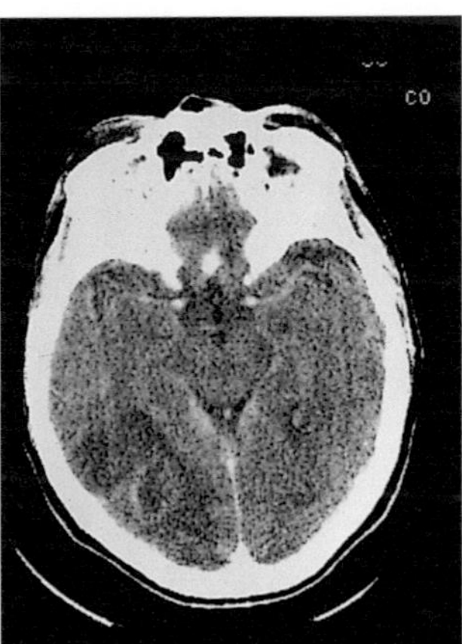

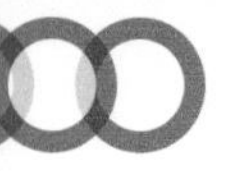

Case 20: ANSWERS

A20.i The film shows spherocytosis, polychromasia, thrombocytopenia and lymphocytosis.

A20.ii The 'indolent form of leukaemia' in this case was chronic lymphocytic leukaemia (CLL), which became complicated by autoimmune haemolytic anaemia (AIHA). (This is a recognised association.) Direct anti-globulin test, reticulocyte count, lymphoid cell flowcytometric analysis and bone marrow examination are required to confirm this. Flowcytometry analysis will show these cells to be positive for B-cell markers [CD19, 20, 21 and 23] and to have low density of surface membrane immunoglobulin [SmIg] with predominance of one light chain, either kappa or lambda. B-CLL cells also characteristically and aberrantly express the T-cell marker, CD5.

A20.iii The scan shows a low attenuation area in the right parieto-occipital area. There is no evidence of midline shift. This is not consistent with acute bleeding, but suggests infection, inflammation or infarction.

A20.iv He requires urgent lumbar puncture. In this case, it showed intracellular Gram-positive rods, consistent with Listeria meningitis. The low platelet count suggests possible disseminated intravascular coagulation (DIC), which frequently complicates meningitis.

He was treated with intravenous ampicillin, chloramphenicol and metronidazole. His AIHA responded to high-dose intravenous steroids (dexamethasone was chosen to reduce cerebral oedema) and blood transfusion. Fludarabine is best avoided as its use has been associated with an increased risk of AIHA in CLL patients. Other immunosuppression for the AIHA may include rituximab, which may have a beneficial effect on the CLL. Splenectomy will increase the risk of infection.

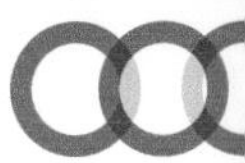

CASE 21

QUESTIONS

Q21.i Comment on the abnormalities in the blood films. The patient's blood count shows

Haemoglobin (Hb)	91 g/L
Mean corpuscular volume (MCV)	62 f/L
White blood cells (WBC) and platelets	Normal

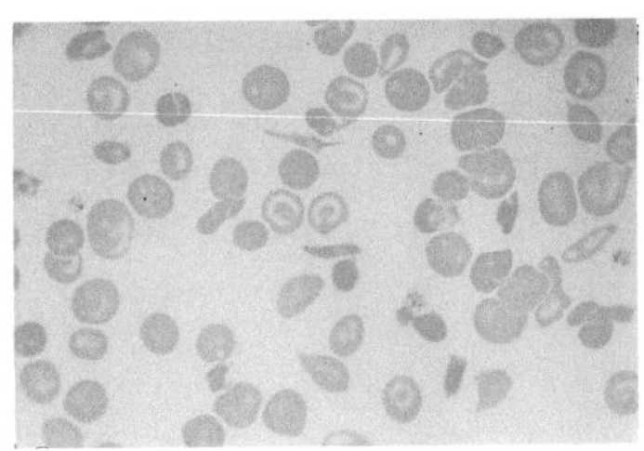

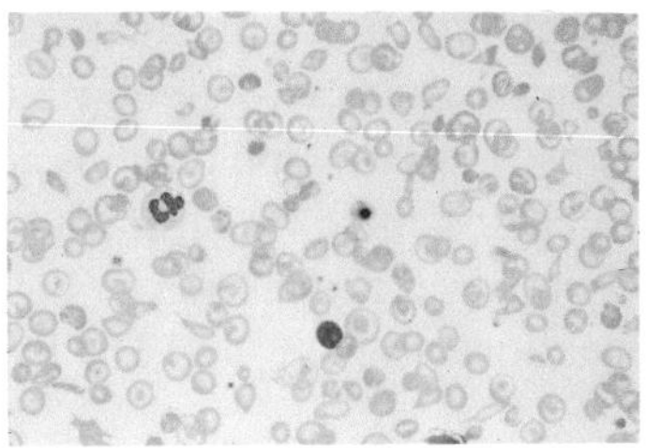

Q21.ii Haemoglobin electrophoresis (Figure 21a) has been performed on

- The patient (lane f)
- His mother (lane e)
- His father (lane d)

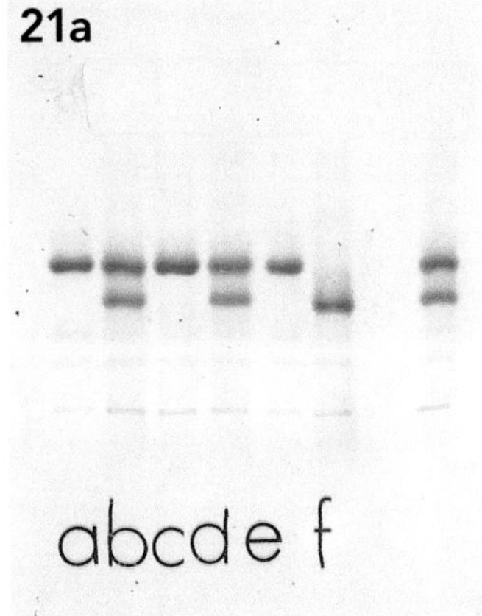

Appropriate controls as follows:

- Lane a: Beta thalassaemia trait
- Lane b: Sickle cell trait
- Lane c: Normal

Quantification of separated haemoglobin bands in the patient shows

- Hb F 9%
- Hb S 86%
- Hb A_2 5%

Quantification of separated haemoglobin bands in his mother shows

- Hb F 3% (NR <1%)
- Hb A 92%
- Hb A_2 5% (NR 1.5%–3.5%)

Quantification of separated haemoglobin bands in his father shows

- Hb A 47%
- Hb S 49%
- Hb A_2 3%

What is the diagnosis in the patient? What is the diagnosis in his mother and his father?

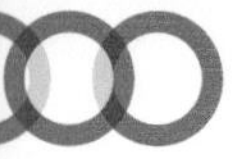

Case 21: ANSWERS

A21.i The blood film shows hypochromic, microcytic cells with target cells and occasional sickle cells. The appearance of these is consistent with sickle beta thalassaemia.

A21.ii The patient has sickle beta thalassaemia. The patient's mother has beta thalassaemia trait. His father has sickle cell trait. In citrate agar electrophoresis (Figure 21a), Hb C migrates to the same position as Hb A_2. Agar gel electrophoresis allows separation of Hb C and Hb A_2. Figure 21b illustrates the expected pattern of migration of normal and abnormal haemoglobins by citrate agar electrophoresis in a diagrammatic form. Hb A is composed of two alpha chains and two beta chains ($\alpha_2\beta_2$); Hb A_2 is composed of two alpha chains and two delta chains ($\alpha_2\delta_2$); Hb F is two alpha chains and two gamma chains ($\alpha_2\gamma_2$). Patients with beta thalassaemia have impaired production of beta chains and compensate by increasing their production of Hb A_2 and Hb F.

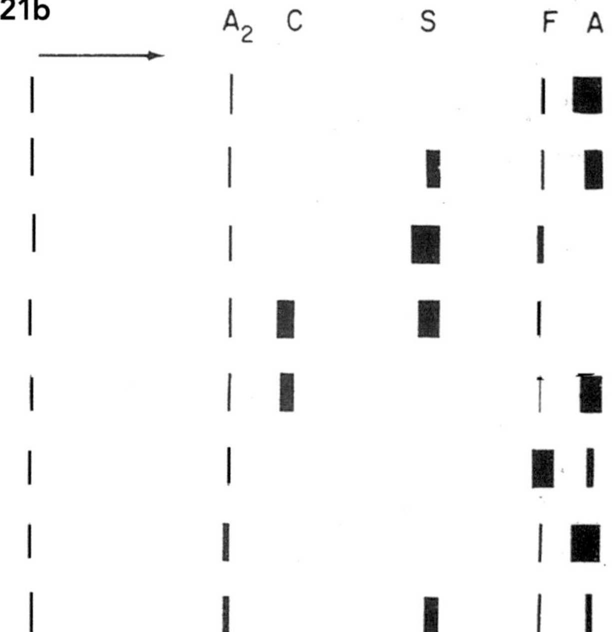

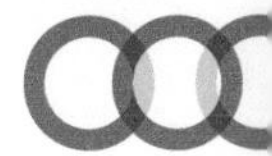

Case 21: QUESTION (Continued)

Q21.iii The patient has decided to marry someone who is a sickle cell trait carrier. What advice would you give?

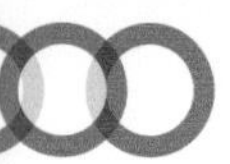

Case 21: ANSWERS (Continued)

A21.iii The patient has sickle beta thalassaemia and the partner is denoted sickle trait (A/S). The possible combinations for their offspring are therefore

- S/A
- S/S
- A/beta thal
- beta thal/S

There is thus a 50% chance of a significant haemoglobinopathy (S/S or S/beta thal). These two conditions have a similar clinical presentation and course. Non-directional, informed counselling should be offered to the couple. Antenatal diagnosis may be offered, with the prospect of genetic diagnosis by DNA analysis of placental tissue at 8–12 weeks of pregnancy. High-performance liquid chromatography (HPLC) appearances for normal AS and S/beta thal are illustrated as Figure 21c through Figure 21e

Peak name	Calibrated area %	Area %	Retention time (min)	Peak area
Unknown	---	0.1	1.02	1486
F	0.4	---	1.09	4401
Unknown	---	1.4	1.23	17859
P2	---	4.6	1.31	60173
P3	---	4.1	1.70	53848
A0	---	86.4	2.48	1121967
A2	3.0	---	3.62	39439

Total area: 1,299,173

F concentration = 0.4%
A2 concentration = 3.0%

Analysis comments:

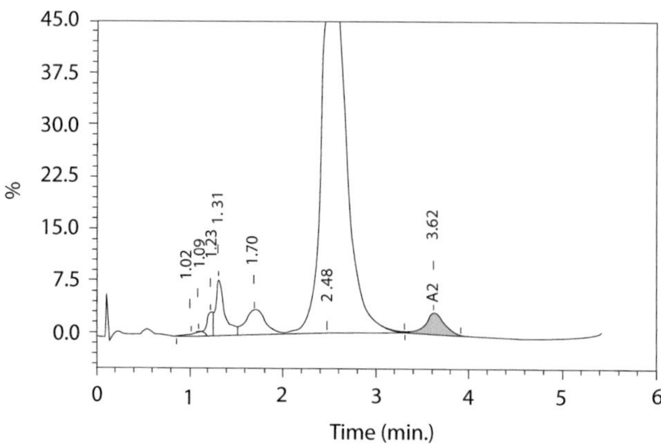

Figure 21c Normal.

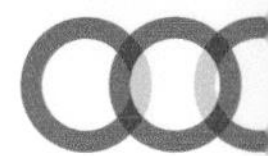

Case 21: ANSWERS (Continued)

Peak name	Calibrated area %	Area %	Retention time (min)	Peak area
F	0.2	---	1.09	4379
Unknown	---	0.7	1.23	13599
P2	---	2.7	1.31	48797
P3	---	2.2	1.68	40361
Ao	---	52.3	2.49	960055
A2	2.5	---	3.63	46364
S-window	---	39.3	4.45	720569

Total area: 1,834,125

F concentration = 0.2%
A2 concentration = 2.5%

Analysis comments:

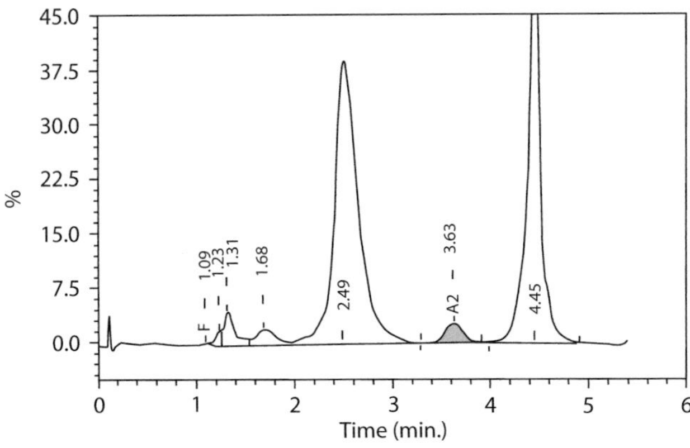

Figure 21d A + S.

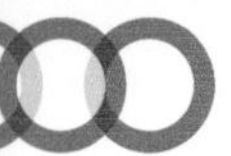

Case 21: ANSWERS (Continued)

Bio-Rad CDM System
Bio-Rad Variant V-II Instrument #1

PATIENT REPORT
V2_BThal

<u>Patient Data</u>

Sample ID: 519896
Patient ID:
Name:
Physician:
Sex:
DOB:
Comments:

<u>Analysis Data</u>

Analysis Performed: 05/07 12:40:28
Injection Number: 4565
Run Number: 223
Rack ID: 0002
Tube Number: 9
Report Generated: 08/07 17:01:45
Operator ID:

Peak name	Calibrated area %	Area %	Retention time (min)	Peak area
F	21.4*	- - -	1.15	350684
Unknown	- - -	0.7	2.10	13160
A0	- - -	1.8	2.26	34292
A2	5.5*	- - -	3.65	98186
S-window	- - -	74.2	4.50	1429406

Total area: 1,925,729

F concentration = 21.4* %
A2 concentration = 5.5* %

* Values outside of expected ranges

Analysis comments:

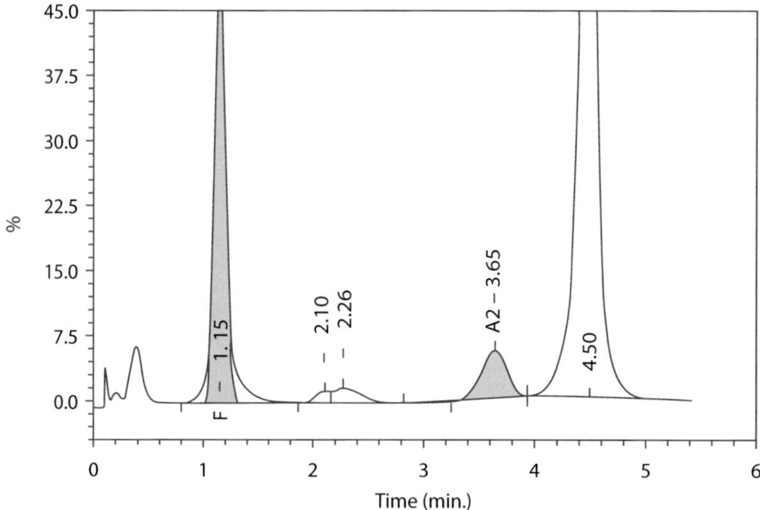

Figure 21e Sickle beta thalassaemia.

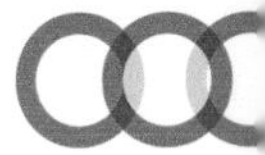

CASE 22

QUESTIONS

Q22.i This blood films is from a 34-year-old woman who has a white blood cell (WBC) count of 63 × 10^9/L. She was initially treated with four courses of intensive chemotherapy and entered complete remission. She relapsed 6 months later, remission was again achieved with chemotherapy and she then received an allogeneic bone marrow transplant from a fully human leukocyte antigen (HLA) compatible sibling. What is the likely diagnosis at presentation? What chromosomal translocation is typically seen?

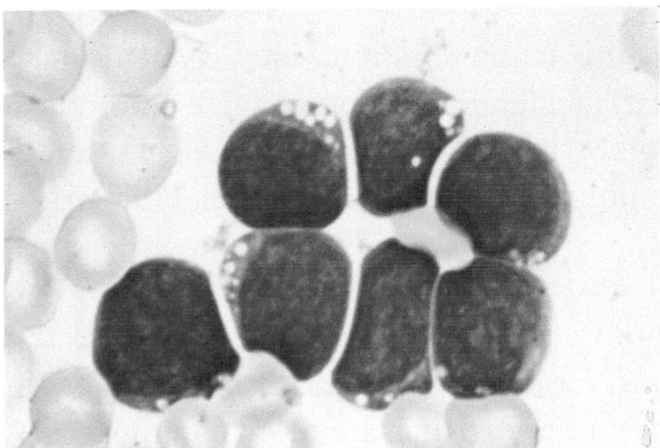

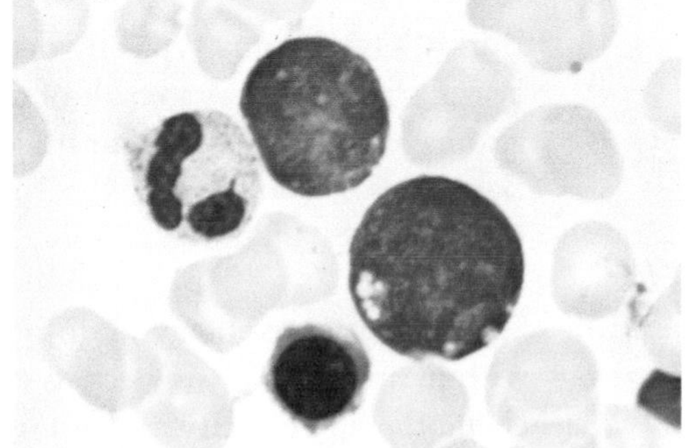

Q22.ii She recovered from the procedure but 9 weeks later she develops increasing shortness of breath. Her chest x-ray is shown below.

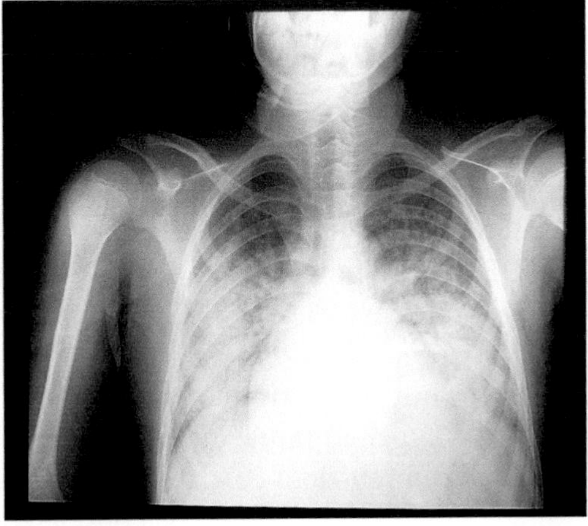

Q22.iii What is the differential diagnosis and how would you manage her?

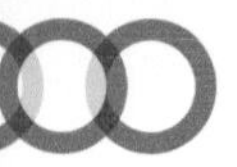

Case 22: ANSWERS

A22.i The blood film shows large numbers of blast cells with intensely basophilic cytoplasm and vacuoles. These features suggest B-cell acute lymphoblastic leukaemia, but an identical appearance is seen in Burkitt's lymphoma. The cells are positive for the presence of monoclonal surface membrane immunoglobulin.

A22.ii Nearly all patients have a chromosomal translocation involving the *c-myc* oncogene (chromosome 8) and one of the loci for immunoglobulin genes (typically the heavy chain locus on chromosome 14). It seems likely that this event is involved in the abnormal and uncontrolled proliferation of primitive B lymphocyte seen in this condition.

Burkitt's lymphoma typically occurs in African children, who have chronic B-cell stimulation as a result of malaria endemicity. Most of these children also have evidence of recent infection by the B lymphotropic virus, Epstein–Barr virus. Although t(8;14) is the commonest translocation, variant forms include t(2;8) and t(8;22).

A22.iii She has developed bilateral diffuse pulmonary infiltrates in association with dyspnoea. Non-infectious causes, for example, pulmonary oedema, chemotherapy toxicity and pulmonary haemorrhage, are more common in the first post-transplant month. However, at 9 weeks, an infectious cause is more likely (e.g. viral – cytomegalovirus [CMV], herpes simplex, varicella zoster and respiratory syncytial virus), *Pneumocystis carinii* (though the use of routine co-trimoxazole or pentamadine prophylaxis has made this less common) and fungal or bacterial infection. CMV seronegative bone marrow transplant recipients should receive CMV-negative blood components.

Blood gas/oxygen saturation analysis and clinical review by an intensive therapy unit (ITU) physician are mandatory. An accurate microbiological diagnosis should be sought, for example, by bronchoalveolar lavage with possible transbronchial biopsy, sputum culture and cytology, blood, tissue and urine cultures particularly for CMV (e.g. by detection of early antigen fluorescent foci [DEAFF] test or polymerase chain reaction), and computed tomography (CT) scan for evidence of fungal or pneumocystis infection.

Empirical broad-spectrum antibiotic and anti-viral therapy (e.g. IV ganciclovir plus CMV hyper-immune globulin) are required and specific anti-pneumocystis (with high-dose co-trimoxazole) and anti-fungal therapy (with IV liposomal amphotericin) should be considered.

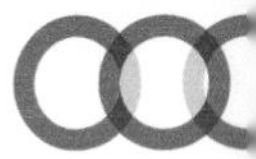

CASE 23

QUESTIONS

A 37-year-old woman of African origin is diagnosed as suffering from tuberculosis. Treatment is commenced with isoniazid (in combination with pyridoxine), rifampicin and ethambutol. After 2 weeks on this regime, she develops bruising over her legs. Her full blood count shows

Haemoglobin (Hb)	111 g/L
White blood cells (WBC)	11.7 $\times 10^9$/L (neutrophils 9.0 $\times$ 10^9/L, lymphocytes 1.8 $\times$ 10^9/L, eosinophils 0.9 $\times$ 10^9/L)
Platelets	6 $\times$ 10^9/L

A bone marrow aspirate is performed.

Q23.i Comment on the appearance of the blood film (Figures 23a and 23b) and the bone marrow aspirate (Figures 23c and 23d).

Q23.ii Why does she have bruising?

Q23.iii Why is she on pyridoxine?

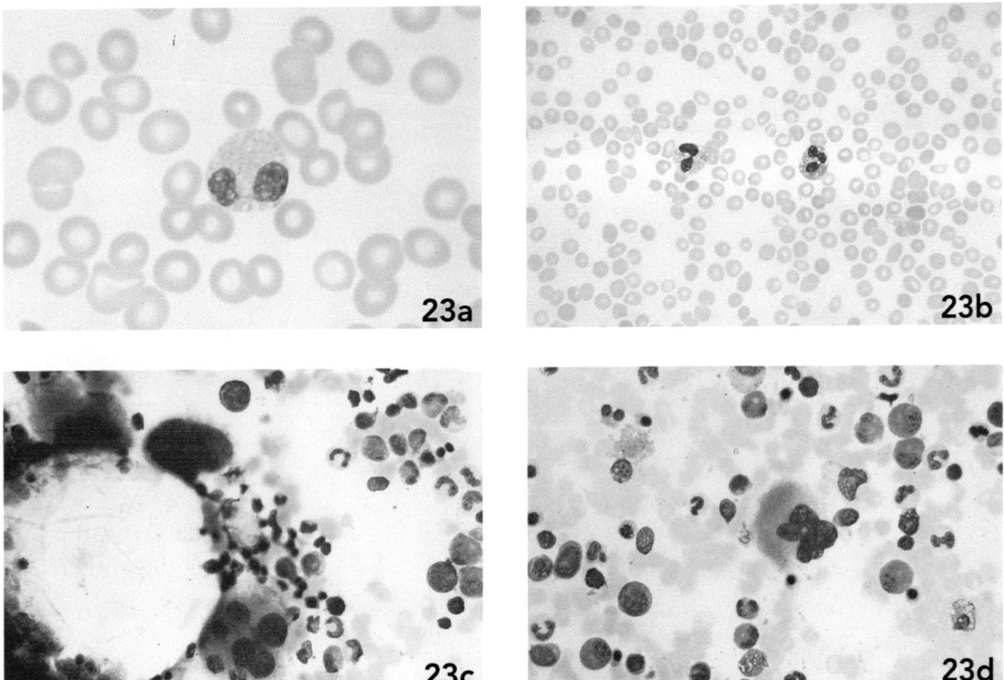

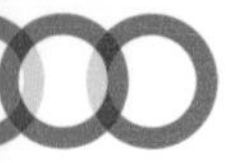

Case 23: ANSWERS

A23.i The blood film shows eosinophils, which may indicate drug allergy. The bone marrow aspirate shows megakaryocytes, and eosinophil precursors are also evident.

A23.ii She has thrombocytopenia. The presence of megakaryocytes in the marrow suggests that platelet production is adequate and destruction must be increased. Immune destruction of platelets is well-recognised as a complication of rifampicin. Other drugs that can have this effect include heparin, sulphonamides and thiazide diuretics. Thrombocytopenia can also occur because of a drug-induced decreased platelet production (e.g. chemotherapeutic and immunosuppressive drugs).

A23.iii Isoniazid therapy can cause sideroblastic anaemia by antagonising the action of pyridoxine (vitamin B_6), thus disturbing haem synthesis. The image below is an iron stain of bone marrow and shows abnormal iron granules in a perinuclear location (ringed sideroblasts).

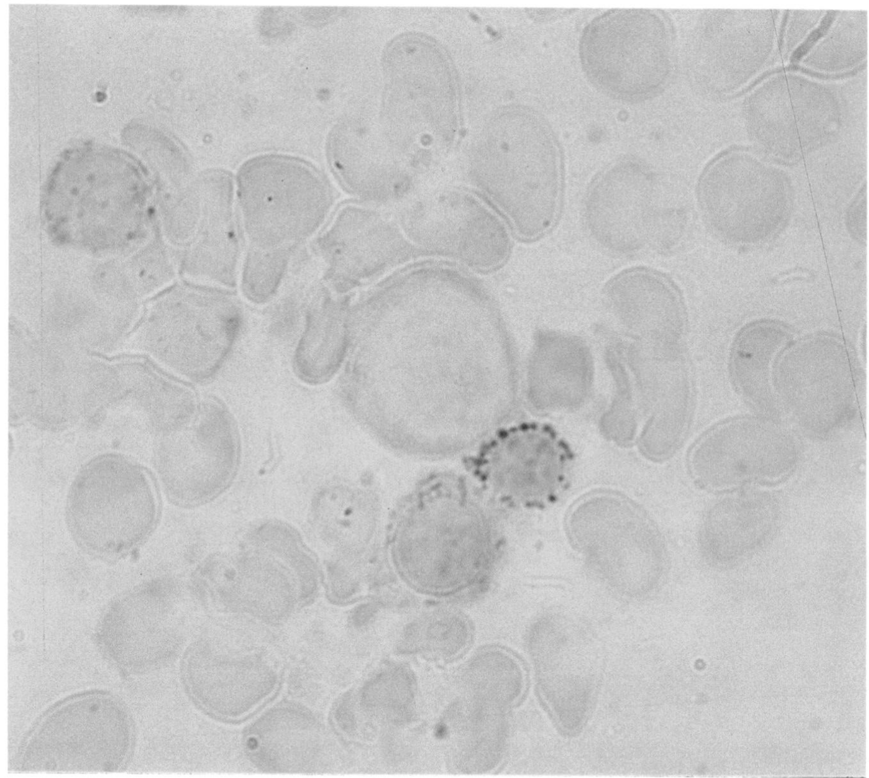

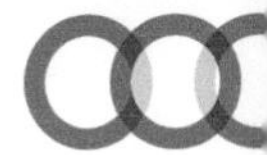

CASE 24

QUESTIONS

A 31-year-old woman returned 3 months ago from a long holiday in the Middle East and North Africa, where she travelled widely and slept in a tent or in cheap hotels. She gives a 2-week history of fever, anorexia and abdominal discomfort. She has taken malaria prophylaxis. There is no history of diarrhoea or constipation. On examination, she is pale but not jaundiced. There is no lymphadenopathy, but the spleen is palpable 8 cm below the left costal margin, and the liver is also clinically enlarged. Investigations show

Haemoglobin (Hb)	93 g/L
White blood cells (WBC)	3.4 × 10^9/L (lymphocytes 40%, neutrophils 55%)
Platelets	74 × 10^9/L
Urea and electrolytes	Normal
Liver function tests	Normal
Stool, blood, urine and throat saliva culture	Negative

A liver biopsy (Figure 24a) was performed.

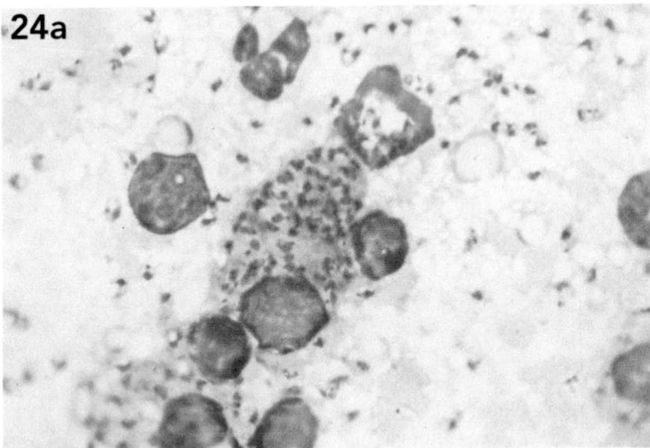

Q24.i What is the diagnosis?

Q24.ii What other features may occur in this condition?

Q24.iii What is the recommended therapy?

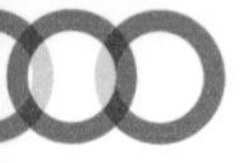

Case 24: ANSWERS

A24.i The bone marrow aspirate (Figure 24c) shows Leishman–Donovan bodies within a macrophage, and the diagnosis is visceral leishmaniasis (kala-azar). Her mild pancytopenia is due to splenic enlargement, though a mild leukopenia can also occur as part of the disease.

A24.ii Infection with *Leishmania donovani*, which is a protozoan, is transmitted by the bite of sandflies, typically from an animal (e.g. dog) reservoir. The reservoir is humans in the Indian form of the disease. Hepatosplenomegaly, sometimes with lymphopenia, is typically seen. Hypergammaglobulinaemia, notably a polyclonal increase in IgM, and a correspondingly raised erythrocyte sedimentation rate (ESR) are other noteworthy features. The peripheral blood film (Figure 24b) showed circulating, reactive plasma cells and rouleaux. Leishman–Donovan bodies are also seen in the bone marrow aspirate (Figure 24c).

A24.iii Pentavalent antimonials, for example, sodium stibogluconate, are the drugs of choice.

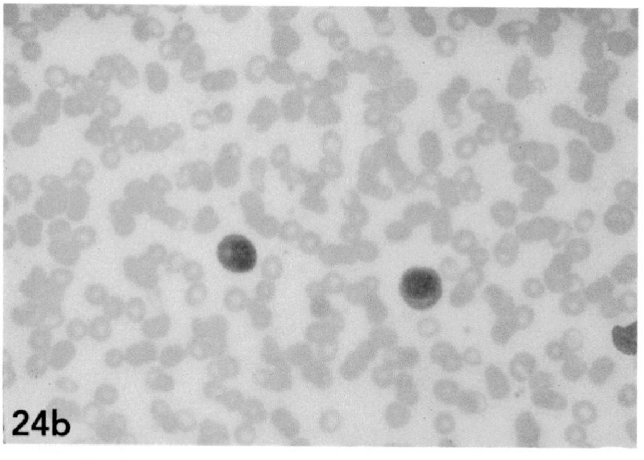
24b

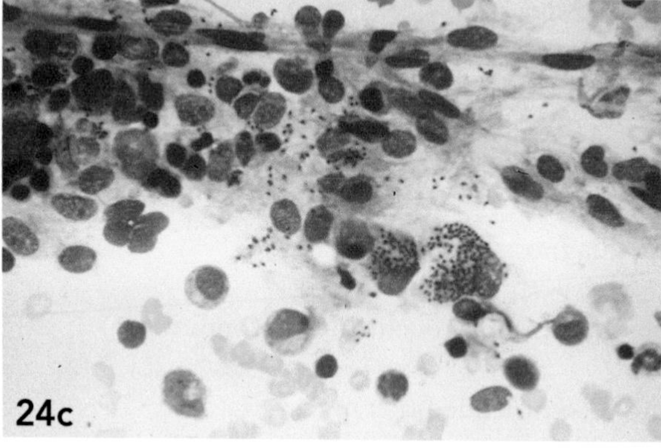
24c

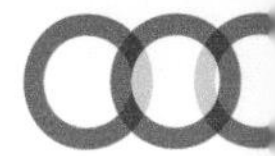

CASE 25

QUESTIONS

A 75-year-old woman presented with a 3-month history of gradually increasing tiredness. She had generalised lymphadenopathy. Abdominal examination revealed a palpable spleen 8 cm below the left costal margin. Her blood count shows

Haemoglobin (Hb)	89 g/L
White blood cells (WBC)	23.7 × 10^9/L (lymphocytes 81%, neutrophils 18%)
Platelets	109 × 10^9/L

Q25.i Comment on the blood film.

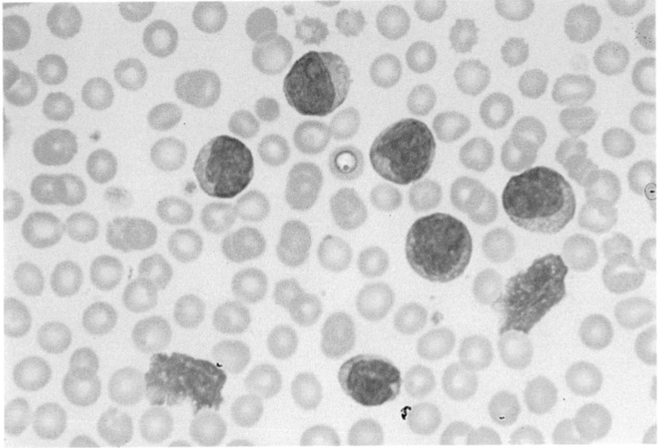

Q25.ii Comment on the bone marrow trephine biopsy.

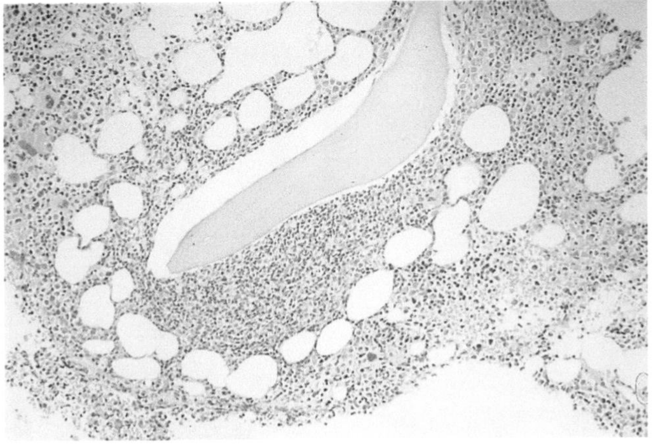

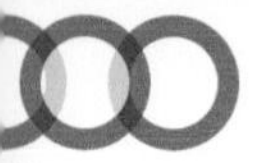

Case 25: ANSWERS

A25.i The film shows circulating atypical lymphoid cells with cleaved nuclei. The mild thrombocytopenia is due to splenomegaly. The count also shows a lymphocytosis.

A25.ii The biopsy shows abnormal deposits of mature lymphoid cells along the bony trabeculae – so-called paratrabecular deposits.

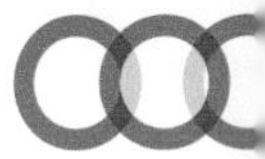

Case 25: QUESTIONS (Continued)

Q25.iii What is the differential diagnosis? How would you confirm it?

Q25.iv The patient developed profound hypothermia and sleepiness 2 years later. There were no focal neurological signs. A computed tomography (CT) scan of the brain was performed. What complication has occurred?

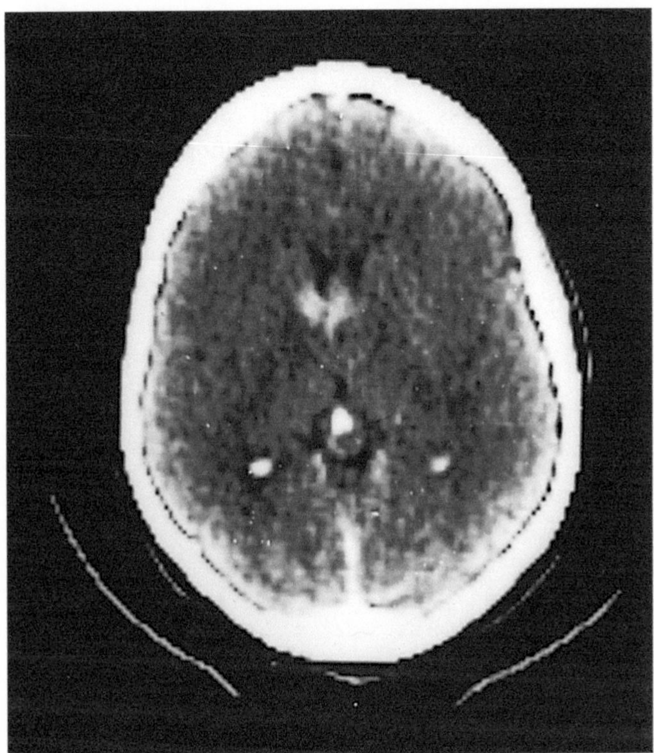

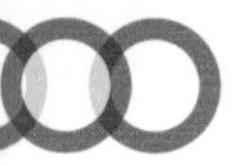

Case 25: ANSWERS (Continued)

A25.iii This patient has a chronic lymphoproliferative disorder. The likeliest diagnosis is low-grade follicular lymphoma, confirmed by lymph node biopsy (Figure 25a). Other possibilities would include chronic lymphocytic leukaemia and its variants (hairy cell leukaemia, splenic lymphoma with villous lymphocytes, prolymphocytic leukaemia). Classification and differential diagnosis of these disorders requires careful clinical assessment, flow cytometric analysis and cytogenetics. Molecular profiling distinguishes germinal centre B-cell (GCB), activated B-cell (ABC) and primary mediastinal B-cell (PMBL) types. The ABC types have constitutive NF-κB signalling and features of arrested plasma cell differentiation. The table below shows the flow cytometric features of lymphoproliferative disorders.

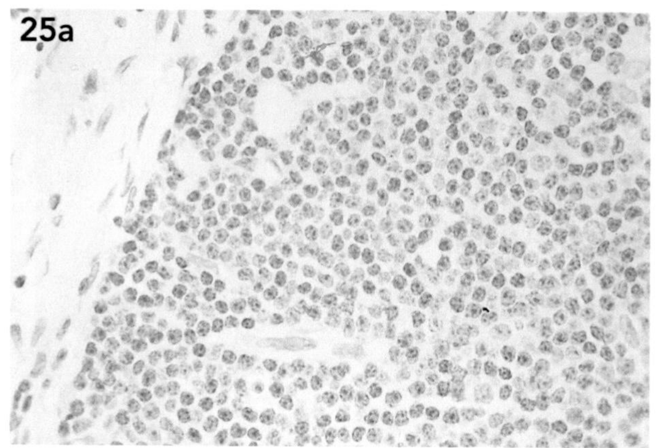

Flow cytometric features of lymphoproliferative disorders

	CD19/20	CD10	CD5	Other
CLL/Small lymphocytic lymphoma	+	–	+	
B prolymphocytic leukaemia	+	+/–	–/+	FMC7+–
Hairy cell leukaemia	+	–	–	*BRAF V600E*
Lymphoplasmacytic lymphoma	+	–	–	CD11c/CD25c, *MY88*
Marginal zone lymphoma	+	–	–	BCL–2+
Follicular lymphoma	+	+/–	–	BCL–2+, t(14;18)
Mantle cell lymphoma	+	–	+	Cyclin D1+ t(11;14)
Diffuse large B-cell lymphoma	+	+/–	–	t(14;18), t(3;4) t(2;5) ALK and NPM genes in anaplastic large cell lymphoma
Burkitt lymphoma	+	–	–	t(8;14) t(8;22)

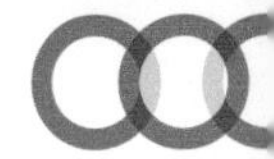

Case 25: ANSWERS (Continued)

Follicular lymphoma is a germinal centre cell tumour. It is histologically categorised into grades depending on the proportion of small cells (centrocytes) to large cells (centroblasts). Grades 1–2 have a high proportion of small cells and tend to have a low proliferation index (<20%); grade 3 has a higher proportion of large cells and a higher proliferation index (>20%).

The Follicular Lymphoma International Prognostic Index (FLIPI) incorporates age (>60 versus ≤60 years), stage (III–IV versus I–II), number of involved nodal groups (>4 versus ≤4), anaemia (Hb <120 g/L versus ≥120 g/L) and serum lactate dehydrogenase (LDH) (>upper limit of normal [ULN] versus ≤ULN).

Cytogenetic analysis showed translocation t(14;18), associated with rearrangement of the *BCL-2* oncogene and characteristic of follicular lymphoma. This translocation increases expression of the anti-apoptotic proto oncogene *BCL-2,* by bringing it into close proximity to the enhancer sequences of the immunoglobulin heavy chain locus. Central nervous system (CNS) prophylaxis is considered in those patients with non-Hodgin's lymphoma (NHL) who are considered 'high risk' – the major risk factors being high grade histology, high International Prognostic Index (IPI) score, involvement of more than one extranodal site, and involvement of testis, epidural space, paranasal sinuses and breast.

A25.iv The CT scan shows a high-density lesion of the hypothalamic region, and this was presumably responsible for her disorder of temperature control and her sleep disorder.

The lesion was not amenable to biopsy but her symptoms responded to local radiotherapy. It is likely that the low-grade tumour had transformed into a high-grade neoplasm. A fungal infection or some other infective process could cause a similar picture. This particular patient also had retroperitoneal lymphadenopathy and subsequently developed renal failure. Her central nervous system lymphoma recurred, and she presented with visual disturbance. A repeat CT scan (Figure 25b) showed a lesion affecting her occipital cortex. Subsequent lymph node biopsies (Figure 25c) showed that her histology had progressed from predominantly small cell to large cell (diffuse large B-cell) lymphoma (Figure 25d). Fluorodeoxyglucose-positron emission tomography (FDG-PET) scans can show areas of residual disease and are helpful in assessing response to treatment. Figure 25e shows pre- and post-treatment scans in NHL.

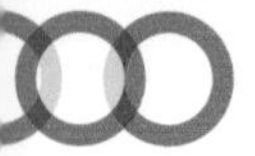

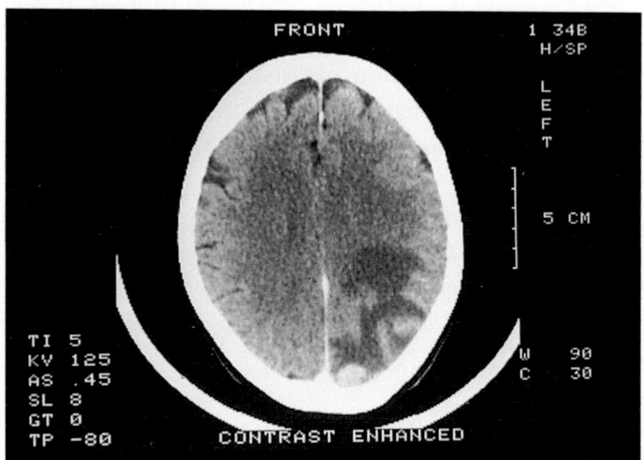

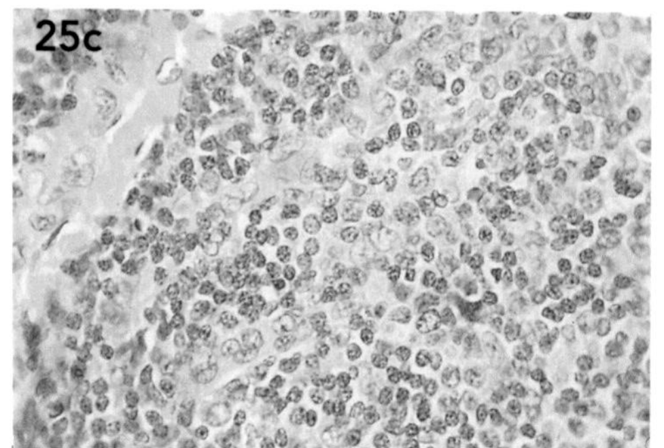

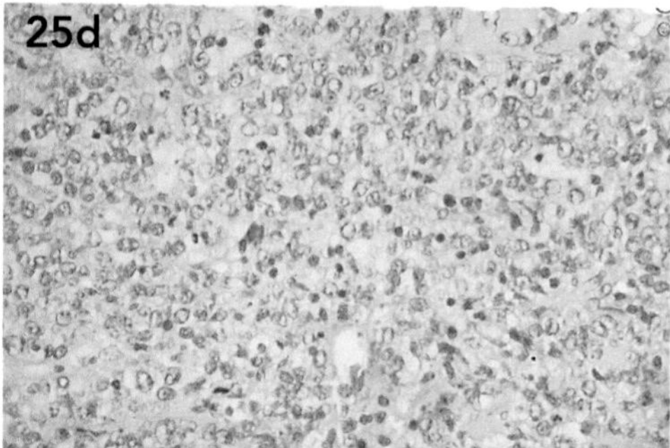

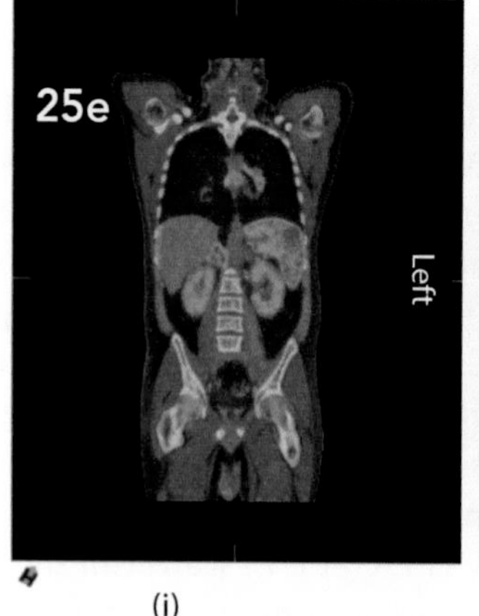

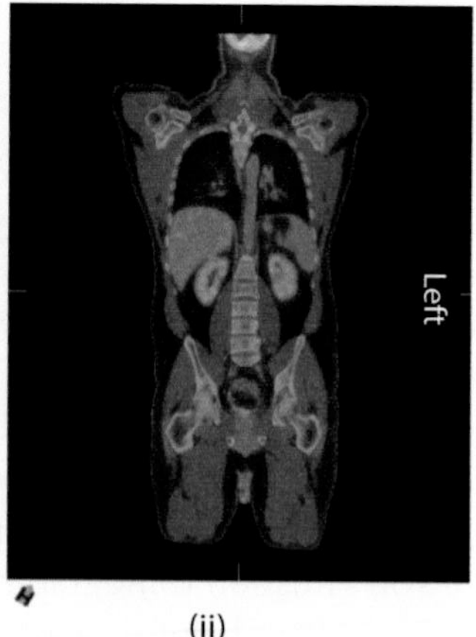

(i) (ii)

Figure 25e Fluorodeoxyglucose–positron emission tomography (FDG–PET) scans in diffuse large B-cell lymphoma. (i) Pre-treatment. (ii) Post-treatment.

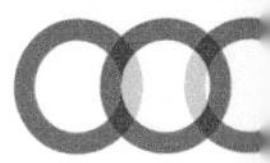

CASE 26

QUESTIONS

A 53-year-old woman, who is a heavy smoker, develops a productive cough and receives oral amoxycillin. Her symptoms persist and 1 week later she develops progressive tiredness and shortness of breath. Her full blood count shows

Haemoglobin (Hb)	87 g/L
Mean corpuscular volume (MCV)	110 fL
White blood cells (WBC)	11.3×10^9/L (neutrophils 71%)
Platelets	305×10^9/L

Q26.i Comment on the chest x-ray.

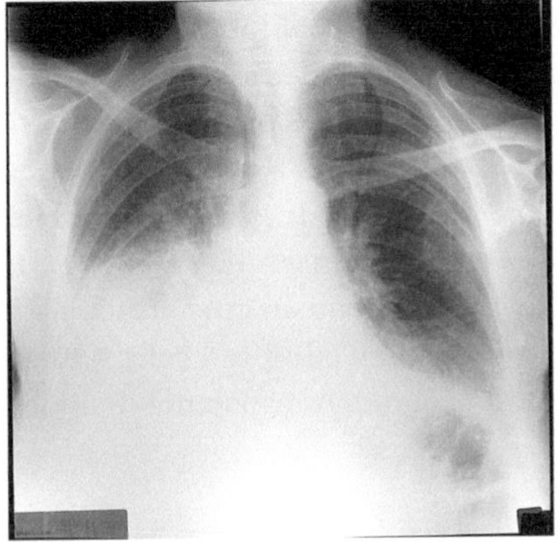

Q26.ii Comment on the blood film.

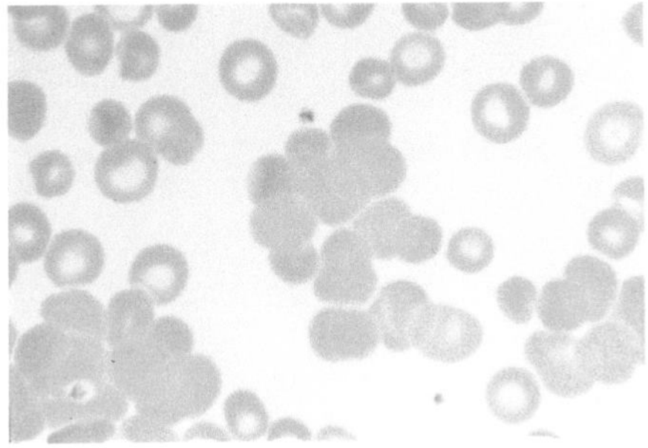

Q26.iii What is the likely diagnosis?

Q26.iv What further investigations are indicated?

Q26.v How would you treat her?

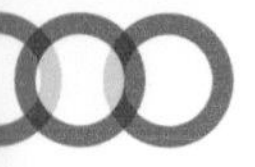

Case 26: ANSWERS

A26.i The chest x-ray shows evidence of a lobar pneumonia affecting the right base.

A26.ii The blood film shows marked auto-agglutination, suggesting the presence of cold agglutinins.

A26.iii Autoimmune haemolytic anaemia with cold agglutinins secondary to *Mycoplasma pneumoniae* infection.

A26.iv A direct anti-globulin (DAT) test was positive, and demonstrated both IgM and complement on the red cell surface. Mycoplasma titres should be assessed.

The blood group should be determined and the cold agglutinin titre should be measured. Autoimmune haemolytic anaemia following *M. pneumoniae* infection is typically associated with an increased titre of anti-I antibodies, which react optimally at 4°C. Patients with cold reactive auto-antibodies often develop acrocyanosis and Raynaud's phenomenon, as the periphery is at a lower temperature than the body core. The suggested mechanism of autoimmune haemolytic anaemia following *M. pneumoniae* infection is that antibodies to the organism cross-react with the I antigen, which is normally expressed on all adult red cells. Other infections that may lead to autoimmune haemolytic anaemia include syphilis and infectious mononucleosis.

A26.v Treatment is with erythromycin.

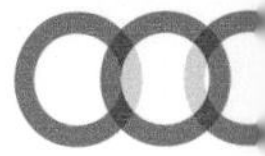

CASE 27

QUESTIONS

A full-term neonate is found to have purpura, ecchymosis and difficulty in breathing. A full blood count shows

Haemoglobin (Hb)	173 g/L
White blood cells (WBC)	16.4×10^9/L
Platelets	4×10^9/L

A computed tomography (CT) scan was performed. The mother has had one previous pregnancy 4 years ago, and there were no complications during the current pregnancy.

Q27.i Comment on the appearance of the CT scan.

Q27.ii What important causes would you consider for the thrombocytopenia?

Q27.iii How should the child be treated?

Q27.iv What advice would you give regarding future pregnancy?

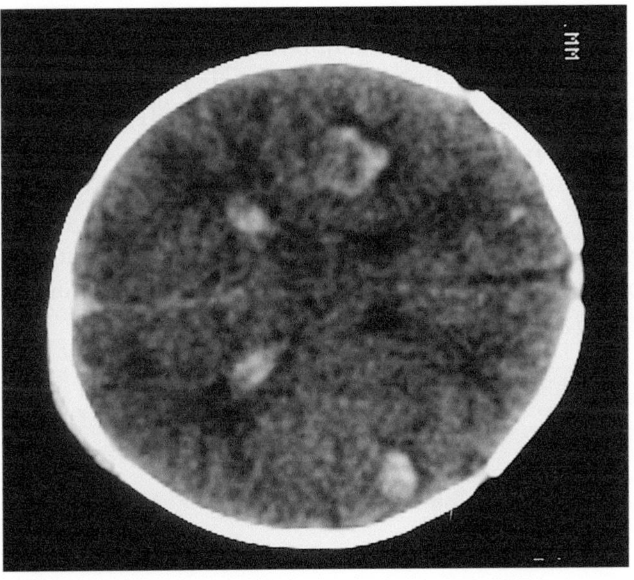

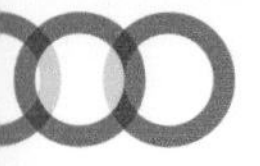

Case 27: ANSWERS

A27.i The CT scan shows evidence of acute haemorrhage.

A27.ii Important causes of neonatal thrombocytopenia are genetic, congenital and acquired. Genetic causes are rare, but include thrombocytopenia with absent radii (TAR) syndrome. Congenital infection (rubella, cytomegalovirus [CMV] and toxoplasmosis) should be excluded by serological tests on mother and culture studies of the neonate. Congenital immune thrombocytopenia may arise through transplacental passage of IgG anti-platelet antibodies in mothers with idiopathic thrombocytopenic purpura, or may present as neonatal alloimmune thrombocytopenia. Mothers who lack certain platelet antigens (most commonly human platelet antigen [HPA]-1a) will make antibodies if sensitised by previous pregnancy or transfusion. Acquired causes include sepsis, disseminated intravascular coagulation and drugs.

A27.iii Maternal serum was found to contain anti-HPA-1A antibodies. The mother's own platelets were HPA-1A negative, and the father and both children were HPA-1A positive (as are more than 95% of people). Thus, a diagnosis of neonatal alloimmune thrombocytopenia was made. The child received transfusion of HPA-1A-negative platelets, which were continued until the child was able to maintain an unsupported count of more than 50×10^9/L. This occurred within 3 weeks as the titre of transplacentally derived antibody fell. High-dose intravenous immunoglobulin may also help to elevate the neonatal platelet count.

A27.iv The partner should be tested and, if he is homozygous HPA-1a positive, as is likely, then future children will be affected. The fetal platelet count can be monitored during pregnancy and, if required, HPA-1a negative platelets can be transfused as prophylaxis against bleeding. Delivery should be by elective caesarean section.

All blood components for intra-uterine transfusion should be CMV negative and irradiated to minimise the risk of graft versus host disease.

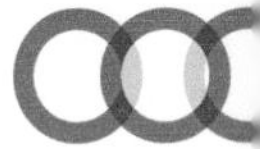

CASE 28

QUESTIONS

Q28.i What abnormalities are shown in this blood film (Figure 28a)? What is the likely diagnosis?

Q28.ii What abnormality is shown (Figure 28b)? What is the likely diagnosis?

Q28.iii What abnormality is shown (Figure 28c)? What is the likely diagnosis?

Q28.iv What abnormality is shown (Figure 28d)? What are the possible causes?

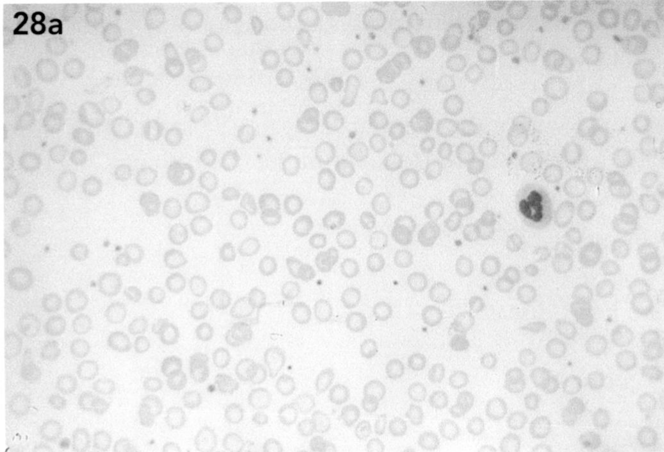
28a

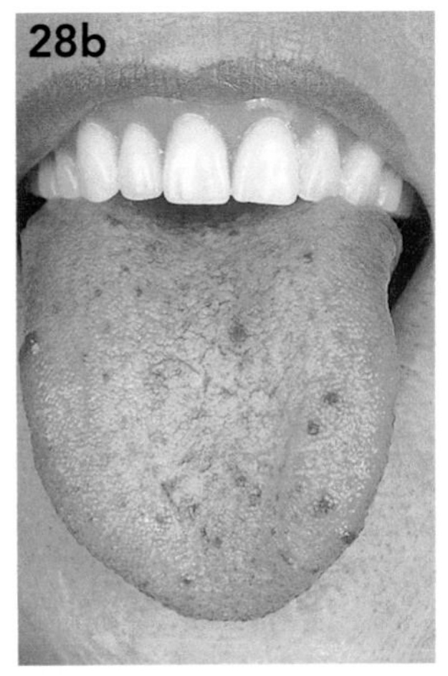
28b

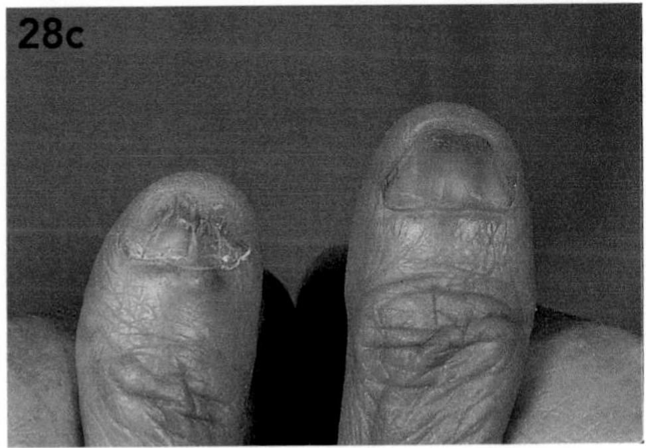
28c

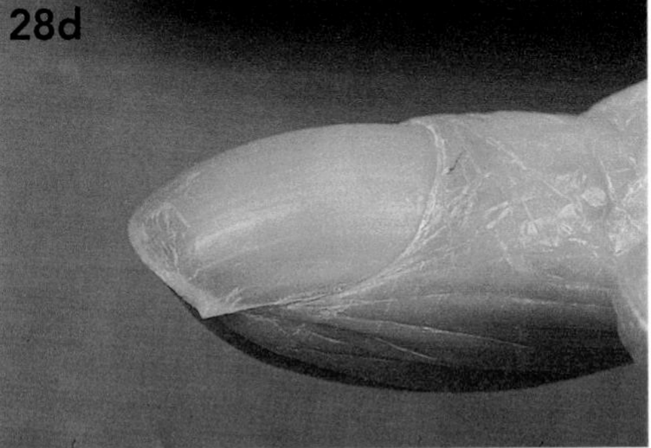
28d

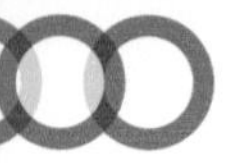

Case 28: ANSWERS

A28.i This blood film shows hypochromic, microcytic red blood cells with occasional target cells. The features suggest iron deficiency.

A28.ii This patient has multiple telangiectasia over the tongue and lips, and suffers from hereditary haemorrhagic telangiectasia (Osler–Weber–Rendu syndrome). Chronic iron deficiency may result from gastrointestinal blood loss. The condition is inherited as an autosomal dominant.

A28.iii The appearance of the nails are those of koilonychia (spoon-shaped nails), which is seen in chronic iron deficiency. Other skin and mucosal changes in iron deficiency include

- Brittle nails
- Angular cheilitis
- Postcricoid and pharyngeal webs (Plummer–Vinson syndrome), which may present as dysphagia

A28.iv Clubbing. This is associated with pulmonary arteriovenous fistulae in hereditary haemorrhagic telangiectasia, as shown in the chest x-ray. Other causes of clubbing include

- Carcinoma of the bronchus
- Suppurative lung disease
- Cyanotic congenital heart disease
- Cirrhosis
- Inflammatory bowel disease

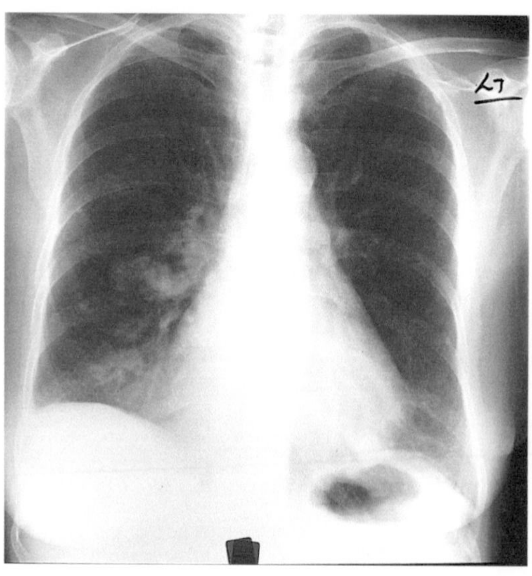

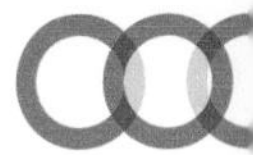

CASE 29

QUESTIONS

This patient gives a 3-month history of gradually increasing tiredness and lack of energy. Her blood count shows

Haemoglobin (Hb)	94 g/L
Mean corpuscular volume (MCV)	100 fL
White blood cells (WBC)	4.7×10^9/L
Platelets	130×10^9/L

Q29.i What is the diagnosis (Figures 29a and 29b)?

Q29.ii What other information should be sought in the history?

Q29.iii What other haematological complications may occur?

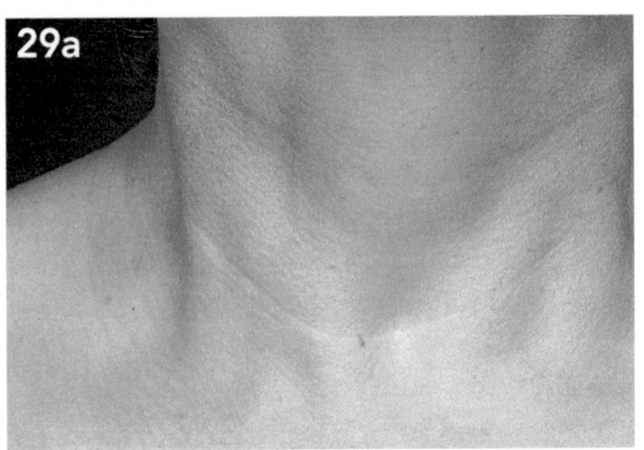

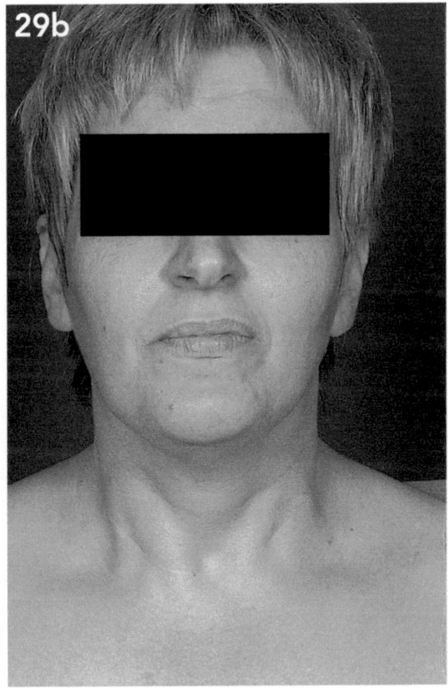

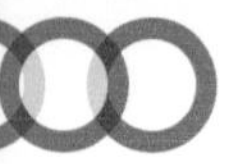

Case 29: ANSWERS

A29.i This patient is suffering from hypothyroidism.

A29.ii This patient had a strong family history of thyroid disease. Voice changes, intolerance to cold, slow mentation and shortness of breath arising through associated congestive cardiac failure (or, less commonly, pericardial effusion) are other frequent symptoms.

A29.iii Both hyperthyroidism and hypothyroidism are associated with mild anaemia, which is usually normochromic and normocytic, though there may be a macrocytosis in hypothyroidism.

Iron deficiency may arise through associated menorrhagia in hypothyroidism, and defective iron utilisation may occur as in the anaemia of chronic disease. There is an increased incidence of pernicious anaemia in patients with autoimmune hypothyroidism, as well as in those with hypoadrenalism, hypoparathyroidism and diabetes mellitus. Mild normochromic normocytic anaemia may also occur in Addison's disease, hypopituitarism and hypogonadism. Phaeochromocytoma is occasionally associated with erythrocytosis.

A neutrophil leukocytosis may occur in Cushing's syndrome and phaeochromocytoma, and diabetes mellitus is associated with impaired neutrophil function. Abnormal platelet function is reported in diabetes mellitus and hyperthyroidism, and hypercoagulability is of clinical significance in diabetes, following oestrogen therapy, and in Cushing's syndrome.

In the anaemia of chronic disease (ACD), the serum iron is low but the iron binding capacity is also low, whereas it is raised in iron deficiency. A low serum ferritin indicates iron deficiency, but ferritin may rise in inflammatory conditions. Assessment of iron status only rarely requires bone marrow examination. Figure 29c shows a Perl's stain with reduced iron stores. Figure 29d shows normal/increased stores. In ACD, iron may be present in stores but absent in developing erythroblasts.

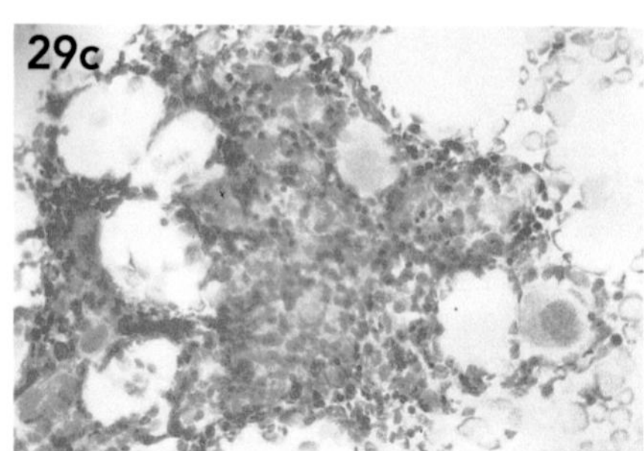

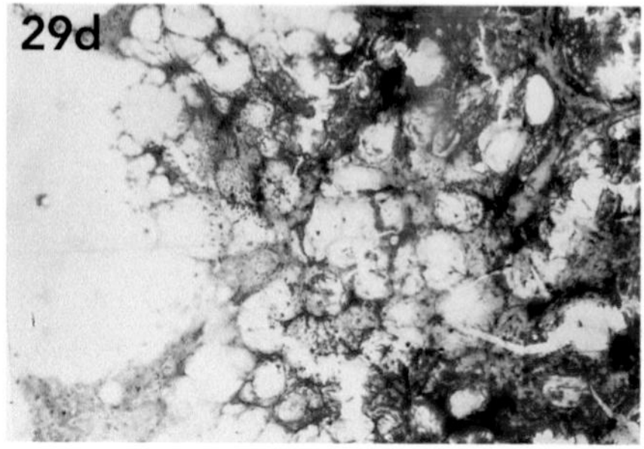

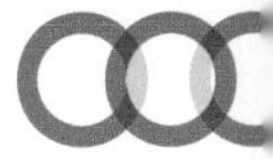

CASE 30

QUESTIONS

A 62-year-old man has progressive onset of pain at the back of the neck. He has also noted weakness of his hands over a 3-week period, and he is having difficulty grasping objects. He reports numbness along the inner aspect of his arm. Investigations show

Haemoglobin (Hb)	94g/L
Mean corpuscular volume (MCV)	87 fL
Platelets	137×10^9/L
Erythrocyte sedimentation rate (ESR)	110 mm/h
White blood cells (WBC)	7.4×10^9/L

Q30.i Comment on the blood film.

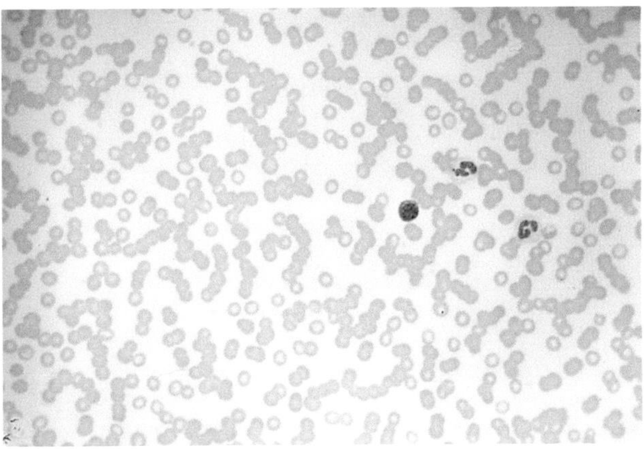

Q30.ii Comment on the photograph of the patient's hands.

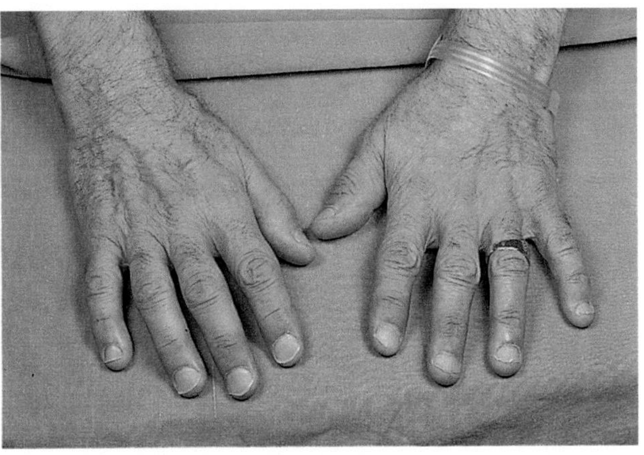

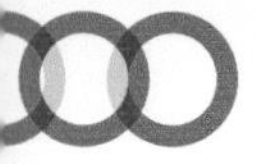

Case 30: ANSWERS

A30.i The blood film shows rouleaux formation. This is frequently seen in association with a raised erythrocyte sedimentation rate (ESR) and should raise suspicion of an underlying disorder of plasma proteins, for example, polyclonal or monoclonal increase in gamma globins.

A30.ii The hands show bilateral changes of muscle wasting, and are consistent with a T1 cord lesion.

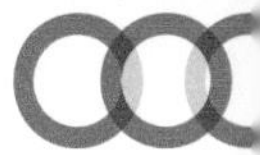

Case 30: QUESTIONS (Continued)

Q30.iii Comment on the computed tomography (CT) scan of his neck.

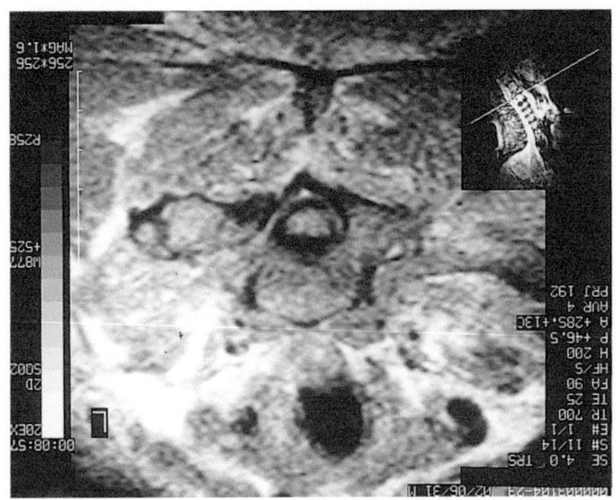

Q30.iv Comment on the protein electrophoretic strip:

- Lane X is from a patient with cirrhosis.
- Lane Y is from the patient.
- Lane Z is a normal control.

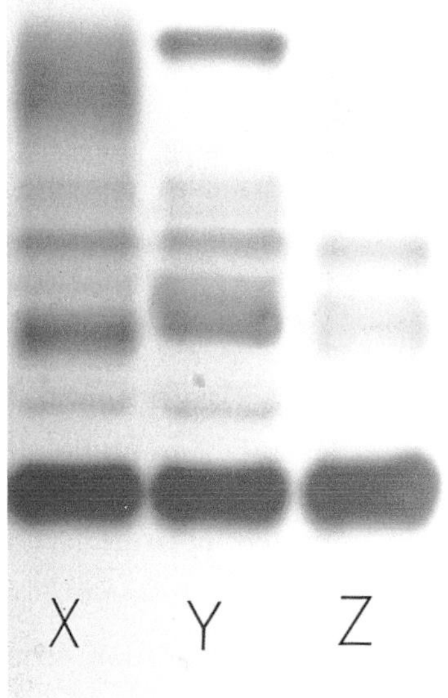

Q30.v What is the diagnosis?

Q30.vi What further investigations are indicated?

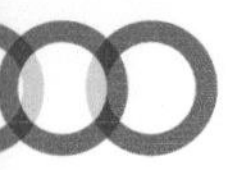

Case 30: ANSWERS (Continued)

A30.iii CT of the neck shows an extradural tumour affecting the cervical spine.

A30.iv Protein electrophoresis on the patient (lane Y) shows a monoclonal band in the gammaglobulin region with a corresponding reduction in the other immunoglobulins. Lane X shows polyclonal hypergammaglobulinaemia. The paraprotein band is further characterised by immunofixation, and clearly reacts with only IgG and kappa antisera.

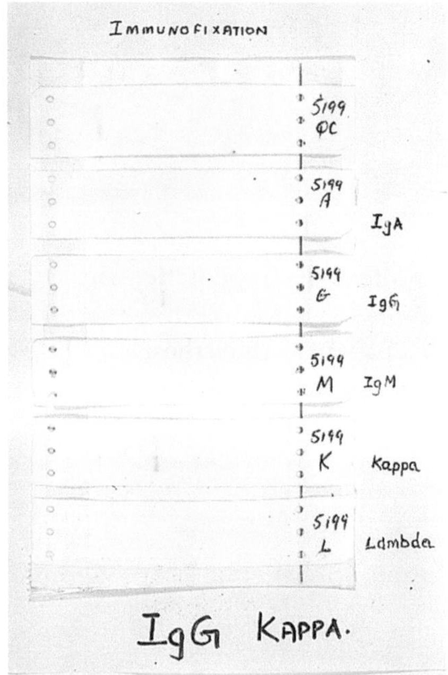

A30.v Multiple myeloma.

A30.vi A full biochemical assessment is needed, including urea, calcium, liver function tests, creatinine clearance, immunoglobulins, paraprotein quantitation in serum and urine, assessment of serum free light chains and screening for Bence–Jones protein in urine.

Bone marrow aspirate and possibly aspirate of the cervical lesion will confirm the diagnosis. A skeletal survey is more sensitive than a bone scan at detecting myeloma deposits and magnetic resonance imaging (MRI) is more sensitive than x-ray. Both the beta-2 microglobulin level and the plasma C-reactive protein give useful prognostic information in myeloma.

Myeloma cells are monoclonal B lymphocytes, and as such have a discrete rearrangement of their immunoglobulin genes. Molecular techniques offer a

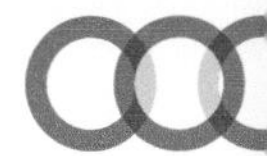

sensitive method for detecting minimal residual disease after chemotherapy. Advanced myeloma is often characterized by complex and evolving cytogentic clones (Figure 30a); and fluorescence in situ hybridization (FISH) is a very useful technique for evaluating these clones (Figure 30b).

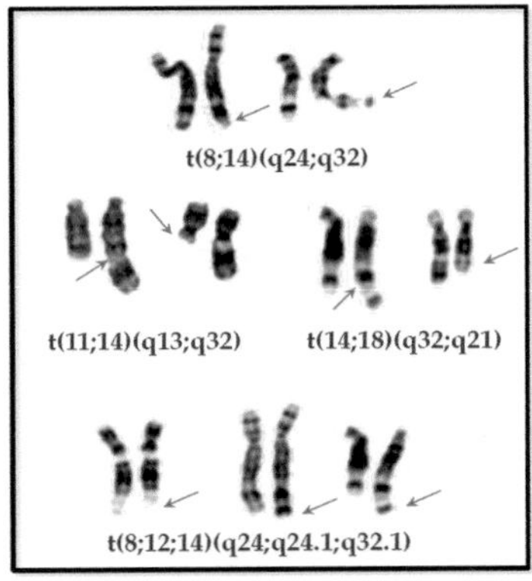

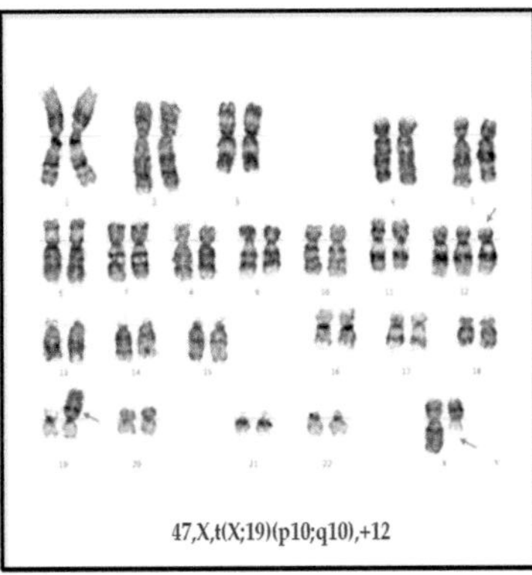

Figure 30a Myeloma – Complex cytogenetics.

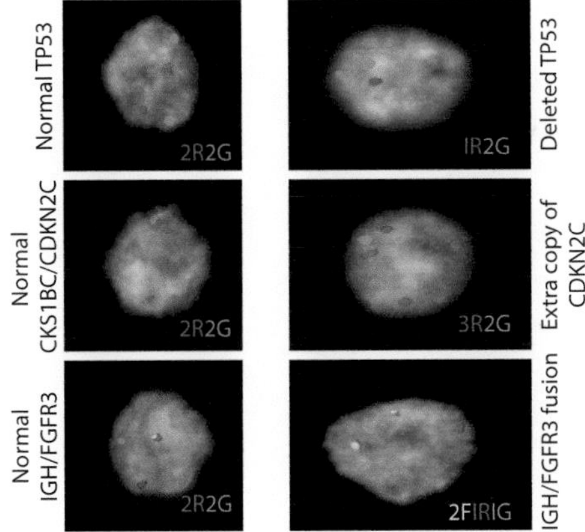

Figure 30b Fluorescence in situ hybridization (FISH) screening for high-risk markers of CD138+ in myeloma.

POEMS syndrome is the association of polyneuropathy with organomegaly, endocrinopathy, a monoclonal gammopathy and skin lesions. The bone marrow aspirate (Figure 30b) shows an increase in plasma cells. Patients with POEMS often have an increased plasma level of vascular endothelial growth factor (VEGF).

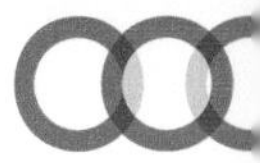

CASE 31

QUESTIONS

A 9-year-old boy presents with a long history of anaemia. It was first noted when he was 4, at that time his blood count showed as follows:

Haemoglobin (Hb)	65 g/L
Mean corpuscular volume (MCV)	56 fL
Mean corpuscular haemoglobin concentration (MCHC)	29 g/dL

Since this initial presentation, he has received blood transfusions on three occasions. He has hepatosplenomegaly.

Q31.i Comment on the blood films. What is the likely diagnosis?

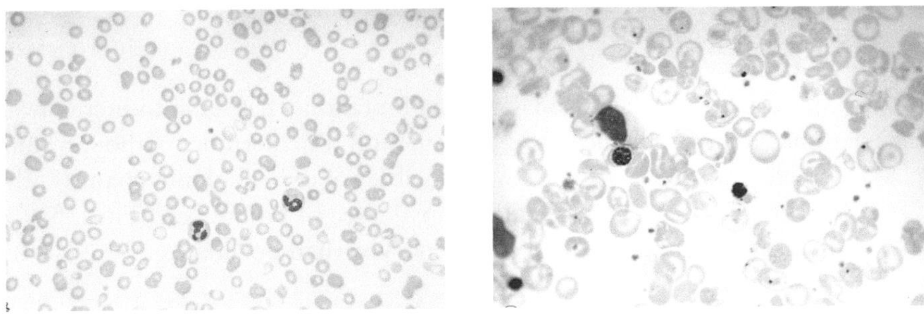

Q31.ii Comment on the boy's facial appearance.

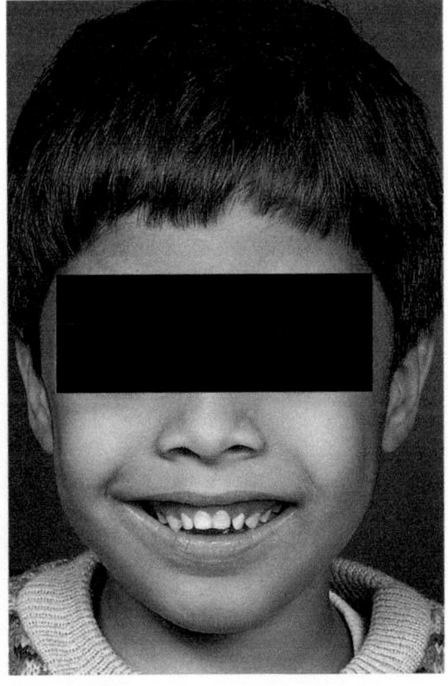

Q31.iii What is the pathogenesis of this condition?

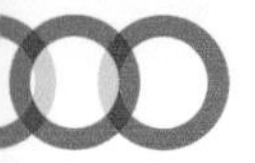

Case 31: ANSWERS

A31.i The blood film shows hypochromic microcytic red cells and occasional circulating nucleated red cells. The likely diagnosis is beta thalassaemia of a severity greater than thalassaemia trait but with an age of onset later than beta thalassaemia major. The patient is able to survive without regular transfusion therapy, suggesting he has beta thalassaemia intermedia.

A31.ii The facial appearance ('chipmunk face') confirms maxillary enlargement due to extramedullary haemopoiesis. Skeletal abnormalities are often prominent in thalassaemia intermedia as a result of chronic extramedullary haemopoiesis.

A31.iii The commonest mechanism of amelioration of beta thalasseamia major is co-inheritance of alpha thalassaemia. This is because excess deposition of alpha chains is an important cause of ineffective erythropoiesis and haemolysis in beta thalassaemia major; the extent of such deposition is lessened if the patient has defective formation of alpha chains by virtue of having alpha thalasseamia trait.

Some patients have additional genetic mutations that serve to increase gamma chain (and hence Hb F) production. Furthermore, although some beta gene mutations lead to complete absence of beta globin chain synthesis (βo), others are compatible with some degree of production. Thus, β+/β+ frequently produces a less severe phenotype than βo/βo.

Splenectomy may be of value, both in reducing splenic pooling of transfused red cells and in reducing haemolysis and extramedullary haemopoiesis. Skeletal abnormalities can be quite dramatic: a paraspinal mass is visible on the plain chest x-ray (Figure 31a), and extramedullary haemopoiesis in the ribs is shown on the magnetic resonance imaging (MRI) scan (Figure 31b).

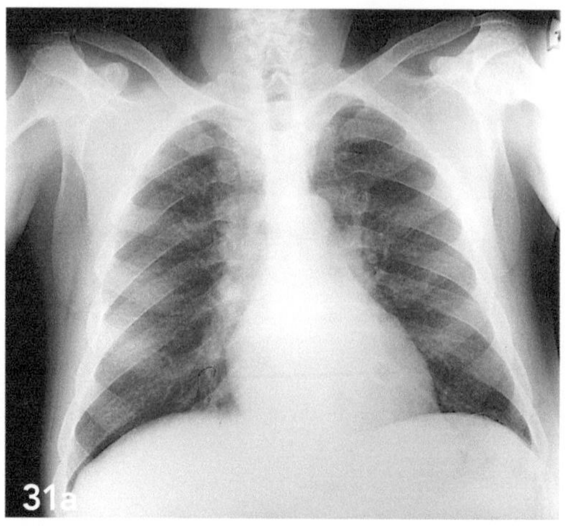

31a

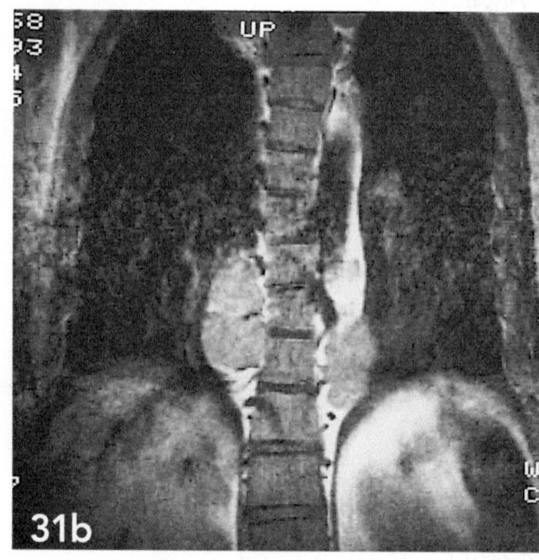

31b

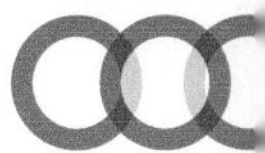

CASE 32

QUESTIONS

A 23-year-old woman gives a 3-month history of progressively increasing tiredness with bruising, malaise and menorrhagia. On examination, she is anaemic and has multiple bruises. Her blood count shows

Haemoglobin (Hb)	69 g/L
White blood cells (WBC)	1.1×10^9/L (neutrophils 0.3×10^9/L)
Platelets	17×10^9/L

Her chest x-ray (posteroanterior [PA] and lateral – Figures 32a and 32b), thoracic computed tomography (CT) scan (Figure 32c) and bone marrow trephine biopsy (Figure 32d) are illustrated.

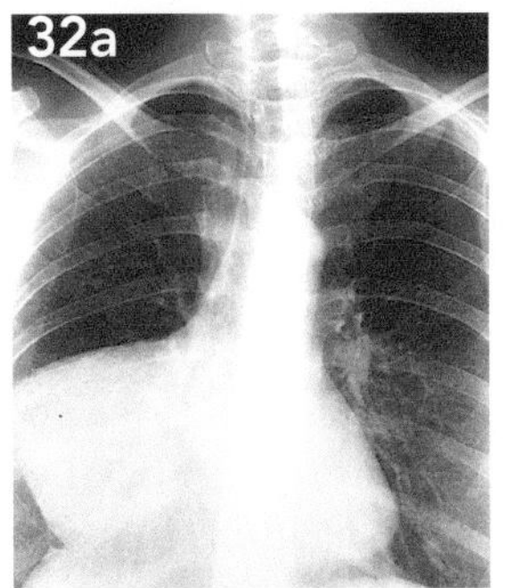
32a

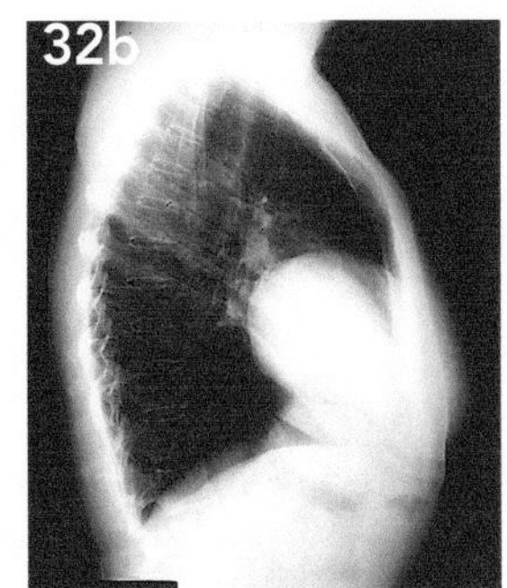
32b

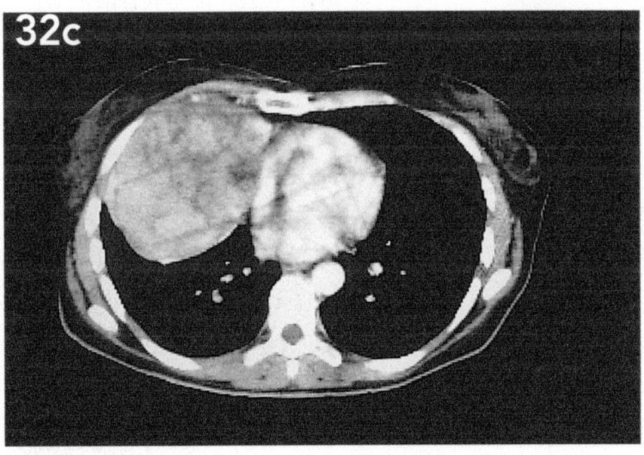
32c

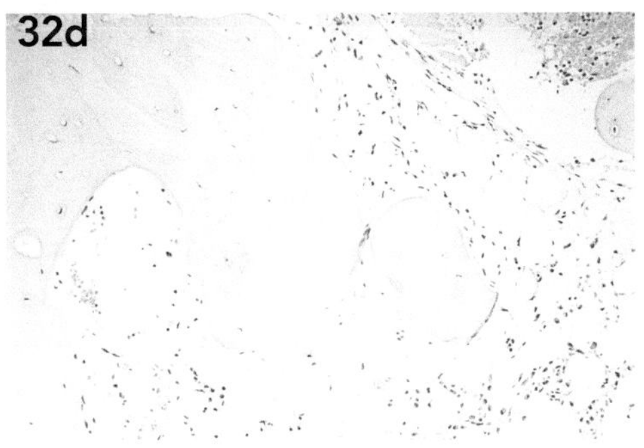
32d

Q32.i What abnormality is shown on the chest x-ray and CT scan?

Q32.ii What abnormality is shown on the bone marrow trephine biopsy?

Q32.iii What further investigations should be undertaken?

Q32.iv What are the treatment options for this condition?

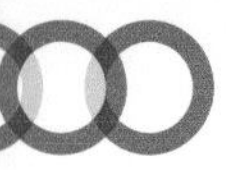

Case 32: ANSWERS

A32.i The chest x-ray shows an abnormal mass in the anterior mediastinum which, notwithstanding the unusual appearance, turned out at surgery to be a thymoma.

A32.ii Her bone marrow trephine biopsy confirms that she has aplastic anaemia (AA). The degree of cellularity is quite variable, not only in normal people but also in patients with AA, and two additional trephine biopsies from aplastic patients demonstrate this.

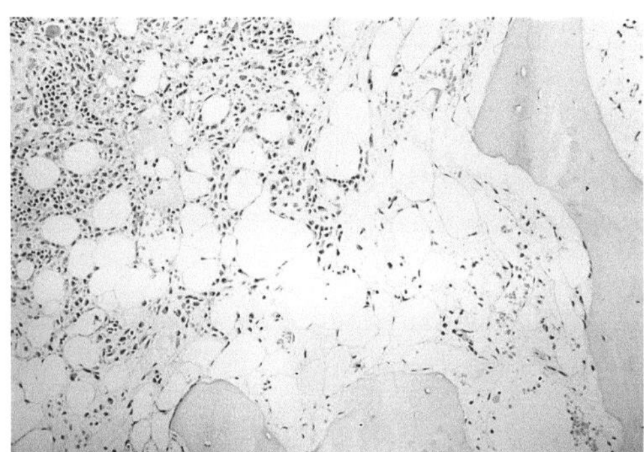

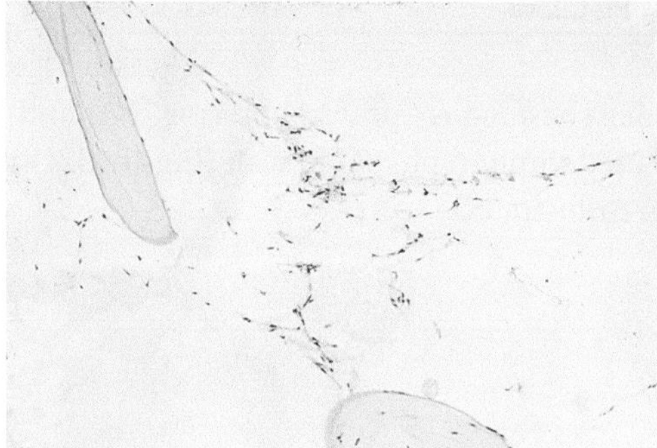

A32.iii Thymoma may be associated with red cell aplasia and was presumably aetiologically related to marrow aplasia in this case. A detailed drug and occupational history is essential. Other investigations that should be performed in AA:

- Anti-nuclear factor, vitamin B_{12} and folic acid levels
- Flow cytometry to exclude coexistent paroxysmal nocturnal haemoglobinuria
- Serology for virus infections including hepatitis, HIV, Epstein–Barr virus (EBV), cytomegalovirus (CMV) and parvo virus
- Immunoglobulins (thymoma may be associated with hypogammaglobulinaemia)
- Cytogenetics on bone marrow to exclude the presence of a clonal proliferation, to aid in distinguishing myelodysplasia from AA; and peripheral blood chromosomal breakage analysis to exclude Fanconi anaemia if patient is under 50 years; gene mutation analysis for dyskeratosis congenital (e.g. DKC1, TERC) is also required

A32.iv This patient underwent thymectomy, though it should be emphasised that thymoma is only very rarely associated with AA and is more frequently associated with isolated red cell aplasia. Supportive care with red cells, platelets and antibiotics and anti-fungal agents is valuable. Recombinant haemopoietic growth factors are of limited value in this condition, but

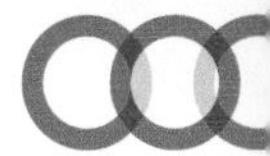

anti-lymphocyte globulin, methylprednisolone and cyclosporin A are beneficial in over 50% of patients. A progestogen (e.g. norethisterone) or the oral contraceptive pill is frequently helpful in controlling menorrhagia.

Allogeneic bone marrow transplantation from a histocompatible sibling, if available, should be considered in any patient under 65 years with severe AA (platelets $<20 \times 10^9/L$, neutrophils $<0.5 \times 10^9/L$) who has a good performance status.

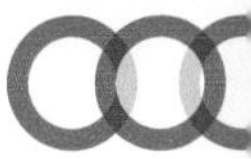

CASE 33

QUESTIONS

A 62-year-old man is generally unwell and complaining of increased tiredness over a 3-month period. He has had two recent episodes of chest infection requiring antibiotic therapy. On examination he is pale. The tip of the spleen is palpable, but there is no jaundice and no lymphadenopathy. His blood count shows

Haemoglobin (Hb)	91 g/L
White blood cells (WBC)	3.9 × 10^9/L (lymphocytes 65%, neutrophils 32%)
Platelets	91 × 10^9/L

A bone marrow aspirate is unsuccessful.

Q33.i Comment on the blood film appearance.

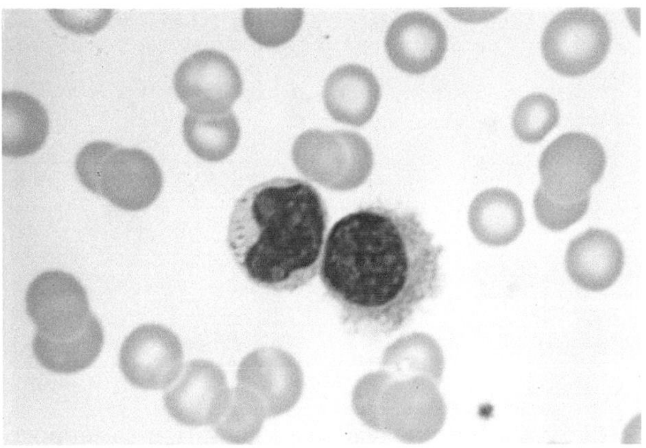

Q33.ii What is the diagnosis?

Q33.iii How would you confirm the diagnosis?

Q33.iv How is this condition treated?

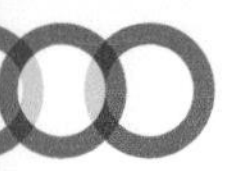

Case 33: ANSWERS

A33.i The blood film shows abnormal circulating lymphoid cells with cytoplasmic projections.

A33.ii The morphology of the circulating cells, history of pancytopenia and splenomegaly and an unsuccessful aspirate strongly suggest hairy cell leukaemia.

A33.iii A marrow trephine biopsy will often show a characteristic appearance of large cells with plentiful cytoplasm. The alkaline phosphatase reaction is usually positive and tartrate resistant (TRAP). Flowcytometric analysis of the lymphocytes will show them to be monoclonal B cells and CD11c positive (T hairy cell leukaemia is exceedingly rare). Nearly all subjects have mutations in the BRAF oncogene.

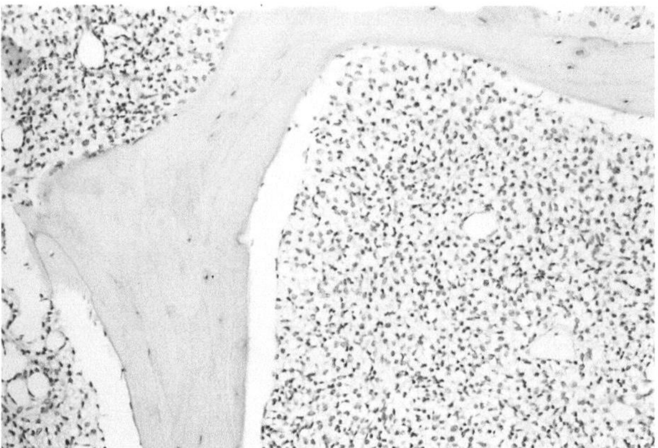

A33.iv A number of treatments are available in addition to supportive care. Effective chemotherapeutic agents include 2-chlorodeoxyadenosine, deoxycoformycin and interferon and rituximab, while splenectomy has an important role in those patients who have good marrow function.

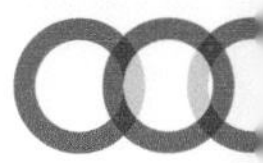

CASE 34

QUESTIONS

A 27-year-old pregnant woman (36 weeks) becomes acutely unwell with fever, purpuric lesions over her limbs and declining consciousness. Her full blood count shows

Haemoglobin (Hb)	75 g/L
Mean corpuscular volume (MCV)	110 fL
Reticulocytes	12%
White blood cells (WBC)	26.4 × 10^9/L (neutrophils 86%)
Platelets	14 × 109/L
Urea	67 mmol/L

Q34.i Comment on the blood film.

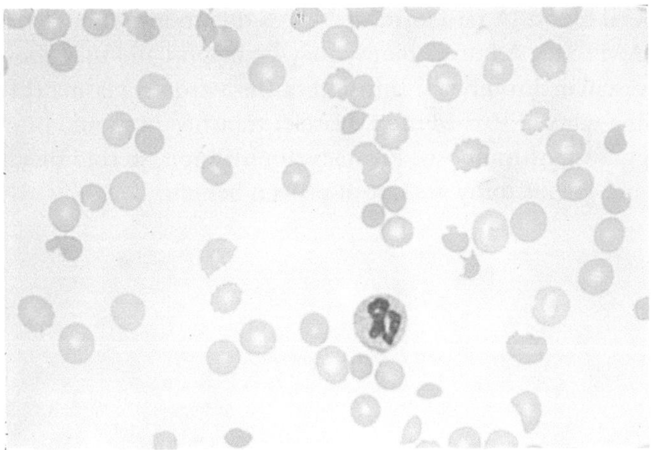

Q34.ii What is the differential diagnosis and what further investigations are required?

Q34.iii What treatment would you recommend?

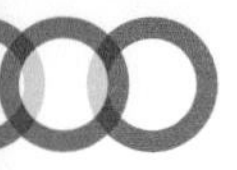

Case 34: ANSWERS

A34.i The blood film shows red cell fragmentation, polychromasia, thrombocytopenia and target cells.

A34.ii The association of fever, fragmentation haemolysis, renal failure, neurological changes and thrombocytopenia suggests thrombotic thrombocytopenic purpura (TTP), which has an increased frequency in pregnancy. It must be distinguished from disseminated intravascular coagulation (e.g. in association with sepsis, amniotic fluid embolism, antepartum haemorrhage and retention of a dead foetus or products of conception), and a coagulation screen is required urgently. This was normal in this case. Liver function tests were normal, differentiating this from haemolytic anaemia, elevated liver enzymes and low platelets (HELLP) syndrome and acute fatty liver of pregnancy. (The image below shows target cells due to coexistent liver disease in a case of TTP.) TTP is caused by the presence of an antibody to a plasma protease ADAMTS13, which normally cleaves von Willebrand factor (VWF). Abnormally high-molecular weight VWF complexes are found in peripheral blood. A rare form of TTP is due to inherited deficient synthesis of ADAMTS13. A buccal biopsy may be helpful and may show evidence of microvascular thrombosis. Infusion of fresh-frozen plasma (FFP), or plasma exchange with FFP, is advised. Platelet transfusion should be avoided, as it may aggravate thrombosis. Prostacyclin infusion, steroid therapy, anti-platelet drugs and splenectomy are not of proven benefit.

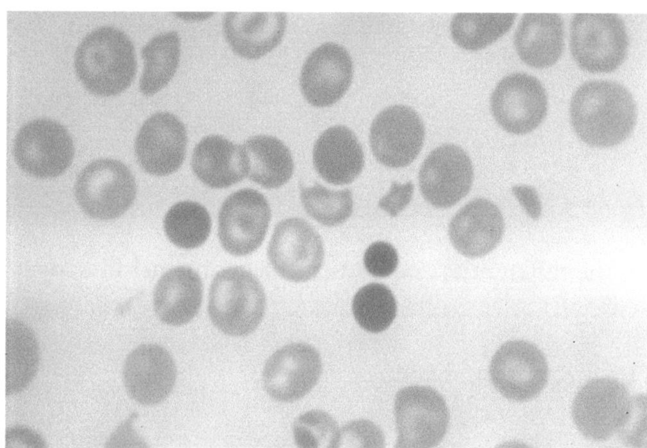

A34.iii Urgent obstetric and haematological review is required, but unlike the situation in disseminated intravascular coagulation, there is no immediate indication to deliver the foetus; indeed, it may be safer to delay this until the mother's condition has been established.

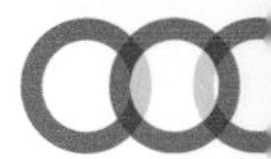

CASE 35

QUESTIONS

A 47-year-old man of Greek–Cypriot origin was noticed to have a hypochromic microcytic anaemia at an insurance medical examination. He was commenced on iron replacement therapy, and this has been continued since, but now, 6 months later, his blood count is unchanged:

Haemoglobin (Hb)	96 g/L
Mean corpuscular volume (MCV)	62 fL
Mean corpuscular haemoglobin concentration (MCHC)	29 g/dL

On examination, he has a palpable spleen.

Q35.i Comment on the blood film.

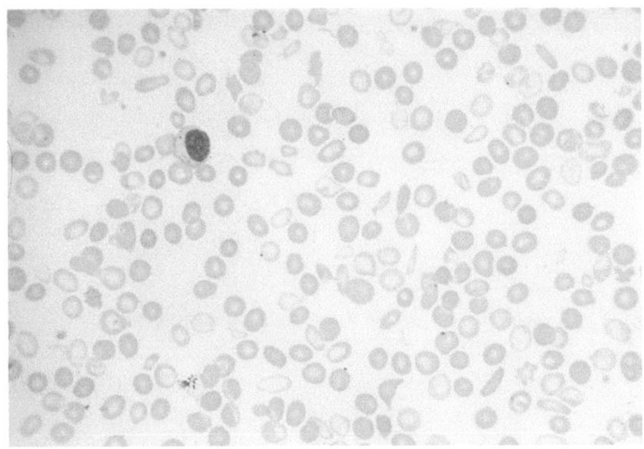

Q35.ii What preparation has been made?

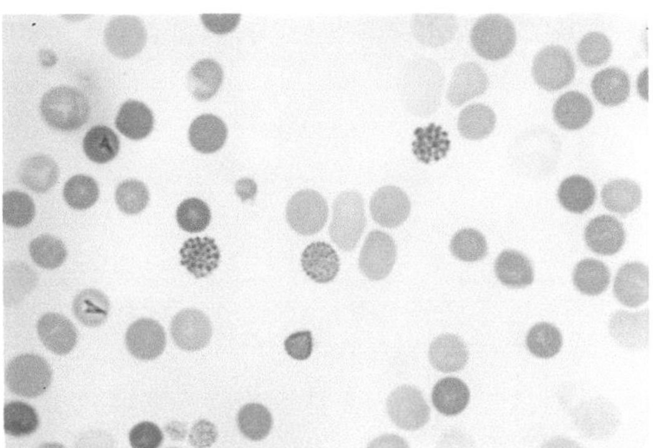

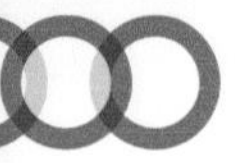

Case 35: ANSWERS

A35.i The blood film shows hypochromic microcytic changes consistent with a thalassaemic disorder. Iron deficiency in a man this age should immediately prompt a search for a cause, for example, gastrointestinal blood loss, and iron replacement therapy should not be commenced until iron deficiency is proven (e.g. by estimation of serum ferritin).

A35.ii This is a 'haemoglobin H' preparation. It shows the characteristic 'golf ball' appearance of red cells, indicating haemoglobin H disease. The inclusions are precipitates of Hb H (B_4, tetramers of beta chains).

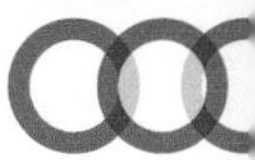

Q35.iii Comment on the haemoglobin electrophoresis result (Y is the patient, Z is an A/S control and X is a normal control).

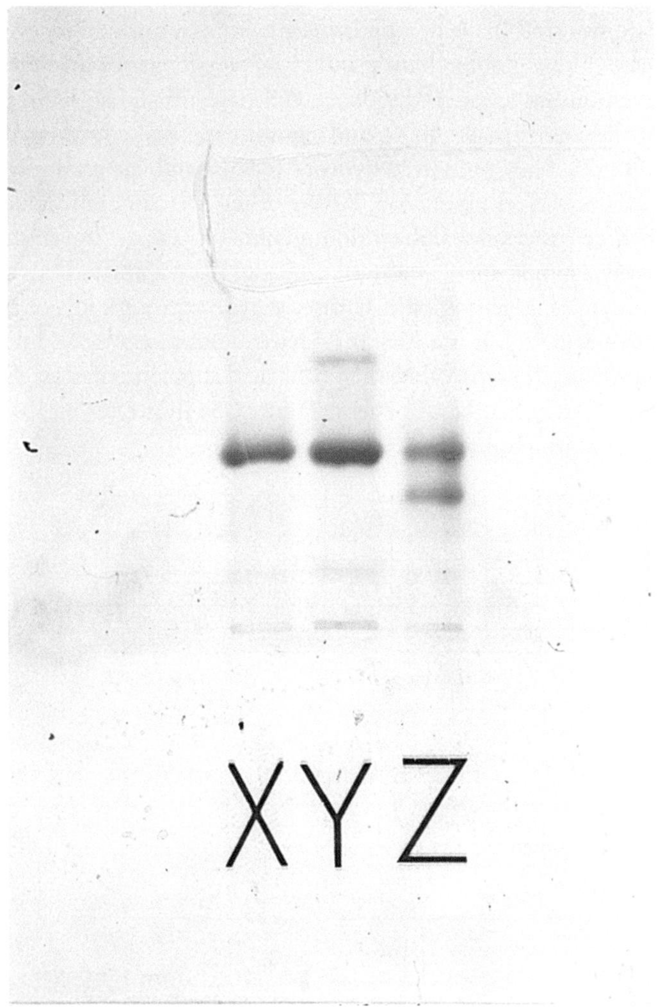

Q35.iv What is the likely diagnosis? What is the pathogenesis of this condition?

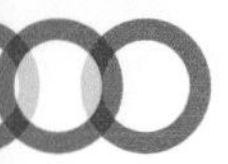

A35.iii There is a fast-migrating band, which is haemoglobin H (tetramers of beta chains).

A35.iv Haemoglobin H disease. Each normal individual has four alpha genes, two on each chromosome 16. Alpha thalassaemia is an autosomal recessive disorder. Absence of alpha globin chain production usually arises through deletion of the corresponding gene. Individuals who have no alpha globin genes have alpha thalassaemia major (–/–), and cannot even make fetal haemoglobin (Hb F, $\alpha 2\gamma 2$). They present as hydrops foetalis and late fetal intrauterine death at 30–34 weeks gestation. At the other extreme, individuals with two or three functional alpha globin genes (–α/αα, α–/α–, or αα/–) are completely asymptomatic and will typically have a normal Hb and a degree of microcytosis. Haemoglobin H disease arises through loss of three alpha globin genes (α–/–). It is a very mild haemoglobinopathy and it typically does not require any therapy other than folic acid supplementation. Erythropoietin supplements may also be of benefit. Figure 35a illustrates high-performance liquid chromatography (HPLC) in this patient.

Peak name	Calibrated area %	Area %	Retention time (min)	Peak area
Unknown	---	0.9	1.26	22787
P2	---	2.7	1.34	65961
P3	---	3.4	1.72	84357
Ao	---	91.8	2.43	2274894
A2	1.4*	---	3.64	29384

Hb H disease

Total area: 2,477,383

F concentration = %

A2 concentration = 1.4* %

*Values outside of expected ranges

Analysis comments:

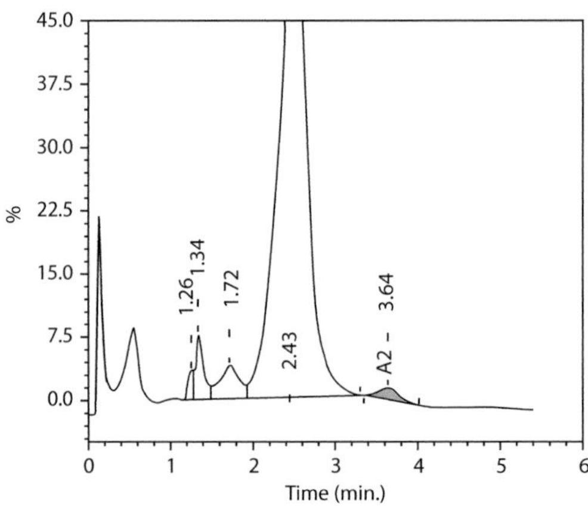

Figure 35a Hb H disease, HPLC.

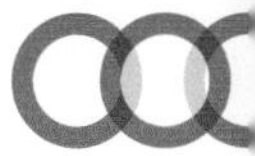

CASE 36

QUESTIONS

A 24-year-old female develops a pruritic rash over her flexor surfaces, at the nape of her back and over her buttocks. The rash is localised, vesicular and intensely pruritic. She has also noted fatigue, weight loss of 3 kg over the preceding 2 months and occasional bouts of central abdominal pain. Her bowels are loose. Her full blood count shows

Haemoglobin (Hb)	91 g/L
Mean corpuscular volume (MCV)	103 fl
White blood cells (WBC)	3.6×10^9/L
Platelets	110×10^9/L

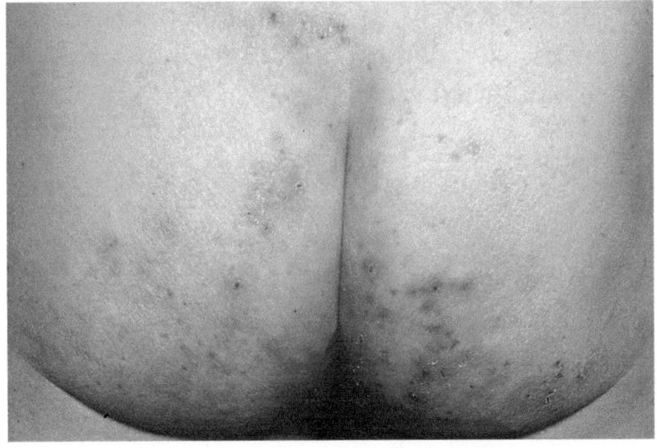

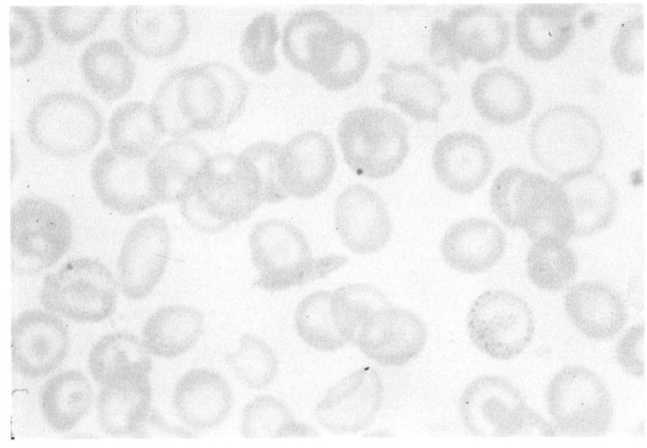

Q36.i What is the dermatological diagnosis?

Q36.ii What abnormalities are seen on the blood film?

Q36.iii What further investigations are required?

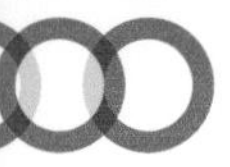

Case 36: ANSWERS

A36.i Dermatitis herpetiformis. Dapsone is the customary therapy, which at high doses can lead to oxidant damage and haemolytic anaemia even in normal individuals.

A36.ii The blood film shows occasional macrocytes, irregularly contracted red cells, target cells and Howell–Jolly bodies. These features suggest hyposplenism.

A36.iii She probably has coeliac disease complicated by dermatitis herpetiformis, hyposplenism and folic acid deficiency secondary to malabsorption.

Her serum and red cell folate levels, calcium, albumin, vitamin D and parathormone level should be estimated. Her serum should be tested for tissue transglutaminase antibodies. She also requires a jejunal or duodenal biopsy to confirm the diagnosis. A duodenal biopsy in coeliac disease (images below) may show subtotal villous atrophy, crypt hyperplasia and inflammatory cells in the lamina propria.

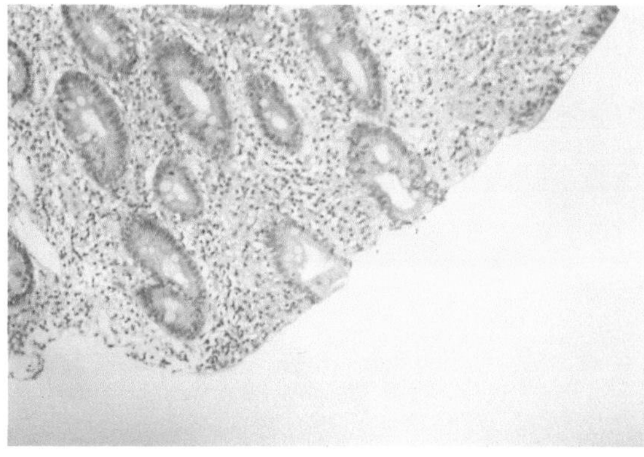

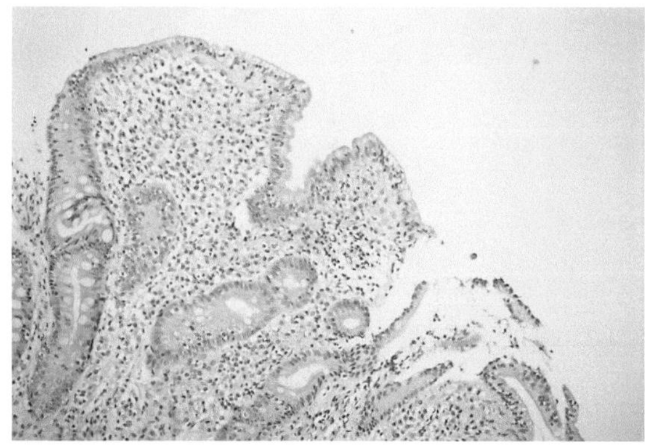

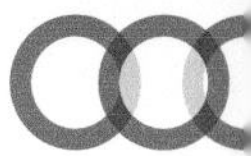

CASE 37

QUESTIONS

A 52-year-old man is found to have an abnormal blood count during the course of routine investigation. He is in good health with no symptoms. He has never suffered excessive bleeding following previous surgery but just before his appointment in the haematology clinic he falls and injures his left arm (Figure 37a). There is no family history of excessive bleeding. On examination, he is found to have a markedly enlarged spleen. Investigations show

Haemoglobin (Hb)	134 g/L
White blood cells (WBC)	51.3×10^9/L
Platelets	147×10^9/L
Liver function tests	Normal
Prothrombin time (PT)	12 seconds (control 11–13 seconds)
Activated partial thromboplastin time (APTT)	74 seconds (control 30–40 seconds)
APTT after 50:50 mix with normal plasma	52 seconds
Factor VIII level	74 IU/dL (normal range 50 IU/dL–150 IU/dL)
Factor IX level	86 IU/dL (normal range 50 IU/dL–150 IU/dL)

His blood film is illustrated (Figure 37b). Figure 37c shows a dual esterase stain on a marrow aspirate.

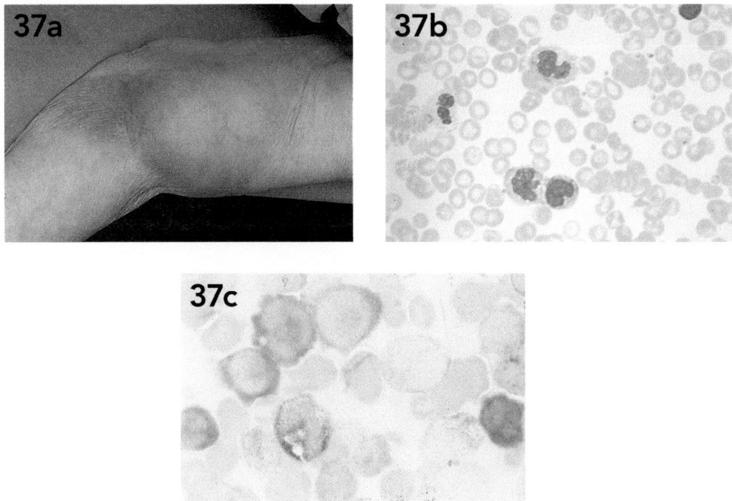

Q37.i What is the likely cause of the elevated white cell count with splenomegaly?

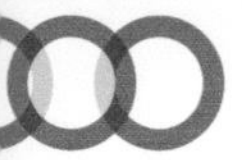

Case 37: ANSWERS

A37.i He has chronic myelomonocytic leukemia (CMML). This is a form of myelodysplasia and abnormal granulocytes accompany increased numbers of mature monocytes. Splenomegaly is usually present. It is unusual to present below the age of 60. Flow cytometry confirmed these cells to be CD 14 positive monocytes.

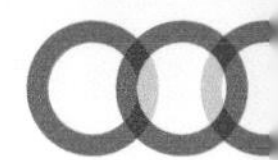

Case 37: QUESTIONS (Continued)

Q37.ii What is the likely cause of his abnormal coagulation?

Q37.iii How are these conditions treated?

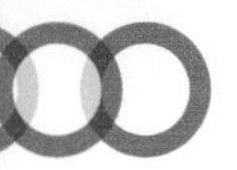

Case 37: ANSWERS (Continued)

A37.ii The isolated prolonged APTT, which corrects well when normal plasma is added, suggests a defect in the intrinsic pathway. As there is a good correction a deficiency is most likely but an acquired inhibitor is a possibility. Further investigations are: assays of Factors VIII, IX, XI and VWF and lupus anti-coagulant. In this case there was an isolated deficiency of Factor XI with a level of 35 U/dL. There was no evidence of an inhibitor to Factor XI. This is an autosomal recessive condition associated with a mild bleeding tendency; it occurs at high frequency in Ashkenazi Jews (approximately 10% are heterozygous carriers). Heterogeneous molecular abnormalities have been identified. Deficiencies of Factor XII, prekallikrein and high-molecular weight kininogen can all lead to an isolated prolonged APTT but are clinically silent.

A37.iii Chronic myelomonocytic leukemia is a slowly progressive condition which is usually treated with oral chemotherapy (e.g. hydroxyurea or etoposide). Splenectomy is helpful if patients become transfusion-dependent or if there are symptoms due to an enlarged organ. Transformation to acute leukemia occurs with a median interval of 18–24 months, but intensive chemotherapy is rarely successful. Younger patients should be considered for intensive therapy, possibly followed by bone marrow transplantation; however, this particular patient did not have a suitable donor 5 azacitidine is often helpful. Recent publications have indicated a role for eltrombopag as an orally active agent.

In mild Factor XI deficiency minor surgery can often be covered with tranexamic acid alone but Factor XI concentrate may be required. In this case subsequent splenectomy was covered with Factor XI concentrate. The two conditions occurred together in this patient by coincidence.

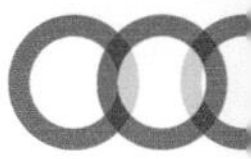

CASE 38

QUESTIONS

A 17-year-old male has been noted to be jaundiced on several occasions. He himself feels completely well. On examination, he is slightly jaundiced. There are no signs of chronic liver disease, but the tip of the spleen is palpable. Investigations show

Haemoglobin (Hb)	134 g/L
Mean corpuscular volume (MCV)	85 fL
Platelets	Normal
Reticulocytes	8%
DAT test	Negative

Q38.i Comment on the blood film.

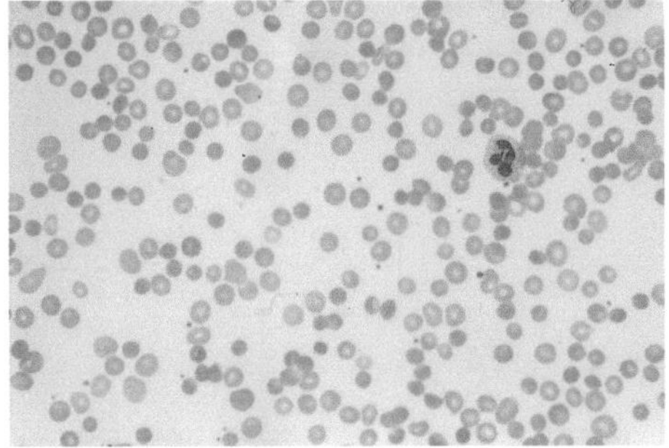

Q38.ii Comment on the results of the osmotic fragility test. How is the diagnosis now made?

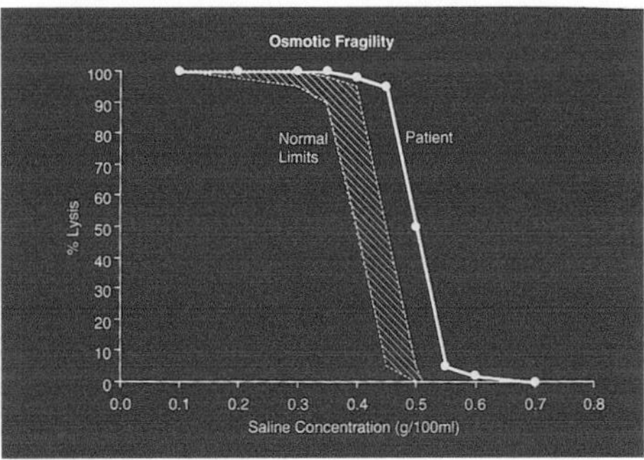

Q38.iii What is the diagnosis?

Q38.iv How should he be treated?

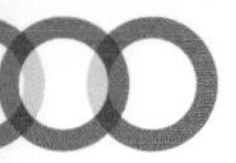

Case 38: ANSWERS

A38.i The blood film shows polychromasia with spherocytes.

A38.ii The graph of his osmotic fragility test shows his red cells to be abnormally susceptible to lysis in hypo-osmolar solution, in comparison with a normal control. This tendency is exaggerated by incubation of his red cells for 24 hours. The diagnosis is now made by flow cytometry showing reduced eosin-5-maleimide in red cells (Figure 38a).

A38.iii With a negative direct anti-globulin test excluding autoimmune haemolytic anaemia, the likeliest diagnosis is hereditary spherocytosis. This is due to an inherited (autosomal dominant) defect in red cell membrane proteins. Hereditary elliptocytosis (Figure 38b) is not usually associated with haemolysis.

A38.iv He should receive folic acid supplements.

Splenectomy (preceded by pneumococcal and *Haemophilus influenzae* B vaccine and followed by long-term prophylaxis with penicillin V) is curative, but recommended only in symptomatic patients or in those with recurrent biliary problems due to pigment gallstones. Parvovirus infection can lead to aplastic crisis.

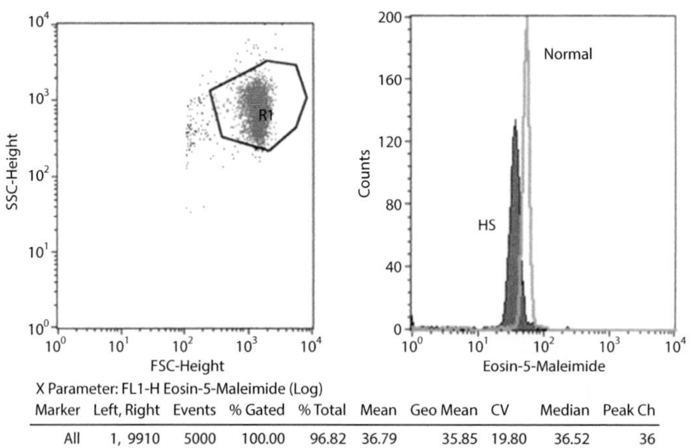

Marker	Left, Right	Events	% Gated	% Total	Mean	Geo Mean	CV	Median	Peak Ch
All	1, 9910	5000	100.00	96.82	36.79	35.85	19.80	36.52	36

Figure 38a Flow cytometry of peripheral blood red cells shows an abnormal population in subjects with HS.

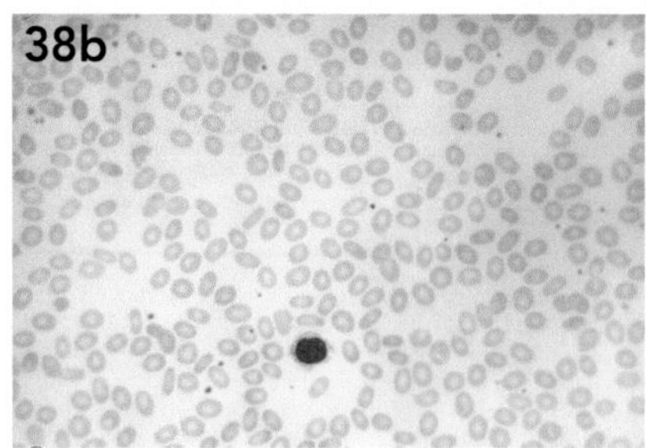

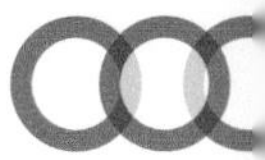

CASE 39

QUESTIONS

A 31-year-old male gives a 2- to 3-week history of fever, bruising and tiredness. There is no palpable splenomegaly. His full blood count shows

Haemoglobin (Hb)	6.7 g/dL
White blood cells (WBC)	$1.3 \times 10/^9/L$ (blasts 12%, neutrophils 61%)
Platelets	$12 \times 10/^9/L$

Bone marrow aspiration is unsuccessful, and a trephine biopsy is performed.

Q39.i Comment on the blood film appearance.

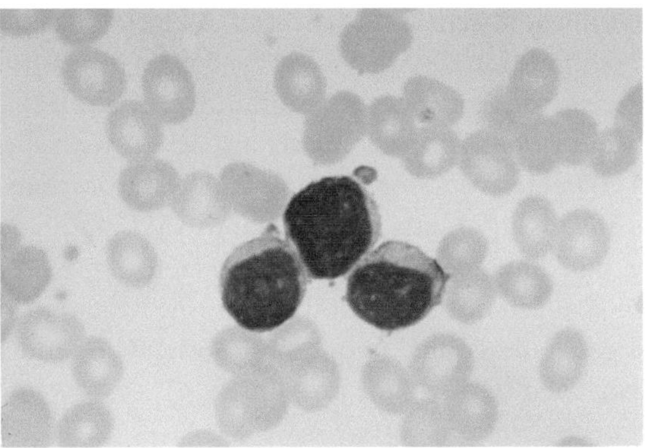

Q39.ii Comment on the bone marrow trephine appearance (on the left). What does the reticulin stain (on the right) show?

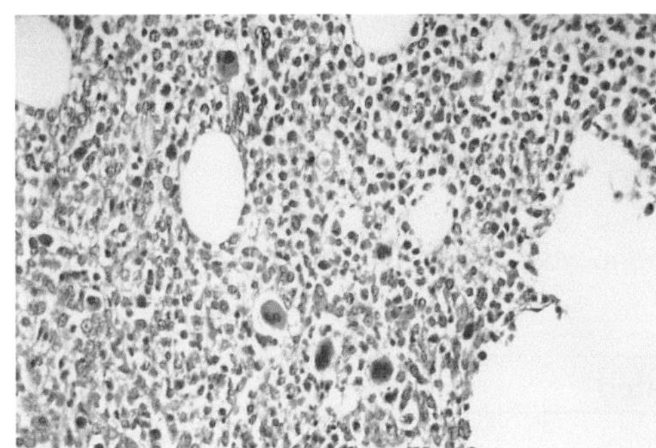

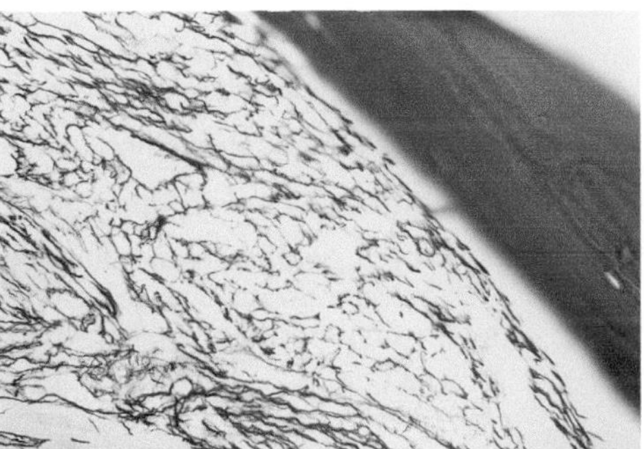

Q39.iii Which further tests may help in making a diagnosis?

Q39.iv What is the likely diagnosis?

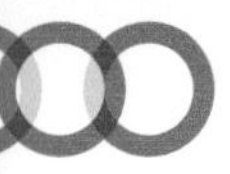

Case 39: ANSWERS

A39.i The blood film shows occasional circulating blasts, presumably leukaemic.

A39.ii The trephine biopsy shows increased numbers of megakaryocytes and scattered foci of immature blasts. The reticulin stains shows increased reticulin fibres, indicating a degree of marrow fibrosis. This fibrosis explains the failure to obtain an aspirate.

A39.iii A full clinical and radiological assessment should be undertaken. The absence of splenomegaly and virtually normal red cell morphology makes chronic myelofibrosis (which is in any event very rare at this age) unlikely. The picture is one of acute myelofibrosis, and further attempts should be made to concentrate and characterise the blast cells with flow cytometry. This may best be done from peripheral blood. The table below shows a simplified classification of acute myeloid leukemia (AML). Cytochemistry is of historic interest only; myeloid cells stain with sudan black (39a) and myelo/monocytic cells can be demonstrated with a combined esterase stain (Figure 39b). The presence of Auer rods indicates myeloid differentiation (Figure 39c). Certain morphological features are particularly associated with specific cytogenetic and clinical characteristics, for example, the translocations t(8;21) and inv 16 are seen with well-differentiated AML and AML with abnormal eosinophils, respectively, both involve the transcription factor core binding factor (CBF) and both are associated with a good prognosis. Mutations in *CEBPA* and *NPM* genes generally confer a good prognosis, while mutations in *FLT3* are generally associated with a poor prognosis.

Simplified classification of acute myeloid leukemia (AML)

Simplified classification of acute myeloid leukemia (AML)
AML with recurrent cytogenetic abnormalities, e.g., t(8:21), t(15;17), inv 16 (with abnormal eosinophils), 11q23 abnormalities, other.
AML with myelodysplasia features
Therapy-related myeloid neoplasms
AML with mutated NPMI or CEBPA
AML not otherwise categorized • E.g., with/without maturation; monocytic, • Monoblastic or myelomonocytic • Erythroid or megakaryoblastic
AML – Biphenotypic or undifferentiated

Myeloid blasts are usually Sudan Black positive, whereas blasts in myelomonocytic leukaemias show positivity for chloroacetate (blue) and butyrate (brown) esterase. Erythroid blasts are usually positive for glycophorin A.

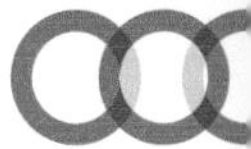

Case 39: ANSWERS (Continued)

A positive platelet peroxidase reaction, visualised by electron microscopy and monoclonal antibody reactivity with anti-glycoprotein IIB/IIIA antibodies are features of megakaryoblastic leukaemia. Light microscopy of the initial Romanovsky stain may show Auer rods, which is pathognomic of AML. The AML subtype with the recurrent cytogenetic manifestation inv 16 was formerly called the M4 Eo variant (myelomonocytic) type is characterised by abnormal eosinophils (Figure 39d). The table gives a simplified classification of AML.

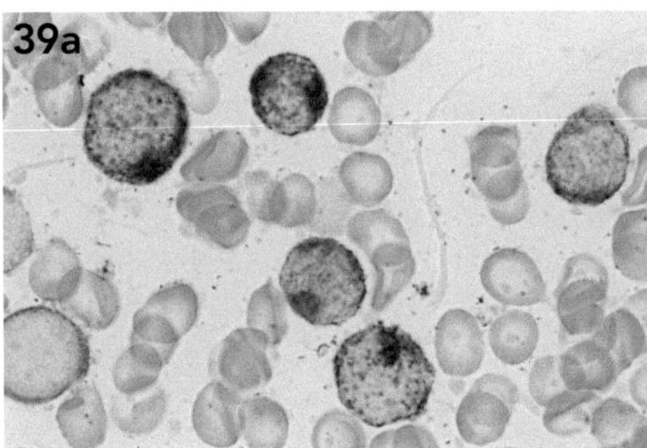

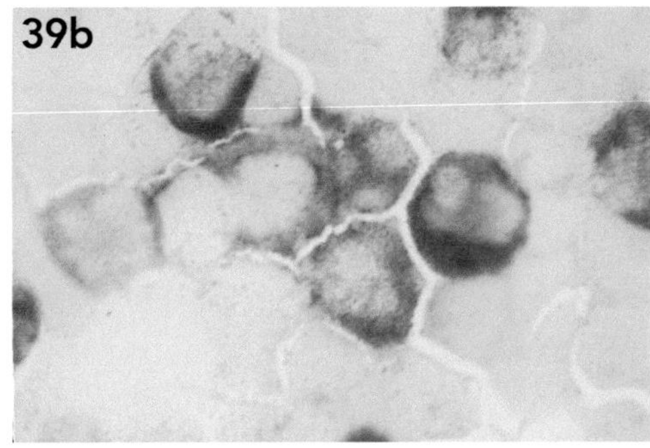

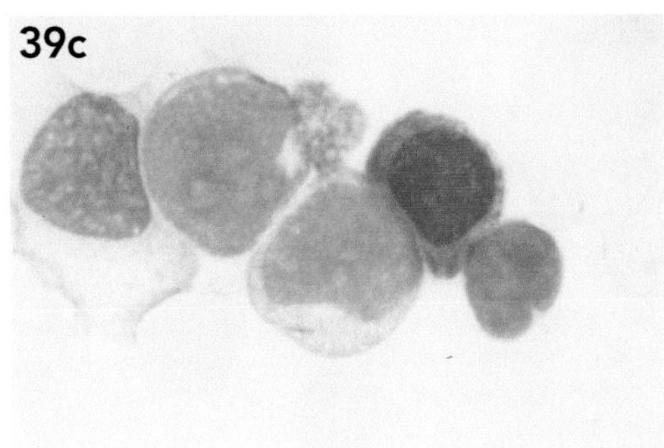

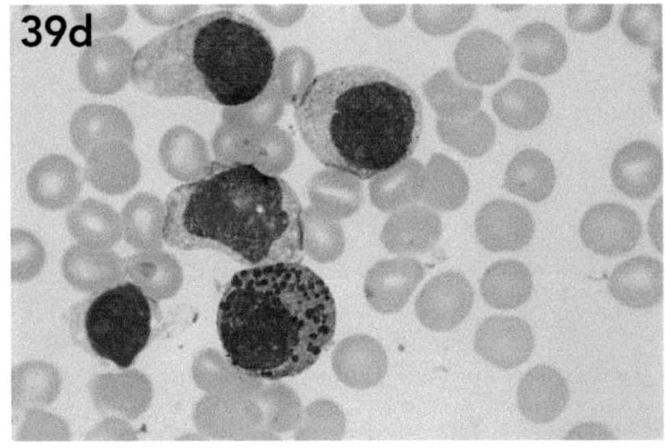

A39.iv The diagnosis in this case of acute onset of myelofibrosis was acute megakaryoblastic leukaemia (AML M7). Other possibilities are myelodysplasia, marrow infiltration by secondary carcinoma or lymphoma, and rarely a non-malignant disorder such as systemic lupus erythematosus. There are no specific cytogenetic changes associated with this type of leukaemia; children with Down's syndrome who develop tis condition often have mutations in the GATA transcription factor. Mutations at 11q23 and 3 p are frequently reported.

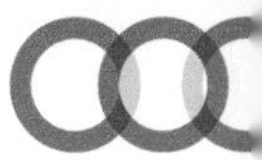

CASE 40

QUESTIONS

A 12-year-old boy has a long history of regular red cell transfusions. These began when he was 1 years old. At that time, he had presented with a blood count:

Haemoglobin (Hb)	3.1 g/dL
Mean corpuscular volume (MCV)	52 fL

His blood films are shown.

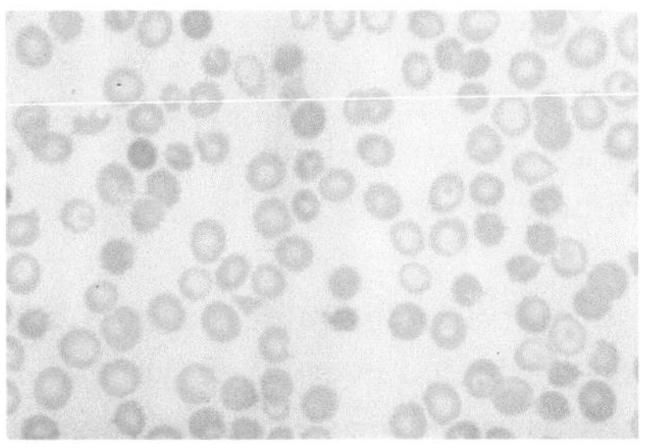

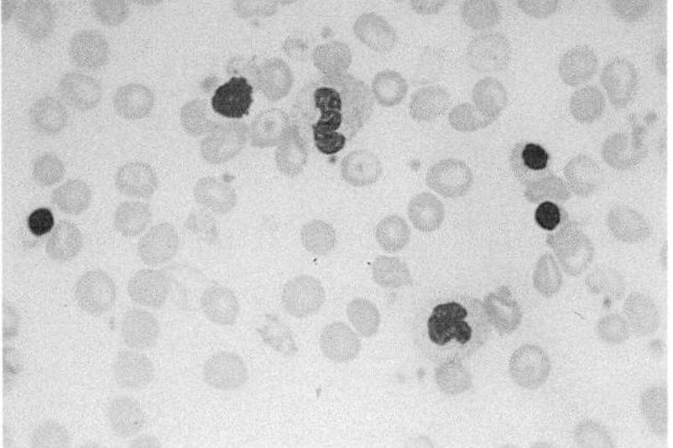

Q40.i What is the diagnosis?

Q40.ii What is the pathogenesis?

Q40.iii What abnormality is illustrated by the skull x-ray?

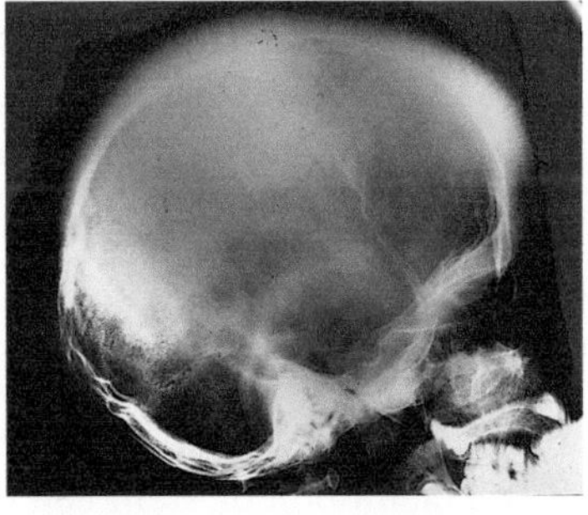

Q40.iv What are the principles of management of this condition?

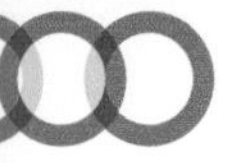

Case 40: ANSWERS

A40.i Beta thalassemia major. There are target cells, hypochromic, microcytic cells and circulating nucleated red cells. There are also transfused red cells.

A40.ii Beta thalassemia major arises through partial or complete failure of synthesis of beta globin chains, and thus causes impaired haemoglobin synthesis and chronic anaemia. Inheritance is as an autosomal recessive condition. The defect in the beta globin gene (situated alongside the gamma and delta genes on chromosome 11) is usually a point mutation affecting expression of the gene or processing of the messenger RNA. A diverse range of mutations is recorded, and this diversity contributes to the variability in the phenotypic manifestations of the condition.

A40.iii The skull x-ray shows a 'hair-on-end' appearance, which is due to extramedullary haemopoiesis.

A40.iv The cornerstone of current management is long-term transfusion therapy. A red cell transfusion is required every 3–5 weeks, and attempts should be made to minimise sensitisation to red cell antigens (by use of genotyped cells) and human leukocyte antigen (HLA) antigens (by use of filtered blood). Splenectomy may be beneficial, but is best delayed until after the age of 5 to reduce the risk of post-splenectomy infection.

A consequence of transfusion therapy is iron overload. Iron deposition in tissues leads to diverse clinical effects on many organs:

- Skin (pigmentation)
- Heart (cardiomyopathy)
- Liver (cirrhosis)
- Endocrine organs and pancreas (diabetes mellitus, growth impairment, delayed puberty)

Iron chelation therapy is usually administered in the form of parenteral desferrioxamine (DFO, typically given by subcutaneous infusion over 12 hours, five nights each week, with oral vitamin C). Side effects of DFO include sensory changes (hearing loss, visual defects), and bone and cartilage abnormalities. The necessity of parenteral administration contributes toward poor compliance. Deferasirox is a once-daily oral iron chelator which can cause renal and gastrointestinal (GI) disturbances but is generally well tolerated. Deferiprone is an oral iron chelator which seems to be particularly effective at removing cardiac iron. Side effects include agranulocytosis (1%), arthralgia and GI disturbances. Cardiac iron is best measured by magnetic resonance imaging (MRI). Haemopoietic stem cell or umbilical cord stem cell transplantation is curative for selected patients.

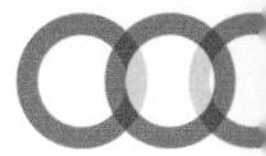

Case 40: ANSWERS (Continued)

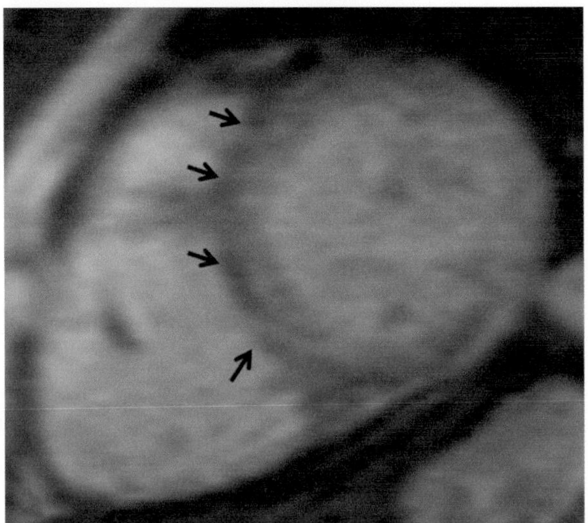

Cardiac magnetic resonance imaging (MRI) to assess iron content; specialised readings on T2 window allow serial quantitation. (Reproduced from Winnie, C.W. et al. *J. Magn Reson Imaging*, 36, 1052–1059, 2012.)

Luspatercept is a agent whch regulates late erythoid differentiation and maturation. It has been shown in trials to reduce transfusion requirement in thalassaemia major by improving erythropoiesis.

Allogeneic stem cell transplantation with reduced intensity conditioning also has an expanding role in thalassaemia major, and the donor could be HLA identical (sibling or unrelated) but could be haplo-identical, with modern conditioning regimes, and could be a thallassaemia carrier without compromising outcome.

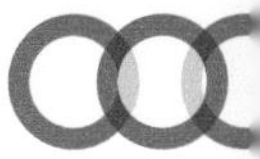

CASE 41

QUESTIONS

A 36-year-old man is referred for investigation of thrombocytopenia. He has recently developed jaundice, tiredness and lack of libido. Investigations show

Haemoglobin (Hb)	93 g/L
White blood cells (WBC)	$3.1 \times 10/^{9}/L$
Platelets	$78 \times 10/^{9}L$
Prothrombin time (PT)	18 seconds (normal range 11–15 seconds)
Partial thromboplastin time with kaolin (APTT)	46 seconds (normal range 30–40 seconds)

Q41.i What abnormalities are shown in the blood film?

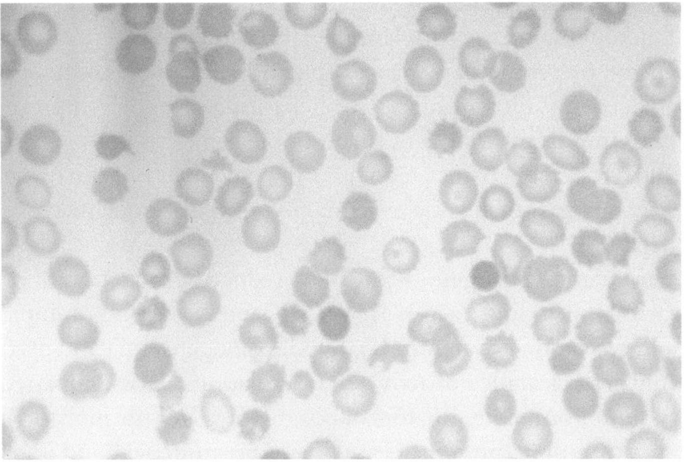

Q41.ii What additional information should be sought in the history and clinical examination?

Q41.iii What other haematological complications may occur?

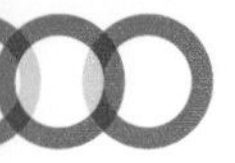

Case 41: ANSWERS

A41.i The blood film shows target cells, macrocytosis, occasional acanthocytes and thrombocytopenia. These findings, together with the presence of jaundice and the abnormal coagulation profile, suggest underlying chronic liver disease.

A41.ii This patient gave a history of travel to the Far East and an attack of hepatitis, which was 5 years previously. He was found to have serological evidence of past infection with hepatitis A and C viruses. He had also been an intravenous drug abuser, and drank alcohol excessively. Examination revealed spider naevi, gynaecomastia, ascites, jaundice and splenomegaly. The probable cause of his pancytopenia is splenomegaly.

A41.iii Haematological complications of liver disease include

- Anaemia – Due to increased risk of gastrointestinal bleeding, dilution through increased plasma volume, sequestration within an enlarged spleen, abnormal erythropoietin metabolism and haemolysis arising from alterations in red cell membrane lipids.
- Leukopenia – Due to splenomegaly, paraproteinaemia in cirrhosis.
- Thrombocytopenia – Due to splenomegaly, autoimmune destruction associated with chronic active hepatitis and impaired production (the liver is an important source of thrombopoietin).
- Pancytopenia – Associated with a hypercellular bone marrow in splenomegaly or aplastic anaemia (hypocellular bone marrow occurs in viral hepatitis).
- Coagulation changes – Principally reduced production of coagulation factors (including Factors II, VII, IX and X because of impaired absorption and activation of vitamin K), hypofibrinogenaemia and dysfibrinogenaemia, impaired clearance of activated coagulation factors, impaired production of inhibitors and regulators of coagulation and fibrinolysis (including anti-thrombin, proteins C and S and plasminogen) and impaired platelet function. Thus, these patients are at increased risk of developing thrombosis, haemorrhage and disseminated intravascular coagulation.
- Treatment-related haematological side effects – for example, transfusion-associated viral infection.

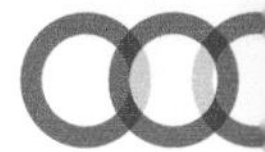

Alcohol ingestion is a common cause of macrocytosis, thrombocytopenia and sideroblastic anaemia. Figure 41a shows vacuolated erythroblasts in the marrow aspirate of a patient with alcohol-related anaemia. Acanthocytosis (Figure 41b) also occurs in abetalipoproteinaemia.

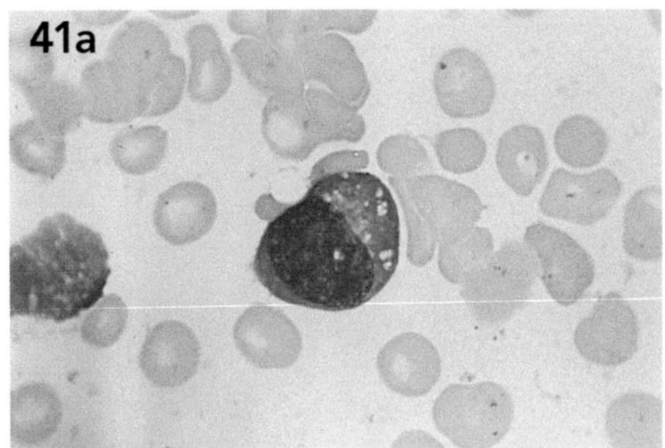

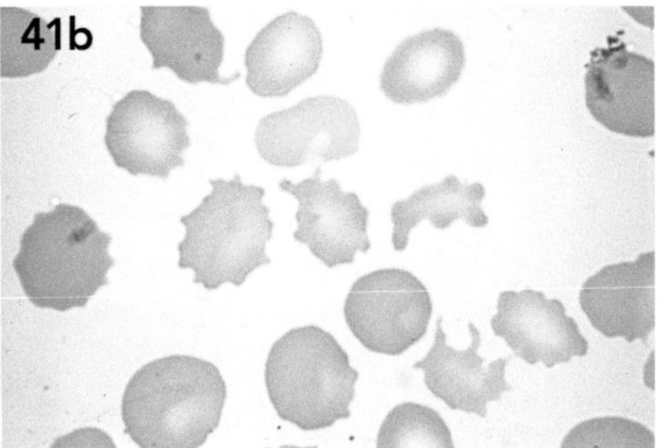

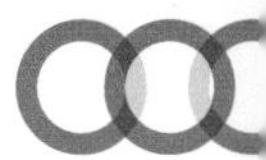

CASE 42

QUESTIONS

A 9-year-old boy presents with a long-standing history of anaemia, renal impairment, growth retardation and skeletal deformity. His full blood count shows

Haemoglobin (Hb)	91 g/L
Mean corpuscular volume (MCV)	103 fL
White blood cells (WBC)	2.1 × 10/⁹/L (neutrophils 47%)
Platelets	90 × 10/⁹/L

A clinical photograph, an x-ray of his hands and a bone marrow trephine biopsy are shown below.

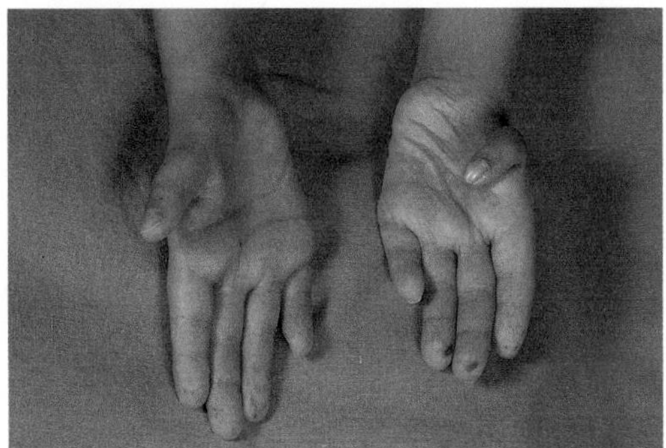

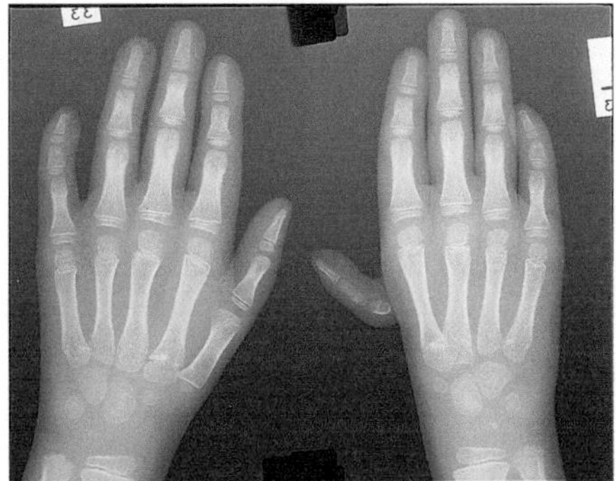

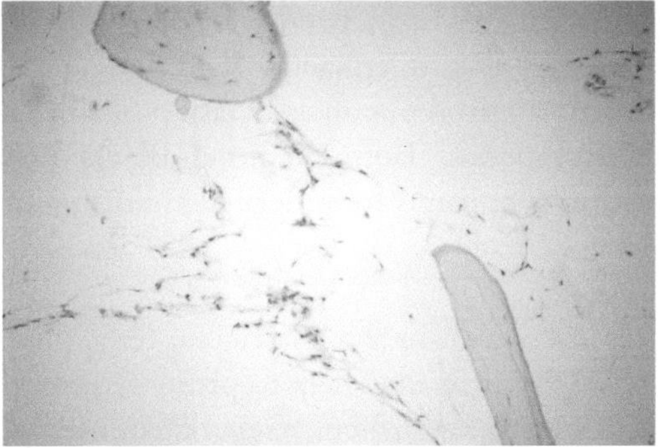

Q42.i What is the diagnosis?

Q42.ii What further tests are indicated to confirm the diagnosis?

Q42.iii What other conditions may cause this haematological picture?

Q42.iv How would you treat him?

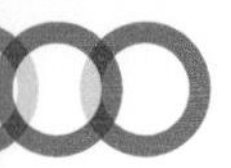

Case 42: ANSWERS

A42.i Fanconi's anaemia. This is an autosomal recessive condition in which increased DNA fragility leads to multiple random chromosomal breaks; this in turn leads to aplastic anaemia. The trephine biopsy shows hypocellularity of the marrow. Multiple skeletal changes may occur, such as hypoplasia of the thumb, the development of abnormal metacarpal bones and an incurved little finger and absent radii. There can also be structural anomalies of the renal tract.

A42.ii The diagnosis is confirmed by cytogenetic (chromosome) analysis of stimulated cultures of haemopoietic cells from the bone marrow. An intravenous pyelogram (IVU) should also be undertaken.

A42.iii Aplastic anaemia may occur secondary to drugs (chloramphenicol, sulphonamides, phenylbutazone and other non-steroidal anti-inflammatory drugs, gold, anti-thyroid drugs, tetracyclines, tricylic anti-depressants, chlorpromazine) and toxins and chemicals (e.g. benzene).

Reversible myelosuppression is inevitably associated with chemotherapy and radiotherapy. Certain viral infections (principally hepatitis, both A and B as well as non-A, non-B and, usually, non-C) are occasionally complicated by aplasia. Approximately 50% of cases are idiopathic, and immune mechanisms may operate.

Other congenital causes of bone marrow failure include dyskeratosis congenital, ataxia telangiectasia and Bloom's syndrome, which, like Fanconi's anaemia, are associated with defects in DNA repair. They also have an increased risk of leukaemia as well as aplastic anaemia. Diamond–Schwachmann syndrome is an association of aplastic anaemia with exocrine pancreatic dysfunction. Both Diamond–Blackfan anaemia and Diamond–Schwachmann syndrome are inherited abnormalities of related ribosomal protein genes.

A42.iv He requires assessment by a pediatrician, renal physician and endocrinologist. Androgen supplements may help to promote growth, and he may need treatment for renal impairment. Genetic counselling should be offered, as this is an autosomal recessive condition. The pancytopenia is mild and may respond to oral oxymetholone. Surgery (e.g. dental therapy) will need to be covered by platelet transfusion, and infections will require antibiotic therapy. Definitive treatment (e.g. allogeneic stem cell transplant) is only indicated if the counts deteriorate. These patients are at increased risk of malignancy, especially acute myeloid lymphoma (AML).

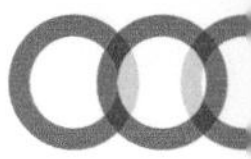

CASE 43

QUESTIONS

A 67-year-old female has bone pain affecting her spine and limbs. Two years ago she suffered a fracture of her lower femur, which has failed to heal properly. She complains of easy bruising and on examination has splenomegaly. Investigations show

Haemoglobin (Hb)	10.1 g/dL
Mean corpuscular volume (MCV)	82 fL
White blood cell (WBC)	3.4 × 10^9/L (differential normal)
Platelets	110 × 10^9/L

Q43.i What abnormalities are shown in the x-ray of her femur?

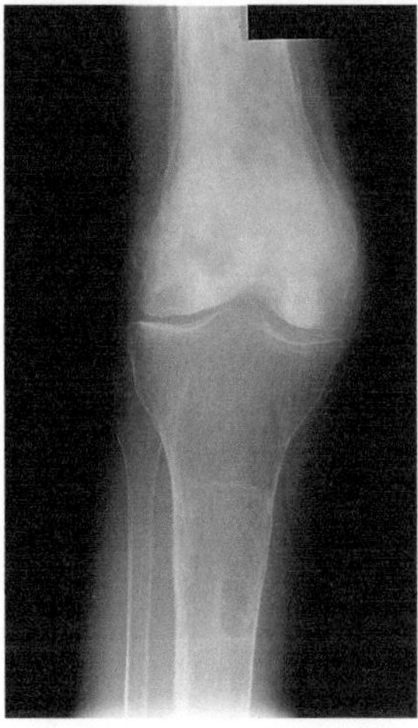

Q43.ii What diagnosis is revealed by the bone marrow aspirate (on the left) and trephine biopsy (on the right)?

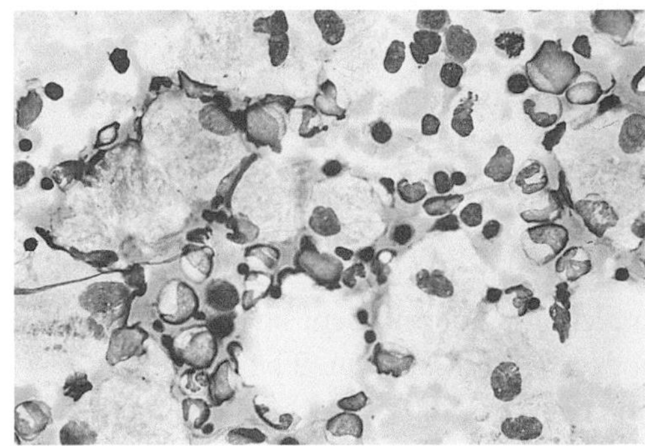

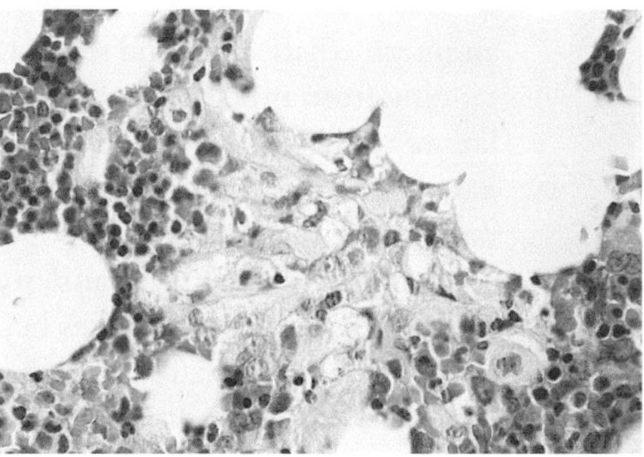

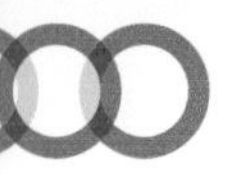

Case 43: ANSWERS

A43.i The x-ray shows loss of bony texture, and the magnetic resonance imaging (MRI) (Figure 43a) demonstrates replacement of the medullary cavity by abnormal tissue with multiple infarcts. The femoral appearances are those of the Erlenmeyer flask deformity in Gaucher disease.

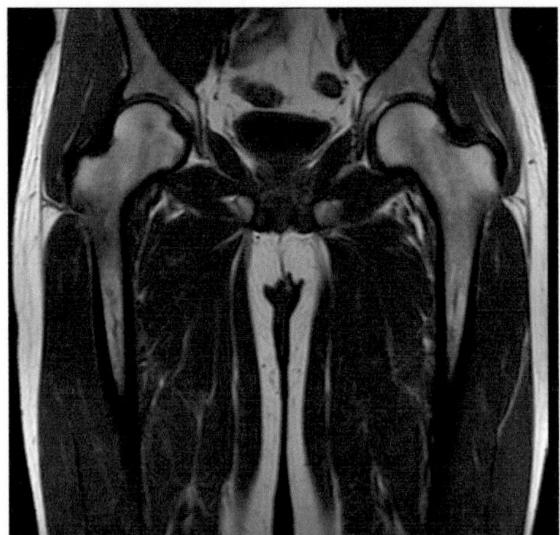

Figure 43a Gaucher disease – early changes of substrate deposition in the right femur.

A43.ii Bone marrow aspirate and trephine biopsy show macrophages laden with lipids – typical Gaucher cells – suggesting she is suffering from Gaucher disease of the chronic adult type (type I). Types II and III Gaucher disease also affect the central nervous system. Gaucher disease is due to mutations within the glucocerebrosidase gene, which causes a deficiency of lysosomal beta-glucocerebrosidase. This in turn leads to accumulation of glucocerebroside in tissues. The different types of Gaucher disease have different degrees of residual enzyme activity. Type II disease has zero or extremely low activity and is incompatible with life – subjects die in utero or within the first year of life and have severe visceral disease and neurological impairment presenting as impaired consciousness, seizures and severe motor abnormalities. Type III is an intermediate form and subjects have variable neurological manifestations, ranging from mild ophthalmoplegia to cognitive impairment with seizures and failure to thrive. Type I Gaucher is the most common form. The condition has an increased prevalence among the Ashkenazi Jewish population (carrier rate approximately 1:12 and population incidence approximately 1:900). The enzyme deficiency manifests principally in reticuloendothelial cells and substrate accumulation causes hepatosplenomegaly and deposition of substrate in the bone marrow (reducing haemopoiesis) and skeleton. The overall incidence of the condition is approximately 1:30,000 individuals and it is one of the most common lysosomal storage disorders.

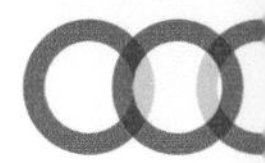

Case 43: QUESTIONS (Continued)

Q43.iii How should she be treated?

Q43.iv What complications can occur?

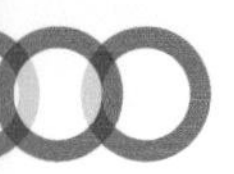

Case 43: ANSWERS (Continued)

A43.iii Although splenectomy may lead to haematological improvement, it can also lead to increased deposition of cerebroside in other tissues such as the skeleton. It is not advised.

Enzyme replacement therapy (ERT) with recombinant glucocerebrosidase has been available for over 20 years and has a proven safety and efficacy record. The infused enzyme does not cross the blood brain barrier and neurological manifestations are not improved. However, intravenous enzyme given every 2 weeks will improve the blood counts, reduce the size of the liver and spleen, and improve skeletal measures such as bone pain, the risk of pathological fracture and bone mineral density. A very recent development for patients with type I Gaucher disease is the availability of substrate reduction therapy (SRT). Such treatment is oral and reduces substrate accumulation by reducing substrate production, whereby residual enzyme can gradually reduce the substrate burden. SRT is widely available and is comparable in efficacy to ERT. Furthermore, the oral formulation of a small molecule allows better tissue distribution than ERT. Gene therapy approaches are under active investigation. Allogeneic stem cell transplantation has been performed successfully in young patients, and this approach warrants further study in countries where ERT and SRT are not available due to the expense of the treatment.

A43.iv Important complications of Gaucher disease are bone pain and pathological fracture due to skeletal disease. Patients may bleed as a result of the thrombocytopenia; and platelet function is abnormal in Gaucher patients. Fatigue is a common symptom, often out of proportion to the degree of anaemia. Gall stones and hepatobiliary disease is common in Gaucher patients and splenomegaly, pancytopenia and cirrhosis can all occur. Gaucher patients are at an increased risk of malignancy – this includes hepatobiliary tumours, gastrointestinal tumours and both myeloid and lymphoid malignancy. The risk of developing a monoclonal gammopathy is increased tenfold in Gaucher and the risk of myeloma is increased fivefold. An intriguing recent observation is that Gaucher patients and carriers have a markedly increased risk of Parkinson's disease. Figure 43a shows early changes of Gaucher disease in the femur; this is reversible with ERT, whereas the features shown in Figure 43b are irreversible and require joint replacement surgery.

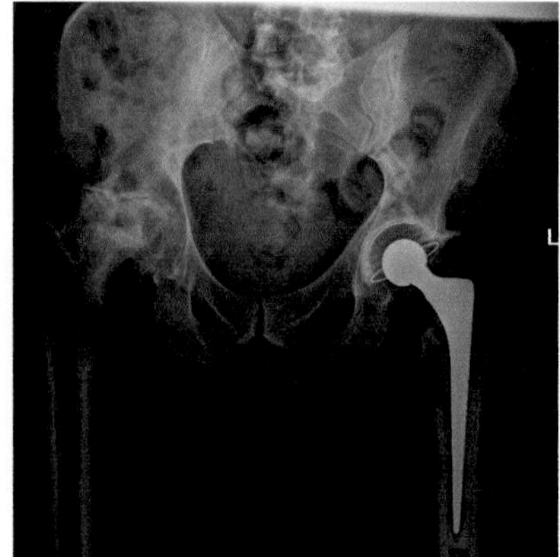

Figure 43b Advanced Gaucher disease.

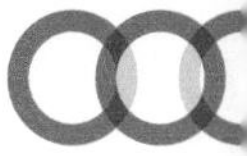

CASE 44

QUESTIONS

A 66-year-old woman has a 4-week history of gradually increasing tiredness. Examination reveals a markedly enlarged spleen, palpable 12 cm below the left costal margin. Investigations show

Haemoglobin (Hb)	9.6 g/dL
Mean corpuscular volume (MCV)	81 fL
White blood cell (WBC)	4.1×10^9/L (differential normal)
Platelets	161×10^9/L

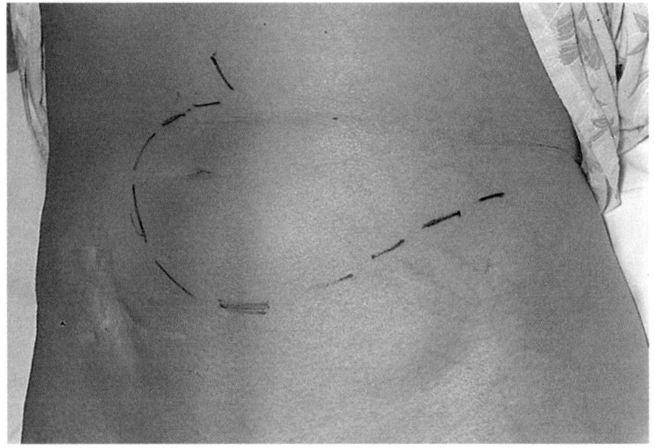

Q44.i Comment on the blood film.

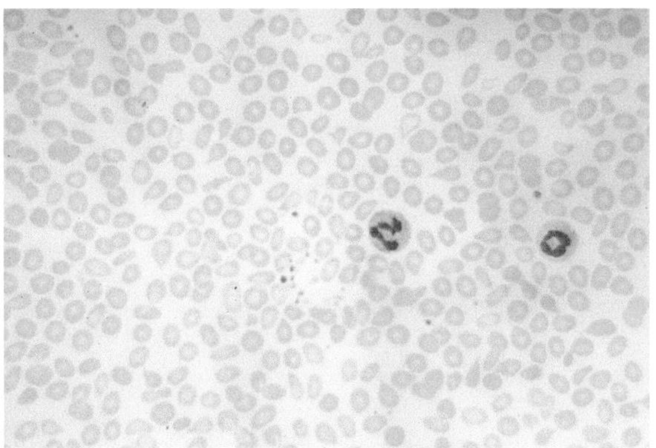

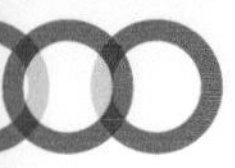

Case 44: ANSWERS

A44.i The blood film shows marked anisocytosis and poikilocytosis with macrocytes and occasional teardrop forms.

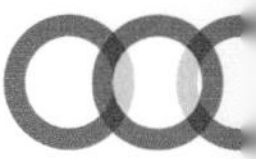

Case 44: QUESTIONS (Continued)

Q44.ii Comment on the haematoxylin and eosin (on the left) and reticulin (on the right) stains of the bone marrow trephine biopsy.

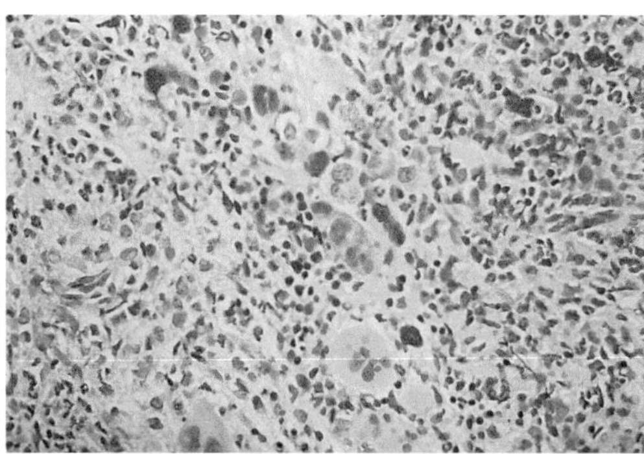

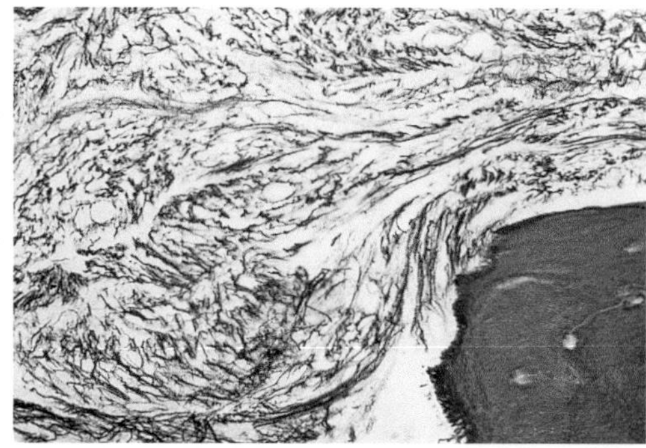

Q44.iii A splenectomy is performed 1 year later. Comment on the spleen histology.

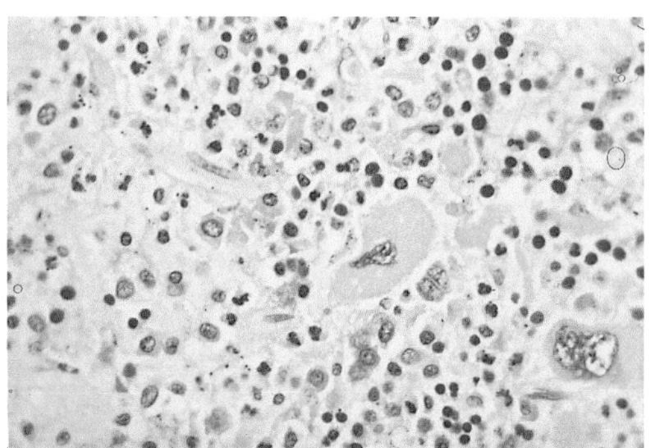

Q44.iv What is the diagnosis? What further investigations are helpful?

Q44.v How is this condition generally treated?

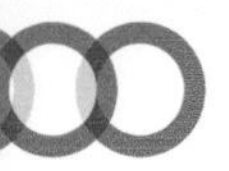

A44.ii Bone marrow reticulin is increased, indicating marrow fibrosis.

A44.iii Megakaryocytes, granulocytic cells and erythroid cells are seen indicating extramedullary haemopoiesis.

A44.iv Chronic idiopathic myelofibrosis. The plasma lactate dehydrogenase (LDH) level is increased. Approximately one-third of patients have a mutation in the Janus kinase 2 (*JAK2*) gene and a higher proportion have a mutation in the calreticulin (*CALR*) gene. Other genes that may be mutated include Ten-Eleven-Translocation2 (*TET2*) and myeloproliferative leukemia (MPL). Bone marrow cytogenetic will typically show abnormalities – commonest are deletions of 20q and 13q, trisomy 8 and abnormalities of chromosomes 1, 5, 7 and 9.

A44.v Treatment is unsatisfactory. Younger patients may be suitable for an allogeneic stem cell transplant; but such approaches have unacceptable morbidity and mortality risks for subjects >50 years.

The marrow fibrosis is a reactive phenomenon, and the precise cause of increased fibrosis in this (and other) myeloproliferative disorder(s) is unknown. A proportion of patients with myelofibrosis have a preceding history of polycythaemia rubra vera. Oral chemotherapy (e.g. hydroxyurea) usually does not reduce fibrosis, but it can lead to a reduction in splenic size and will control the white cell count when the disease is in the proliferative phase. Folic acid is frequently helpful.

Supportive care, with red cell transfusions and occasionally platelet transfusions, is usually required. Splenectomy is usually needed at some point as progressive splenomegaly contributes to an increasing transfusion requirement. Splenectomy should be preceded by pneumococcal and *Haemophilus influenzae* type B (Hib) vaccinations and long-term penicillin prophylaxis is required after splenectomy. Splenic radiotherapy is worth trying in patients who are unfit for splenectomy.

The JAK2 inhibitor ruxolitinib has recently been approved. It has side effects including anaemia and thrombocytopenia and erythropoietin therapy may be required. Its use is associated with improved survival and it is generally well-tolerated.

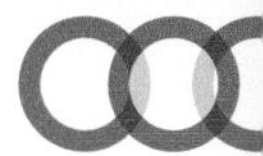

A range of new scoring systems are being introduced for myelofibrosis. These are based on the age of the patient, the baseline level of haemoglobin, the presence of leukocytosis, constitutional symptoms and the presence of cytogenetic changes in the marrow. The baseline level of blast cells in peripheral blood, the need for transfusion and the presence of thrombocytopenia are also indicative of prognosis. Transformation to acute leukaemia (often with a population of megakaryoblasts, image below), occurs in the terminal stages.

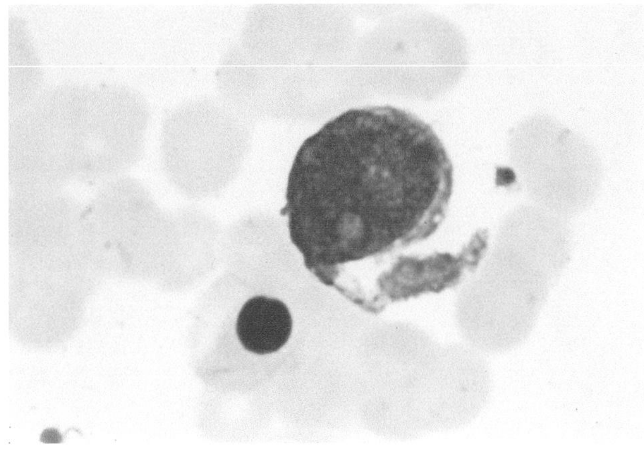

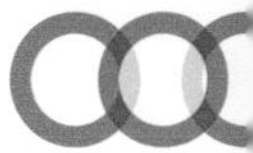

CASE 45

QUESTIONS

A 65-year-old woman presented for investigation of easy bruising. Investigations showed

Haemoglobin (Hb)	95 g/L
Mean corpuscular volume (MCV)	81 fL
White blood cells (WBC)	9.2×10^9/L
Platelets	137×10^9/L
Prothrombin time (PT)	12 seconds (control 11–13 seconds)
Activated partial thromboplastin time (APTT)	38 seconds (control 30–40 seconds)
Ivy template bleeding time	10.5 minutes (control 2–10 minutes)

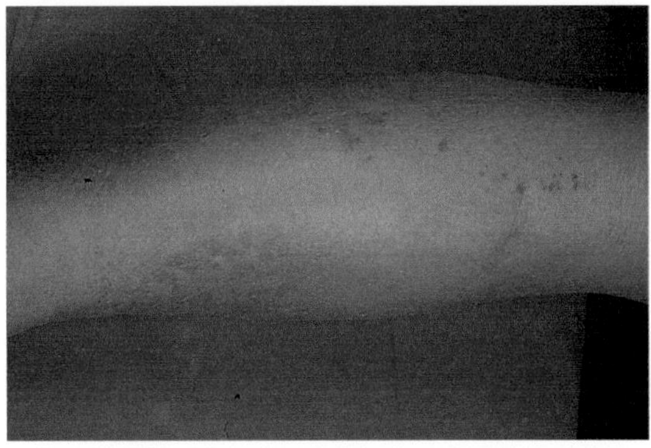

Q45.i Comment on the facial appearance.

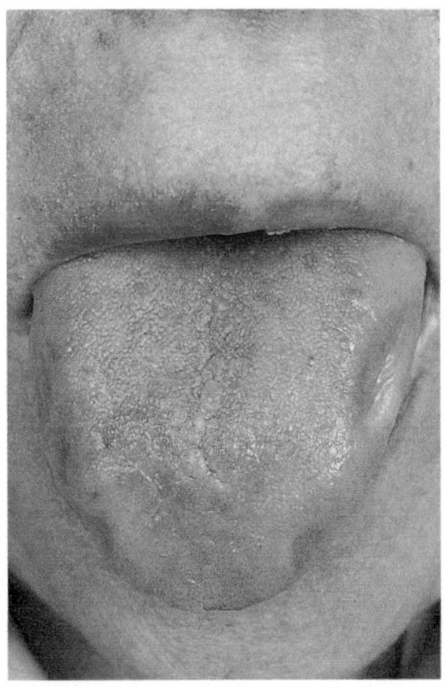

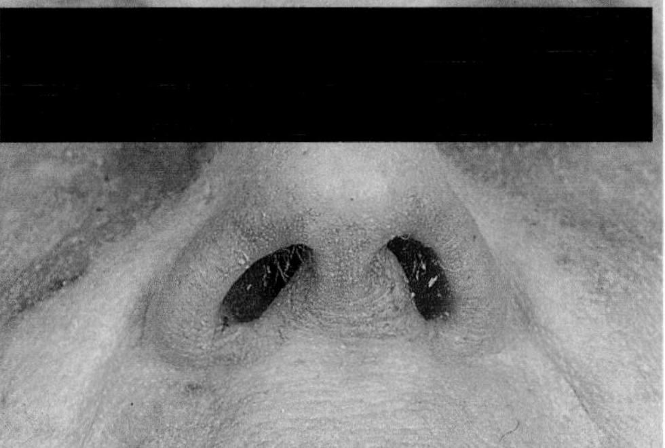

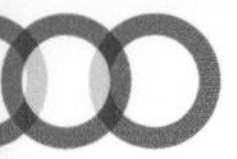

Case 45: ANSWERS

A45.i She has abnormal skin infiltration around the nose and eyes and an enlarged tongue. The history of excessive bruising with inconclusive coagulation profile (marginally prolonged bleeding time) suggests a disorder of skin or connective tissue, for example, amyloidosis.

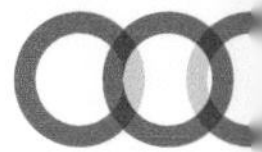

Q45.ii Comment on the bone marrow trephine biopsy.

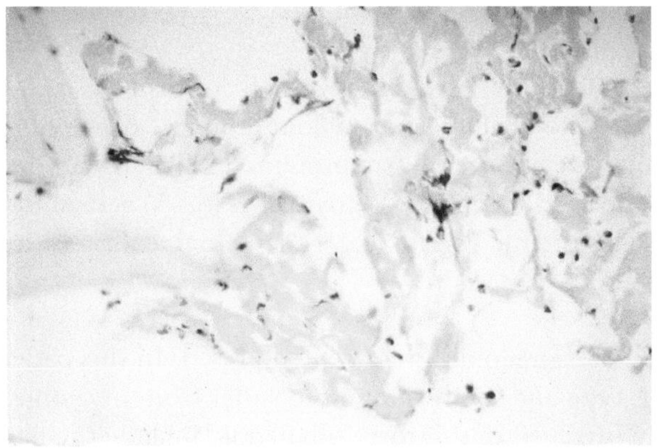

Q45.iii What is the diagnosis?

Q45.iv What further investigations are required?

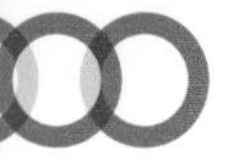

Case 45: ANSWERS (Continued)

A45.ii The bone marrow shows amyloidosis – homogenous pink-staining material (haematoxylin and eosin stain) or red-staining material (Congo red stain), which is birefringent to polarised light.

A45.iii Systemic amyloidosis. A skin biopsy will confirm this and blood tests should be undertaken to characterise amyloid proteins. Amyloid light chains (AL) are seen in association with paraproteins and in primary amyloid, whereas protein A derived from serum amyloid-A (SAA) is seen in amyloidosis reactive to a systemic disease (e.g. rheumatoid arthritis, chronic suppurative infection).

A45.iv A cause for the amyloid should be established. In this patient, the amyloid was of AL type and she was found to suffer from myeloma. Other organs frequently involved in this form of amyloid include the heart, kidneys, liver, spleen and nerves.

Reactive systemic amyloidosis typically affects the liver, spleen, kidneys and marrow, but not usually the skin, tongue, heart or nervous system.

An excess number of plasma cells are frequently present in the marrow aspirate (image below). The level of paraprotein and serum free light chain is a good marker of the response of the clone to chemotherapy. This woman was treated with chemotherapy as for multiple myeloma, including combinations of bortezomib and lenalidomide with steroids. Thalidomide is best avoided because of its cardiac toxicity in this setting. This patient underwent cardiac magnetic resonance imaging (MRI) and was found to have cardiac amyloid. Unfortunately, she developed cardiac arrhythmia and died.

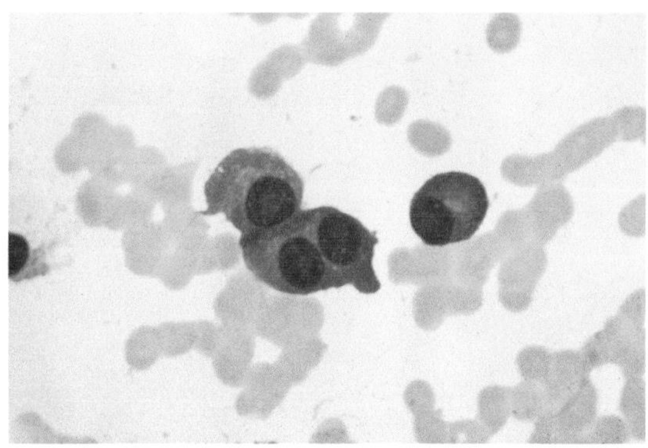

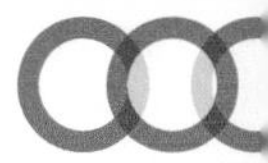

CASE 46

QUESTIONS

A 7-year-old boy of Greek parents gives a 4-day history of fever, sore throat and abdominal pain. He has passed dark urine. He has been taking amoxycillin suspension for 2 days. There is no relevant family history and he has had no similar attacks previously, though his mother reveals that he did have prolonged neonatal jaundice. On examination, he is clinically jaundiced and anaemic. Liver and spleen are not palpable. His full blood count shows

Haemoglobin (Hb)	6.1 g/dL
Mean corpuscular volume (MCV)	110 fL
White blood cells (WBC)	17.3 × 10^9/L (lymphocytes 46%, neutrophils 52%)
Platelets	307 × 10^9/L
Reticulocytes are raised at 18%	

Q46.i What is the diagnosis and how would you confirm it (blood film)?

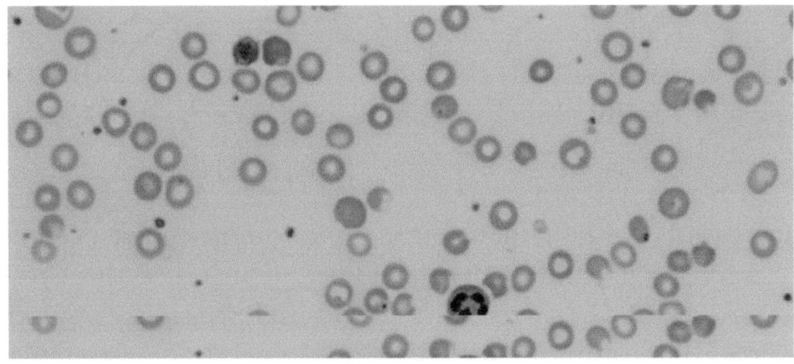

Q46.ii What precipitants are recognised?

Q46.iii How would you manage this patient?

Q46.iv What complications occur in the neonatal period in this condition?

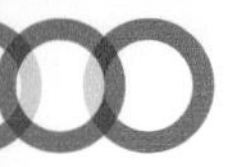

Case 46: ANSWERS

A46.i The blood film shows polychromasia, anisocytosis and 'bite' cells, in which haemoglobin is separated from the red cell membrane.

A46.ii Acute haemolysis in an individual with glucose-6-phosphate dehydrogenase (G6PD) deficiency. G6PD deficiency is X-linked and is the commonest inherited disease, with wide prevalence in Africa, Asia, the Middle East and around the Mediterranean. Confirmation is by red cell enzyme assay or by performing a fluorescent screening test that detects nicotinamide adenine dinucleotide phosphate (NADPH) production. G6PD is the first enzyme in the hexose monophosphate pathway, and it generates NADPH as an important source of reducing power for the red cell. G6PD deficiency renders the red cell susceptible to oxidant stress. Infection (probably viral, as evidenced by the lymphocytosis) is the likely precipitating factor in this case, but other precipitants include the neonatal period, drugs (not amoxycillin, but principally sulphonamides, anti-malarial nalidixic acid and nitrofurantoin) and ingestion of fava beans (broad beans).

A46.iii He requires supportive management with encouragement towards oral fluid intake, intravenous fluids and transfusion of packed red cells. Once the diagnosis is confirmed, he should receive a card informing which drugs and precipitants to avoid. He should also receive oral folic acid 5 mg/day, though haemolysis is usually only intermittent and is frequently very well compensated. Family studies will show his mother to be a carrier and 50% of his male siblings are likely to be affected.

A46.iv Neonatal jaundice. G6PD deficiency is the commonest red cell enzymopathy to cause neonatal haemolysis and jaundice. Neonatal erythrocytes have an increased susceptibility to oxidative haemolysis (since they may have reduced concentrations of glutathione reductase, catalase and vitamin E) and this, combined with hepatic immaturity and G6PD deficiency within hepatocytes, predisposes to jaundice. This usually appears in the first to fourth day of life and unconjugated hyperbilirubinaemia may even lead to kernicterus. Phototherapy and exchange transfusion may be required.

The vast majority of individuals with G6PD deficiency suffer no symptoms unless challenged. Some 350 variant forms of the enzyme have been described, resulting from as many (usually single base) mutations within the gene. Individuals – especially heterozygous females for this gene – enjoy a degree of protection against *Plasmodium falciparum* malaria, as do heterozygotes (but emphatically not homozygous individuals) for sickle cell anaemia and thalassaemia.

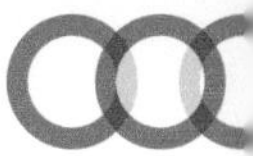

CASE 47

QUESTIONS

A 69-year-old male presents to an ophthalmologist with sudden onset visual loss. The ophthalmologist finds that he has a retinal vein thrombosis (branch occlusion). He also notices an enlarged gland on the right side of the neck. He has no other abnormal physical signs. He is generally in good health

A full blood count shows	Hb 98 g/L
	WBC 7.6 x 10(9)/L
Other tests show	ESR 110 mm/hr
	Total protein 94 g/L
	Protein electrophoresis shows a paraprotein identified as IgM kappa (36 g/L)

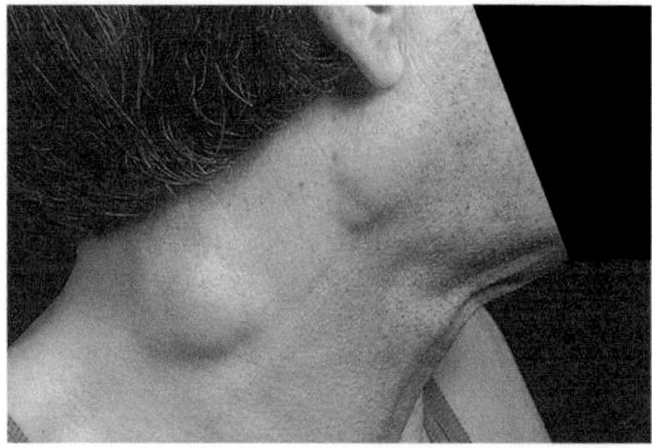

Bone marrow is demonstrated in the image below.

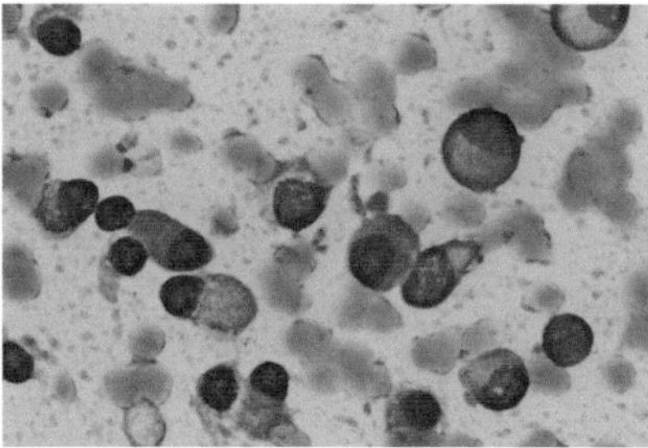

Q47.i What is the likeliest diagnosis?

Q47.ii What confirmatory investigations would you do?

Q47.iii How is the condition treated? Is there a staging system?

Q47.iv What complications can occur?

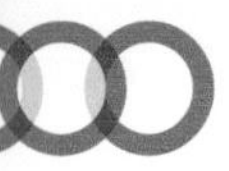

Case 47: ANSWERS

A47.i The likeliest diagnosis is lymphoplasmacytic lymphoma, formerly known as Waldenström's macroglobulinaemia. The bone marrow shows lymphoplasmacytic cells.

A47.ii Flow cytometry of the cells confirms they are CD 19 and CD 20 positive, negative for CD 5 and CD 10, positive for CD 11c and CD 25, and positive for IgM and kappa.

The cells showed a mutation in MYD 88 (L265P). This is known to induce activation of Bruton tyrosine kinase.

The plasma viscosity was elevated.

The LDH was raised. Beta 2 (β2) microglobulin was elevated at 4.2 mg/L.

A CT scan of thorax and abdomen showed his spleen to be enlarged at 15 cm in its longest measurement and lymph nodes were present in the paraortic region.

A47.iii Plasma exchange was commenced and he received three cycles over the first 6 days. His vision was already beginning to improve prior to the procedure and the ophthalmologist fell that the prospects for long term recovery were excellent.

A47.iv The International Prognostic Scoring System for Waldenström's macroglobulinemia (IPSSWM) is a predictive model to characterise long-term outcomes. Predictors of a poor outcome include:

Age > 65 years
Hemoglobin ≤ 11.5 g/dL
Platelet count ≤ 100 × 10(9)/L
β2-microglobulin > 3 mg/L
Serum monoclonal protein concentration > 70 g/L

The risk categories are:

Low: ≤ 1 adverse variable except age
Intermediate: 2 adverse characteristics or age > 65 years
High: > 2 adverse characteristics

This patient has high-risk disease and warrants chemotherapy. A combination of rituximab with bendamustine and dexamethasone is effective. Rituximab can also be used with bortezomib and dexamethasone; some regimes include fludarabine or cladribine; and cyclophosphamide. Ibrutinib is active in this disease.

Other complications include fever, night sweats, weight loss; peripheral neuropathy, amyloidosis, renal failure and cryoglobulinuria.

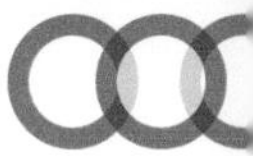

CASE 48

QUESTIONS

Q48.i What abnormality is seen on this blood film (Figure 48a)?

Q48.ii What abnormality is seen in the patient's mouth (Figure 48b) and what are the possible causes?

Q48.iii What further investigations would you carry out?

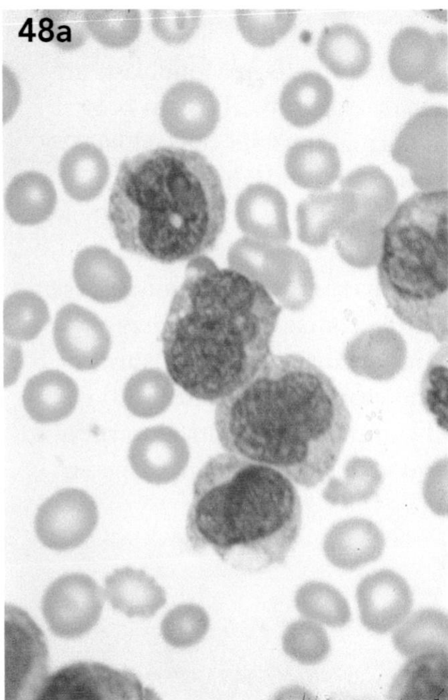

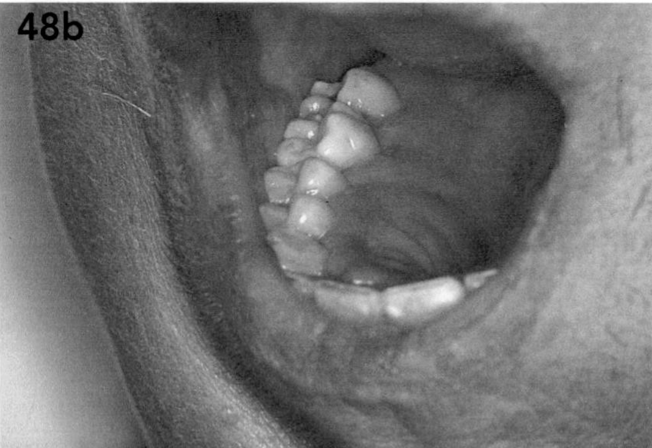

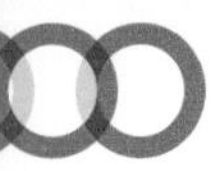

Case 48: ANSWERS

A48.i There are large numbers of atypical blast cells, suggesting a diagnosis of acute leukaemia. These cells have prominent nucleoli, plentiful grey cytoplasm with vacuoles and sparse granules. These features are characteristic of monoblasts, and this is acute monoblastic leukaemia.

A48.ii She has leukaemic infiltration of her gums. Acute myeloid leukaemia (AML) with monoblastic differentiation is often associated with tissue infiltration and in addition, lymphadenopathy, hepatosplenomegaly and nervous system involvement are all more common than in other types of acute leukaemia. Phenytoin (Figure 48c) and cyclosporin therapy are other causes of gum hypertrophy.

A48.iii She clearly needs bone marrow examination (Figure 48d). Monoblasts are usually positive for butyrate esterase (the majority of the cells stain brown on this dual esterase stain; the blue cell is a normal myeloid cell, which is chloroacetate positive). Monoblasts will also stain with the cluster of differentiation 14 (CD14) monoclonal antigen.

Treatment: All forms of acute leukaemia, in patients thought suitable for intensive therapy, are treated with at least three courses of combination chemotherapy. Each course typically contains an anthracycline (daunorubicin or idarubicin), cytosine arabinoside and etoposide and lasts 7–10 days. Supportive care with antibiotics and blood components is critical to success, and most patients have an indwelling central venous (Hickman) catheter.

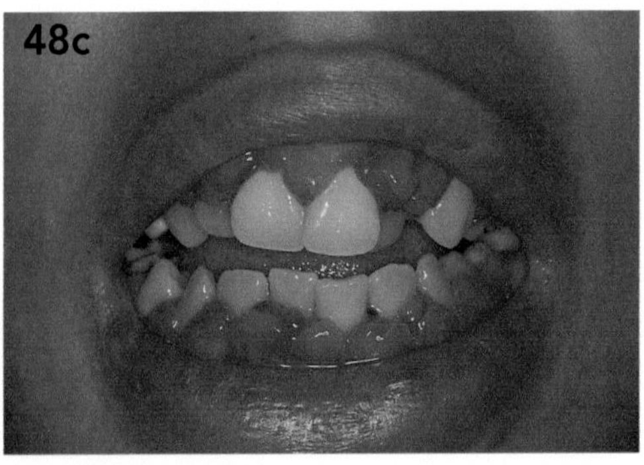
48c

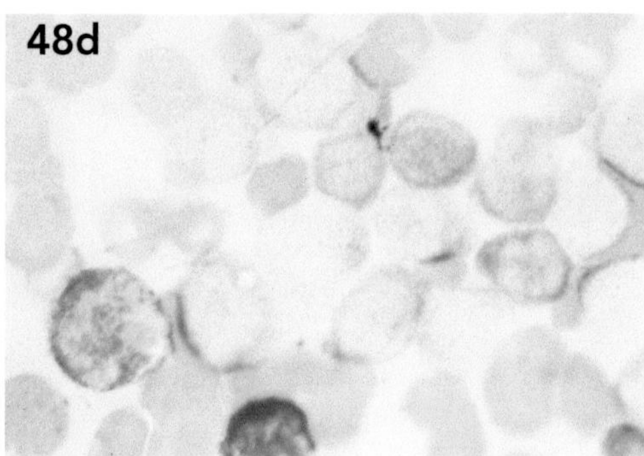
48d

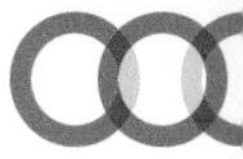

CASE 49

QUESTIONS

A 7-year-old boy gives a 7-day history of a brief febrile illness with nausea, vomiting and diarrhoea. Over the past 24 hours, he is noted to have developed purpuric spots over his limbs and to have become anaemic. Investigations show

Haemoglobin (Hb)	70 g/L
White blood cells (WBC)	23×10^9/L (neutrophils 83%)
Platelets	11×10^9/L
Urea	49 mmol/L
Creatinine	437 mmol/L
Prothrombin time (PT)	12 seconds (control 11–13 seconds)
APTT	31 s (26–36)
Fibrinogen	3.5 g/L (1.5–4.0)

Q49.i Comment on the blood film (see Figure 49a below).

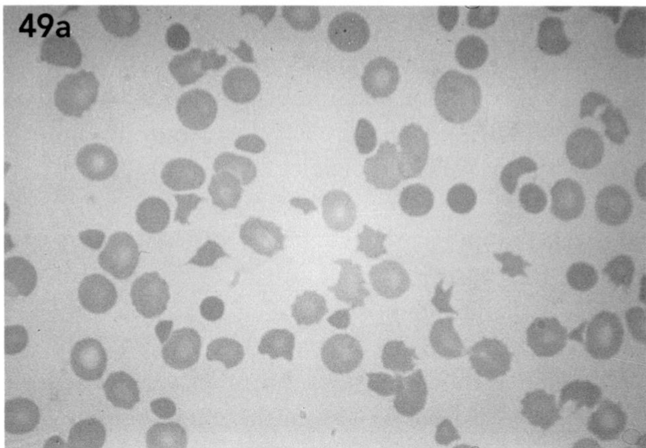

Q49.ii What is the likely diagnosis?

Q49.iii What is the pathogenesis of this disorder?

Q49.iv How should the child be treated?

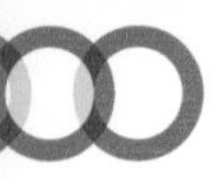

Case 49: ANSWERS

A49.i The blood film shows marked red cell fragmentation, polychromasia and thrombocytopenia.

A49.ii Haemolytic uraemic syndrome (HUS). Henoch–Schönlein purpura is a vasculitis associated with a normal platelet count.

A49.iii The essential features that define this syndrome are renal microangiopathy, haemolytic anaemia and platelet destruction leading to thrombocytopenia. It is commonest in childhood, and the classic form follows an infection with verotoxin-producing strains of *Escherichia coli*, but it is also associated with infections with *Shigella*, *Salmonella* and *Streptococcus*. Bacterial toxins cause endothelial damage, platelet activation and microangiopathic haemolytic anaemia (MAHA). Sporadic cases are described in association with autoimmune diseases, pregnancy, the contraceptive pill, radiation nephritis, immune deficiency disorders and after haemopoietic stem cell bone marrow transplantation. The toxin binds to lipid components, for example, globotriaosylceramide, which is the substrate that accumulates in Fabry disease (alpha galactosidase A deficiency) and triggers a succession of events. These lead to apoptosis of endothelial cells, binding of leucocytes to the cells, activation of the coagulation cascade and also to inactivation of the metalloproteinase ADAM metallopeptidase with thrombospondin type 1 motif, 13 (ADAMTS13) (deficiency of which is the underlying feature of the closely related condition, thrombotic thrombocytopenic purpura [TTP]). Reduced ADAMTS13 activity leads to formation of multimers of von Willebrand factor (VWF) and platelet activation.

A49.iv Early and careful supportive management of renal failure and red cell transfusion are the most important aspects of therapy. Infusions of fresh frozen plasma as therapy or plasma exchange should only be instituted if there is diagnostic uncertainty between HUS and TTP. Platelet transfusions should be avoided as they can cause thrombosis and may have an adverse effect. Isolated reports have supported the use of heparin and anti-platelet drugs. Steroids are not of proven value. Complete recovery is seen in about two-thirds of children, but onset in adulthood usually carries a worse prognosis.

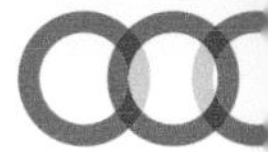

Other causes of red cell fragmentation with haemolysis and thrombocytopenia include disseminated intravascular coagulation (excluded by the normal clotting screen) and MAHA, which can occur in severe hypertension or in association with disseminated malignancy. Fragmentation haemolysis without thrombocytopenia may occur as a result of mechanical damage to red cells – for example, due to a prosthetic heart valve (Figure 49b). Atypical HUS (aHUS) is a condition characterised by dysregulated activation of the alternative pathway of complement activation. It is inherited in almost 70% of patients. Mutations have been reported in complement factors H and I, membrane co-factor protein and complement C3. Antibodies to complement regulatory proteins can also lead to aHUS. Treatment with the monoclonal antibody eculizumab, as for paroxysmal nocturnal haemoglobinuria, may be of value in these patients.

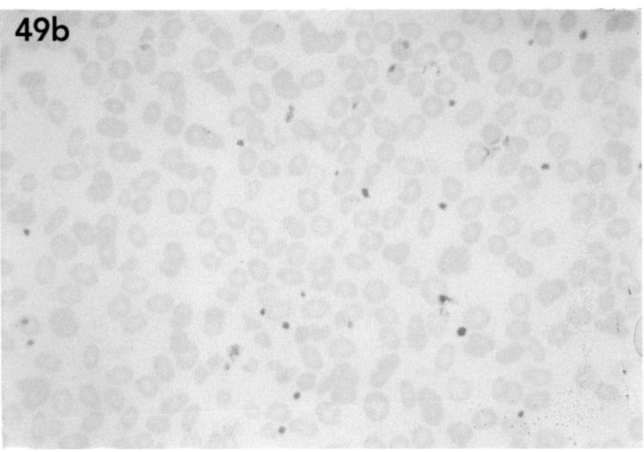

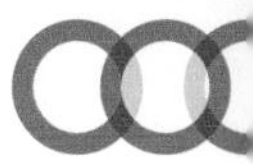

CASE 50

QUESTIONS

A 36-year-old man gives a 3-week history of tiredness, fever and easy bruising. Physical examination shows widespread purpuric lesions. His blood count shows

Haemoglobin (Hb)	76 g/L
White blood cells (WBC)	33.5 × 10^9/L
Platelets	5 × 10^9/L

His bone marrow aspirate is shown in the images below. He receives three courses of intensive chemotherapy and is then monitored. He relapses 2 years later. He receives further reinduction chemotherapy (two courses) followed by allogeneic bone marrow transplantation from a fully histocompatible sibling. He is well but 12 days post-transplant he develops weight gain, painful hepatomegaly with jaundice, ascites and renal impairment. He becomes refractory to platelet transfusions.

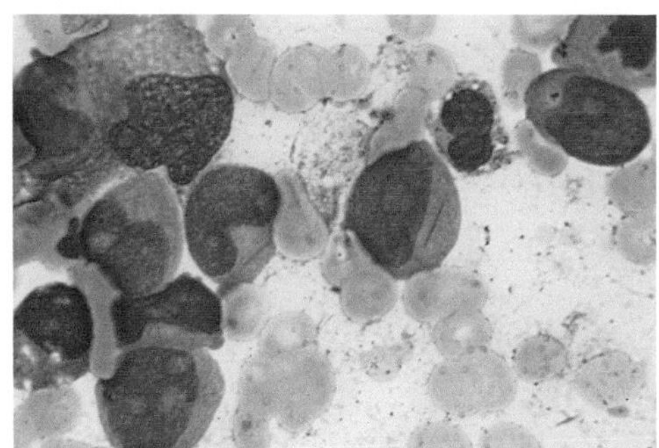

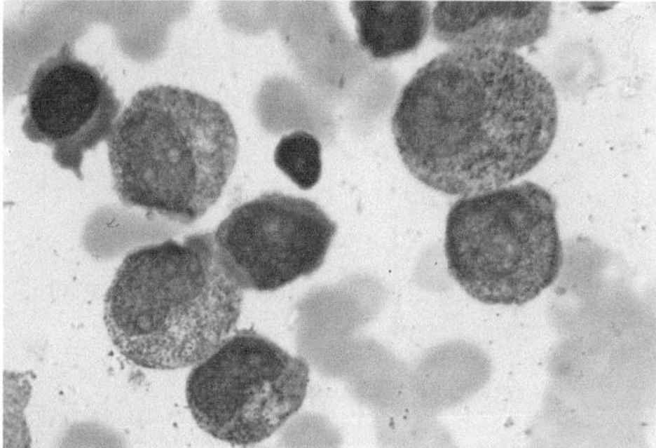

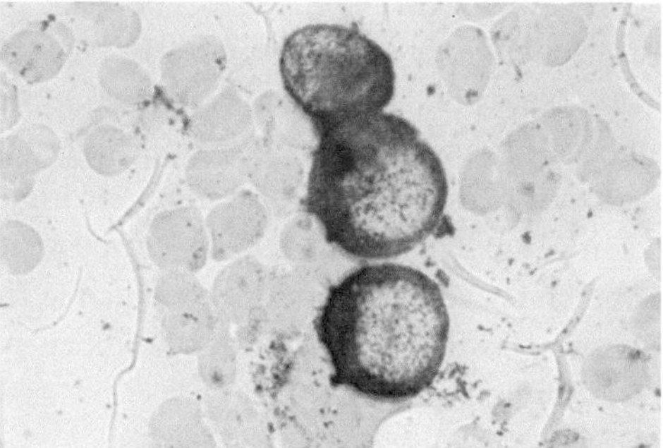

Q50.i What is the presentation diagnosis?

Q50.ii What cytogenetic changes characteristically occur in this disease? How is treatment monitored?

Q50.iii What is the likely cause of his post-transplant complication?

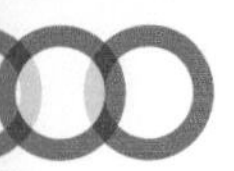

Case 50: ANSWERS

A50.i He has acute myeloid leukaemia (AML). There is evidence of differentiation of myeloid cells, with granule formation and Auer rods.

A50.ii This patient had translocation t(8:21), which is associated with a good prognosis in AML. This condition would be classified as AML with recurrent cytogenetic translocation in the World Health Organization (WHO) classification and AML with differentiation (AML M2) in the French–American–British (FAB) classification. Other cytogenetic changes in AML include t(15:17) in AML M3 (acute promyelocytic leukaemia), inversion 16 (AML M4 with abnormal eosinophils), trisomy 8 and the Philadelphia chromosome t(9:22) in transformed chronic granulocytic leukaemia (CGL). Treatment is monitored by molecular monitoring for the abnormal mRNA transcript generated by the novel fusion gene resulting from the translocation. The level of the transcript falls with treatment; it often persists, but relapse would be characterized by a rising transcript level with falling blood counts and clinical deterioration.

Treatment of AML is with Daunorubicin 60 mg/m^2 for 3 days plus cytosine arabinoside 300 mg/m^2 for 10 days. There is evidence that the addition of the anti-cluster of differentiation 33 (CD33) monoclonal antibody myelotarg reduces the relapse rate; and also evidence that the addition of cladribine may be beneficial in higher risk patients. The FLAG-IDA regimen utilizes fludarabine, cytosine arabinoside, granulocyte colony-stimulating factor (G-CSF) and idarubicin; it is commonly used to reinduce remission in the relapse setting.

A50.iii He has developed veno-occlusive disease. The peak incidence is in the first 2–3 weeks post-allogeneic bone marrow transplant (BMT) and overall incidence is 20%–25%. The cause is unknown, but important risk factors are pre-existing liver disease, a previous myeloablative transplant, large doses of previous cytoreductive chemotherapy or high-intensity pre-transplant conditioning. Treatment is largely supportive but defibrotide has been shown to be effective and steroids are valuable in selected patients. Recombinant tissue plasminogen activator has been successfully used to lyse the intrahepatic blood clot.

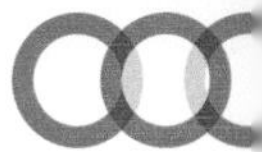

Acute graft versus host disease (GVHD) also typically presents in the early post-transplant phase. Skin rash, often affecting palms and trunk, diarrhoea and abnormal liver function tests occur, but oedema and ascites are uncommon.

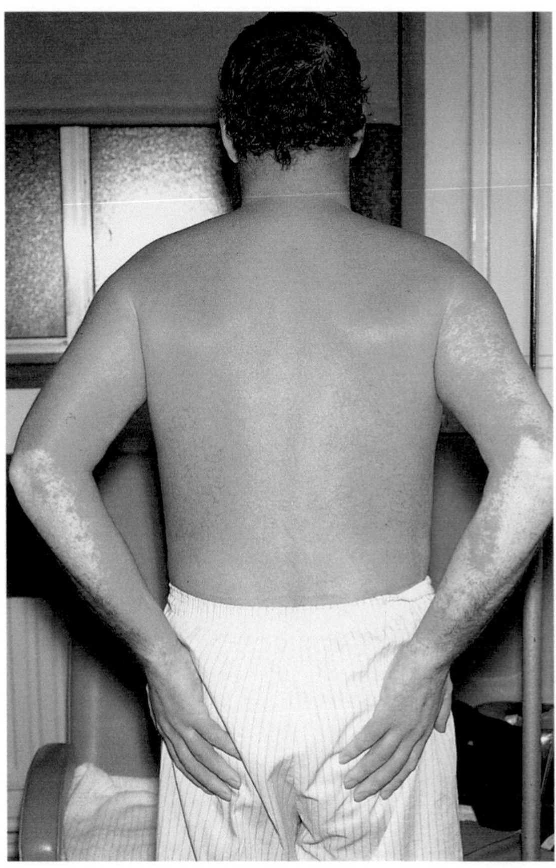

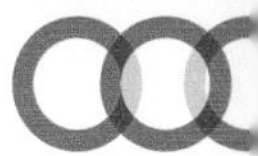

CASE 51

QUESTIONS

A newborn male child is found to be jaundiced and pale at birth. Examination also reveals him to have an easily palpable spleen. The pregnancy was uneventful, even though mother had not attended regularly for antenatal care. She has had one previous uneventful pregnancy. The cord blood count shows

Haemoglobin (Hb)	95 g/L
White blood cells (WBC)	23.4×10^9/L
Platelets	303×10^9/L

The direct anti-globulin test on cord blood is positive.

Q51.i What abnormalities are seen on this child's blood film?

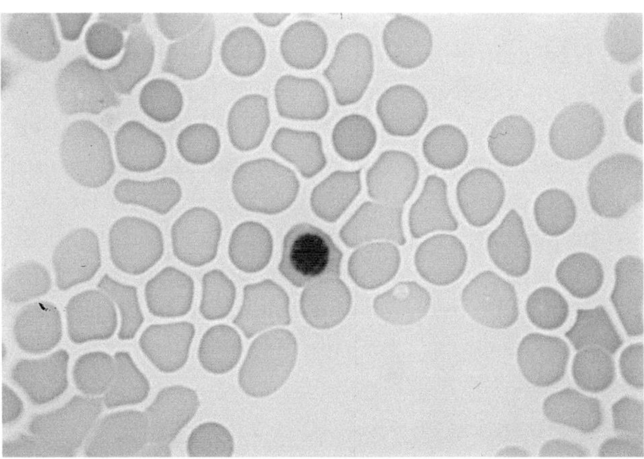

Q51.ii What further tests should be performed?

Q51.iii What is the diagnosis?

Q51.iv How is this condition prevented?

Q51.v How is this condition treated?

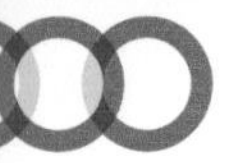

Case 51: ANSWERS

A51.i The blood film shows polychromasia, spherocytes, nucleated red cell and thrombocytopenia, all consistent with an immune haemolytic anaemia. Jaundice at birth is not physiological. The mother's failure to attend for antenatal care means that any atypical red cell antibodies would not have been detected in her serum. Splenomegaly may be normal at birth, but the neonatal haemoglobin (Hb) should be 160–190 g/dL.

A51.ii The child's blood group was found to be O Rh(D) positive, while the mother was O Rh(D) negative with a high titre of anti-D antibodies in her serum. The child's direct antibody test (DAT) is positive, and elution of antibody from child's cells confirmed it to be anti-D. The mother's previous child and the father are both Rh(D) positive, confirming that the mother was sensitised during her previous pregnancy. The child's liver function tests and bilirubin should be assessed, and cytomegalovirus (CMV) and rubella infection should be excluded.

A51.iii Haemolytic disease of foetus and newborn, due to transplacental passage of IgG anti-D antibodies from mother to foetus.

A51.iv Prevention is by administration of anti-D to Rh(D) negative females within 72 hours of a potentially sensitising event, for example, labour, antepartum haemorrhage. The dose of anti-D may need to be increased if the Kleihauer test, which is performed on maternal blood to allow quantification of the number of fetal red blood cells in the maternal circulation, shows a large number to be present. Fetal haemoglobin can be distinguished from adult haemoglobin by this cytochemical test – the fetal cells stain more darkly. Fetal cells can also be detected and quantified in maternal blood by flow cytometry.

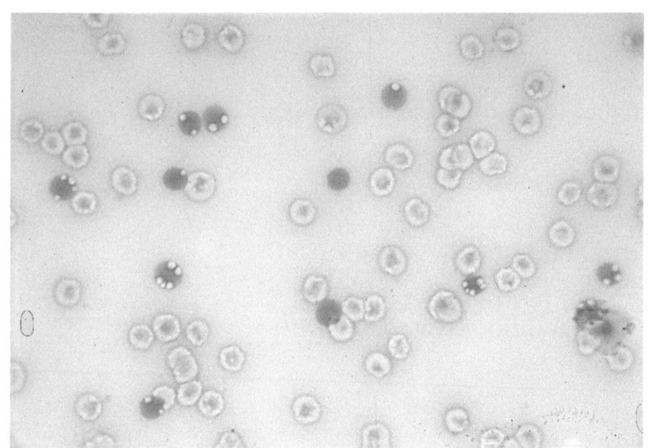

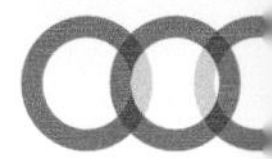

Case 51: ANSWERS (Continued)

A51.v The child may require exchange transfusion with irradiated O Rh(D) negative blood, CMV negative, chosen for compatibility with mother's serum. This will lower bilirubin levels (excessive unconjugated bilirubin in fetal blood may damage the neonatal brain – kernicterus). Phototherapy may promote bilirubin conjugation and may be of value.

All pregnant women should be grouped and have a red cell antibody screen performed at booking. If an antibody is detected, its titre should be monitored, and fetal growth closely monitored if the titre is found to be rising. Amniocentesis can be performed after 16–18 weeks gestation to assess haemolysis. Fetal haemoglobin level can be monitored by sampling the umbilical vein under ultrasound guidance. Intrauterine red cell transfusions can be given from about 23 to 25 weeks gestation – the blood must be irradiated to prevent graft versus host disease, and it must be from a CMV-negative donor. Plasma exchange can be used to lower the maternal antibody titre.

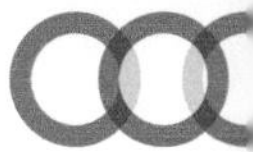

CASE 52

QUESTIONS

A 19-year-old male presented to his general practitioner (GP) with a 3-day history of sore throat. On examination, he has an acutely infected throat with bilateral cervical lymphadenopathy. His GP prescribed a course of amoxycillin, and the patient developed a widespread erythematous rash (Figure 52a). His full blood count shows

Haemoglobin (Hb)	123 g/L
White blood cells (WBC)	7.6 × 10^9/L (lymphocytes 63%, neutrophils 34%)
Platelets	150 × 10^9/L

Q52.i Comment on the blood film (Figures 52b through 52d). What is the diagnosis?

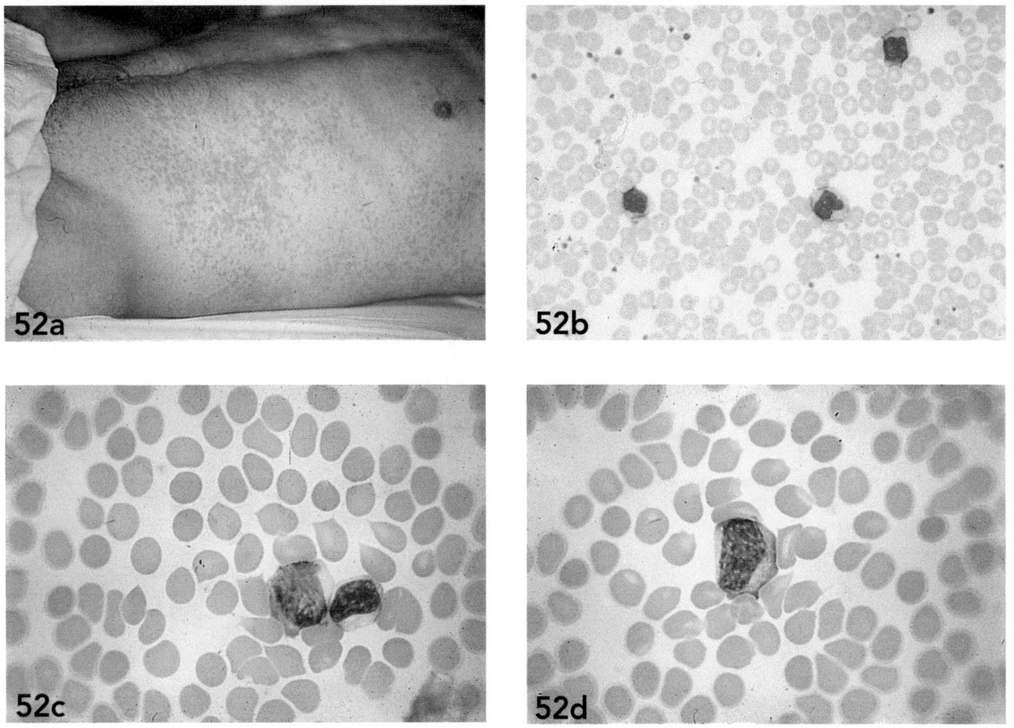

Q52.ii How is the diagnosis confirmed? Indicate the principle involved in the test you describe.

Q52.iii What is the differential diagnosis?

Q52.iv What important complications may occur?

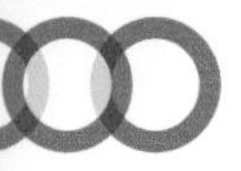

Case 52: ANSWERS

A52.i The blood film shows large activated lymphocytes, and there is a relative lymphocytosis in the blood count. The features suggest infectious mononucleosis. A rash following amoxycillin therapy is characteristic.

A52.ii Infectious mononucleosis (glandular fever) is due to infection by the Epstein–Barr virus (EBV), which infects B lymphocytes; the activated lymphocytes seen in the blood film are reactive T lymphocytes. The Paul–Bunnell screening test or monospot, is a method for detecting a heterophile antibody, which is an antibody that is characteristic of (though not specific for) EBV. This antibody is demonstrated by its failure to be absorbed by guinea pig kidney cells and its ready absorption by ox red blood cells. False-positive results are rare but they can occur, for example, in systemic lupus erythematosus. Detection of IgM antibodies to EBV is a more specific test for recent EBV infection.

A52.iii Cytomegalovirus, toxoplasmosis and adenovirus infections may give a similar blood picture, but they all have a negative monospot.

A52.iv Generalised lymphadenopathy and splenomegaly are often seen in infectious mononucleosis, and spontaneous rupture of the spleen has been reported. Immune thrombocytopenia, immune haemolytic anaemia and hepatitis may also occur.

EBV is implicated in the pathogenesis of nasopharyngeal neoplasia, and it is a co-factor in the development of Burkitt's lymphoma and B-cell lymphomas in immunocompromised people, for example, post-transplant patients, HIV-positive patients. Lymphoma in HIV-positive individuals often affects the central nervous system (CNS) (Figure 52e).

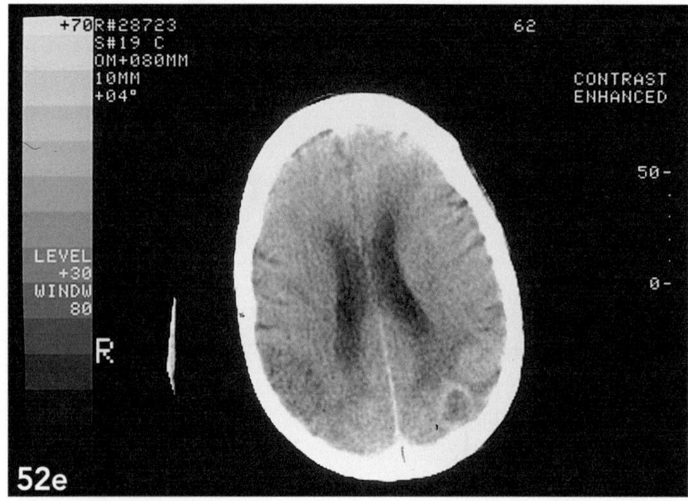

52e

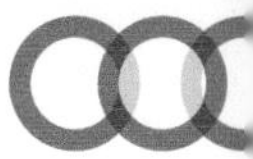

CASE 53

QUESTIONS

A 48-year-old male has noticed a swelling in his left upper abdomen. On examination, he has an easily palpable spleen. There is no history of foreign travel, no jaundice, no drug history and he drinks alcohol only in moderation. There are no signs of chronic liver disease. A full blood count shows

Haemoglobin (Hb)	143 g/L
White blood cells (WBC)	114 × 10^9/L (neutrophils 84%, blasts 1%, myelocytes 4%, promyelocytes 1%, metamyelocytes 5%, lymphocytes 9%)
Platelets	438 × 10^9/L

Q53.i Comment on the blood film.

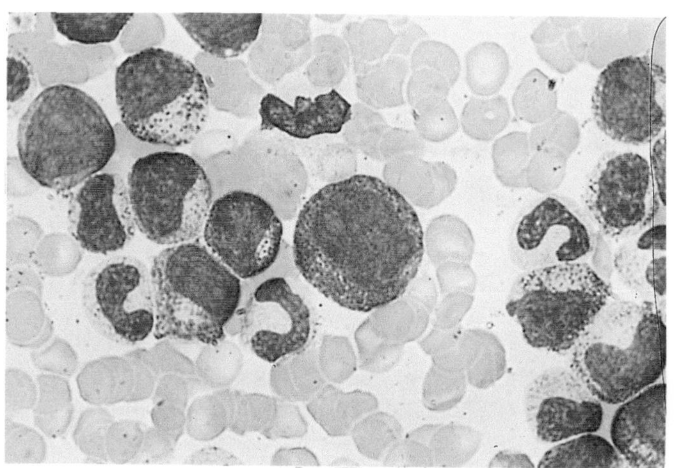

Q53.ii What other tests are indicated?

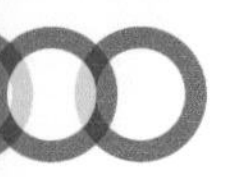

Case 53: ANSWERS

A53.i The blood film shows neutrophil leukocytosis with immature granulocytic cells present. There are no immature erythroid cells, suggesting that this is a myeloproliferative disorder and not a leukoerythroblastic blood film.

A53.ii A bone marrow aspirate should be performed and cytogenetic analysis requested. More than 95% of patients with chronic granulocytic (myeloid) leukaemia have a translocation of chromosomal material from 9 to 22 (t[9;22], Philadelphia chromosome). This means that the Abelson (*ABL*) oncogene is translocated to the breakpoint cluster region (BCR) of chromosome 22 to form a new gene (*BCR-ABL1*) which encodes a chimeric protein with a tyrosine kinase (TK) activity that is many times greater than its normal counterpart. Both aspirate and trephine will show increased cellularity. An abdominal ultrasound is done to confirm splenomegaly. The image below is an illustration of cytogenetics and fluorescence in situ hybridization (FISH) in chronic granulocytic leukaemia (CGL).

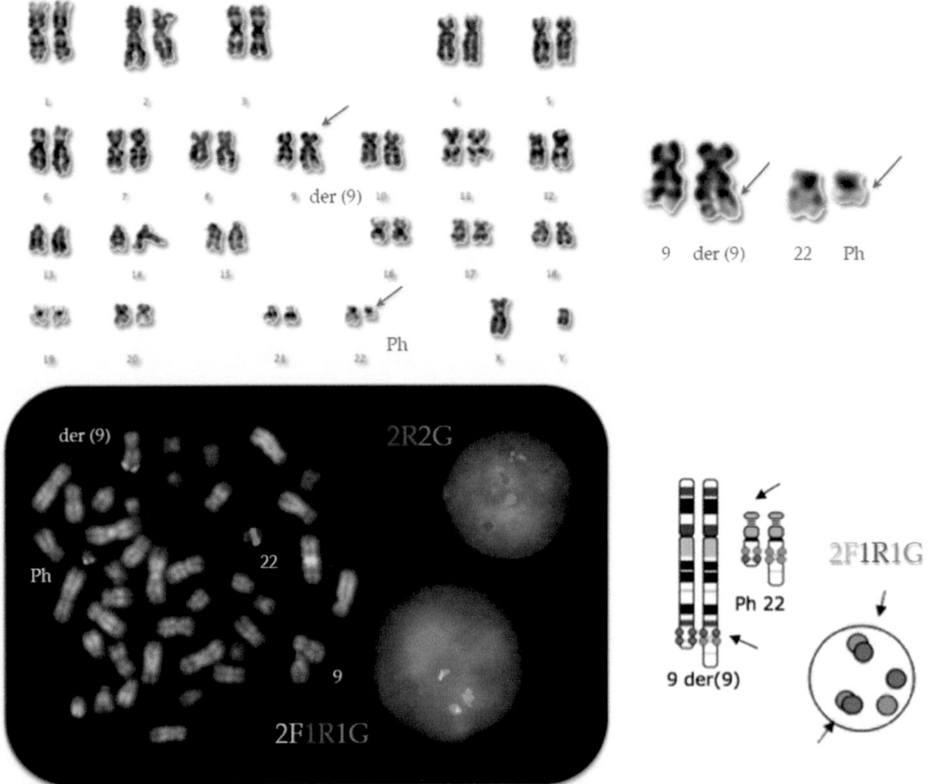

Baseline liver function tests, urea and electrolytes and serum lactate dehydrogenase (LDH) should be carried out.

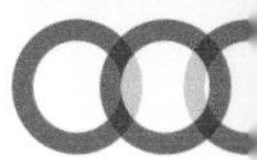

Case 53: QUESTIONS (Continued)

Q53.iii What is the likeliest diagnosis?

Q53.iv How should he be treated?

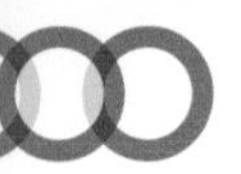

Case 53: ANSWERS (Continued)

A53.iii Chronic granulocytic leukaemia.

A53.iv This condition has a fairly benign chronic phase with a median duration of 2.5 years. During this time, patients are well and the disease is easily controlled with oral chemotherapy (e.g. imatinib). Scoring systems, for example, the Sokal score classify patients into high-, intermediate- and low-risk groups on the basis of age at diagnosis, spleen size, peripheral blood blast count and platelet count. Imatinib is a form of targeted therapy which specifically inhibits the pathological tyrosine kinase and restores normal haemopoiesis. The level of the blood counts gradually improve and spleen size improves as >90% patients achieve a complete haematological response. The majority of patients also achieve normal cytogenetics. The aim of molecular monitoring is to determine the level of the *BCR-ABL1* transcript; at 12 months of treatment, the optimal response is considered to be a 3-log response (<0.1%). Allogeneic haemopoietic stem cell transplantation (SCT) is potentially curative during this phase but the use of tyrosine kinase inhibitor (TKI) therapy has supplanted its use. About 20% of patients demonstrate resistance due to the presence of mutations within the kinase domain of *BCR-ABL1*. Newer TKIs, for example, nilotinib show greater activity than imatinib and are active against many of the resistant mutations. The disease may progress through an accelerated phase toward blast transformation, and it typically becomes less responsive. Newer TKIs, for example, dasatinib, bosutinib, ponatinib may have some activity in this setting, and SCT may also have a role in these later stages. Imatinib and its derivatives are generally well-tolerated but their use is associated with an increased risk of cardiac complications, which may be lower with the newer derivatives. Blast crisis may be myeloid or lymphoid in type, but occasionally blast cells will show biphenotypic features. The cells illustrated below show evidence of both myeloid (cluster of differentiation 33 [CD33], CD13 positive) and lymphoid (CD19 positive, terminal deoxynucleotidyl transferase [TdT] positive) differentiation.

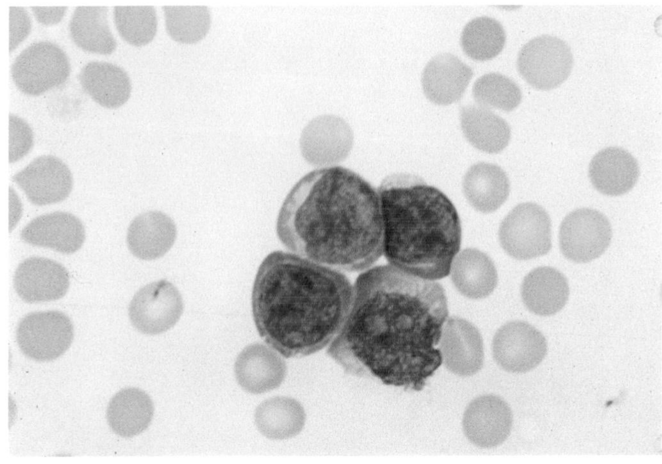

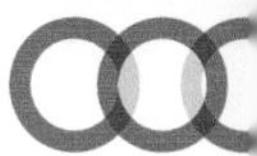

CASE 54

QUESTIONS

A 35-year-old woman has noticed a painless swelling on the left side of her neck, which has been present for over 4 weeks. It is slowly enlarging. There is no relevant past medical history and no history of fever. Physical examination reveals a single small (21 cm × 0.5 cm) mobile lymph node in the left anterior triangle of the neck. There are no other palpable nodes, and the liver and spleen are not palpable. Investigation shows

Haemoglobin (Hb)	119 g/L
White blood cells (WBC)	8.6 × 10^9/L (neutrophils 5.3 × 10^9/L, eosinophils 1.1 × 10^9/L, lymphocytes 2.1 × 10^9/L)
Platelets	165 × 10^9/L

Q54.i Comment on the blood film. What are the important causes of this finding?

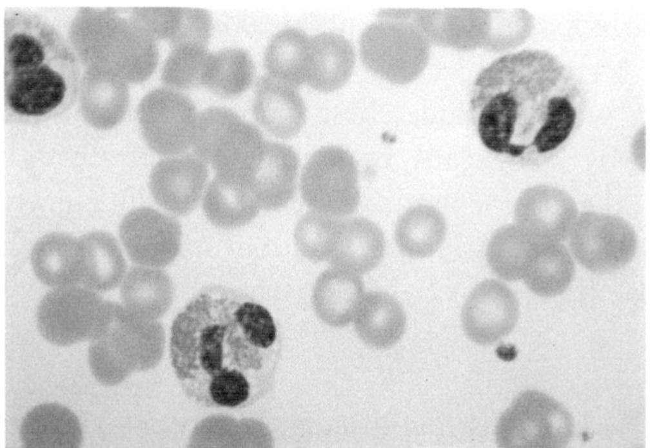

Q54.ii Comment on the lymph node biopsy.

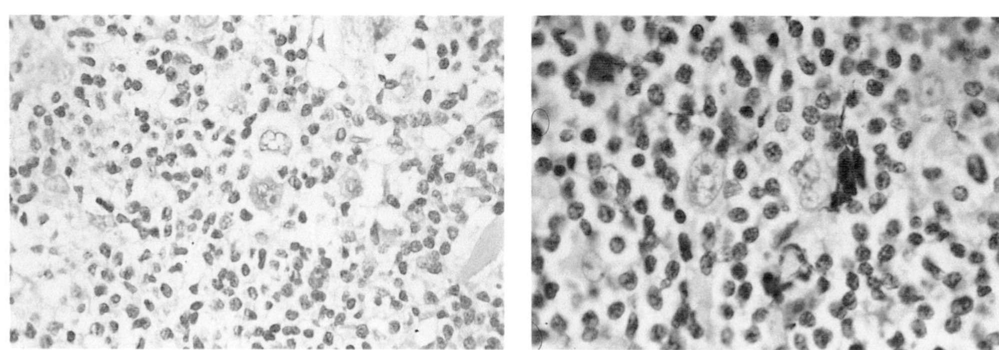

Q54.iii What is the diagnosis?

Q54.iv What further investigations are required?

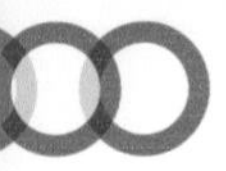

Case 54: ANSWERS

A54.i The film shows increased numbers of eosinophils (normal range $< 0.4 \times 10^9/L$). Important causes of eosinophilia include

- Allergic reactions (drug hypersensitivity, asthma, eczema)
- Parasitic infections
- Collagen vascular disease (e.g. polyarteritis nodosa)
- Granulomatous conditions (sarcoidosis)
- Neoplasms (haematological neoplasms – e.g. lymphoma, acute lymphoblastic leukaemia – and non-haematological neoplasms – e.g. breast, bronchus)
- Idiopathic or primary (e.g. hypereosinophilic syndrome)

A54.ii The lymph node shows a mixed cellular infiltrate with prominent, large Reed–Sternberg cells.

A54.iii Hodgkin's lymphoma.

A54.iv Staging, to include a full history (e.g. 'B' symptoms would be indicated by pruritus, weight loss and fever), physical examination and investigation.

Investigations would include chest x-ray, thoracic and abdominal computerised tomography (CT) scans, bone marrow aspirate and trephine biopsy, full haematological and biochemical screen (to include erythrocyte sedimentation rate [ESR], calcium, immunoglobulins, liver function tests and lactate dehydrogenase [LDH]). A baseline positron emission tomography (PET) scan is performed.

This patient had mediastinal disease (Figure 54a) and received treatment of four cycles of chemotherapy with a four drug combination (adriamycin, bleomycin, vinblastine and dacarbazine [ABVD]) followed by radiotherapy ('upper mantle'). Although the chest x-ray taken 2 years later (Figure 54b) shows continuing remission from Hodgkin's disease, there is evidence of increased shadowing bilaterally in the lower zones, and she had developed radiation pneumonitis that responded to steroid therapy. This could have been avoided if she had received six cycles of chemotherapy. PET scanning is frequently done during the course of treatment for Hodgkin lymphoma and can be used to monitor the extent of residual lymphoma. Thus, a negative PET scan after two cycles would have indicated an excellent response. If it remained negative after six cycles, treatment could have been suspended. Brentuximab is an anti-CD30 monoclonal antibody which has activity in relapsed Hodgkin's disease.

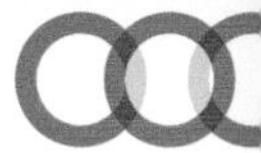

Both autologous and allogeneic transplant have an important role in the treatment of relapsed Hodgkin's lymphoma. Autologous transplant should be considered at first relapse in patients who remain responsive to chemotherapy. Allogeneic transplant carries higher risks and should be considered in second or subsequent relapse.

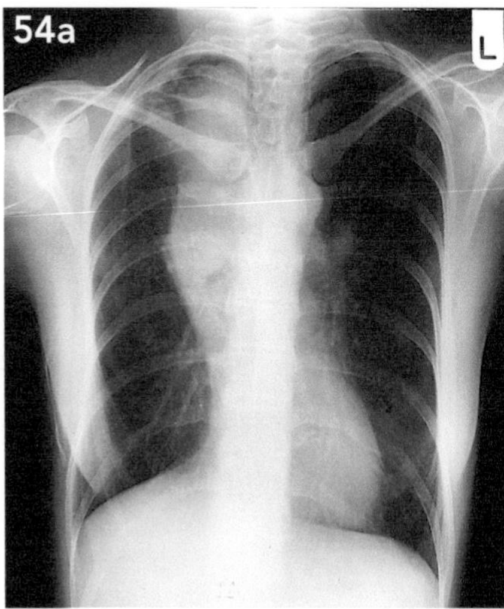

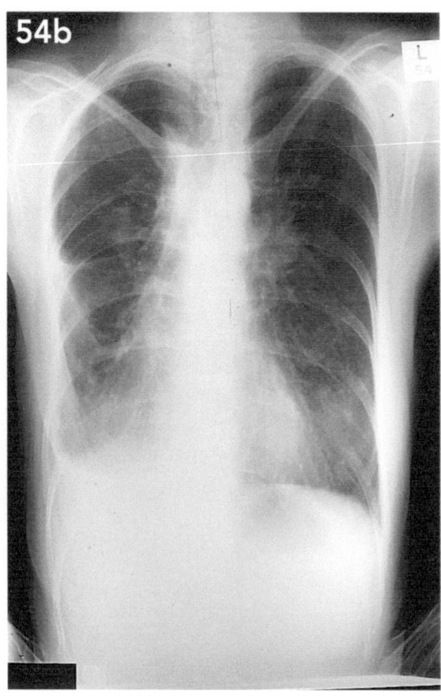

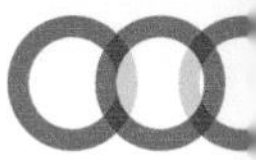

CASE 55

QUESTIONS

A 19-year-old male presents with a 2-week history of bruising and bleeding on brushing his teeth. He has had no serious illness in his past. His girlfriend has noted that over the past few days he has appeared plethoric and his face and eyelids have looked blue, puffy and congested. His full blood count shows

Haemoglobin (Hb)	97 g/L
White blood cells (WBC)	170×10^9/L
Platelets	31×10^9/L

Q55.i Comment on the chest x-ray.

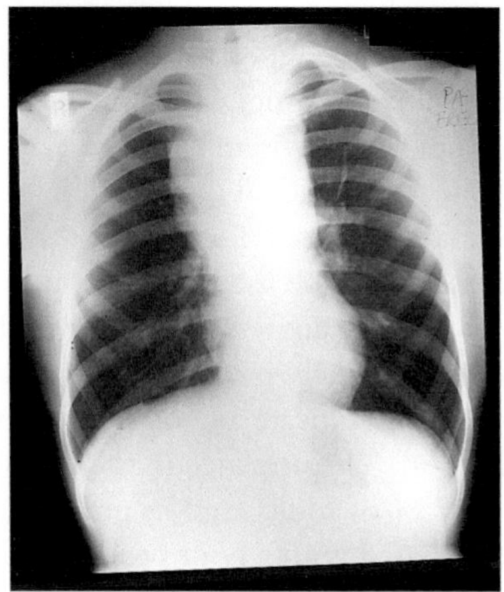

Q55.ii Comment on the blood film (left) and the cytochemistry with acid phosphatase (right). What is the diagnosis? How would you confirm this?

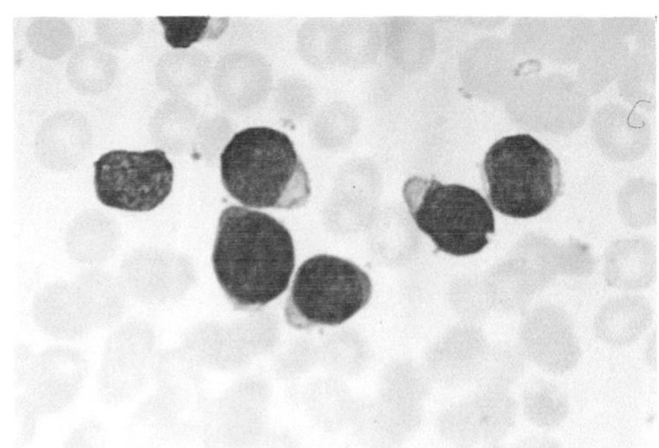

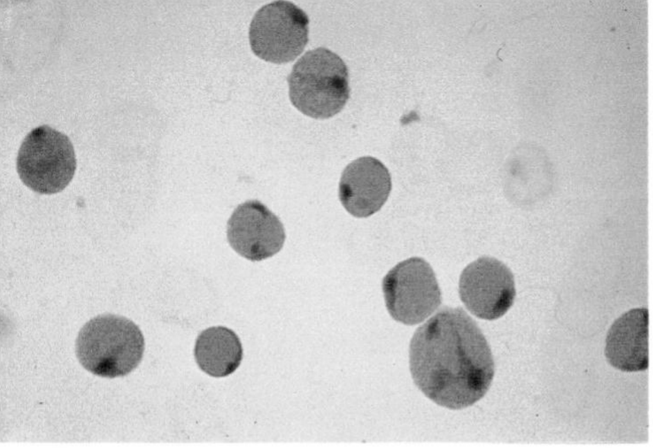

Q55.iii What complications can occur when therapy is commenced, and how would you prevent them?

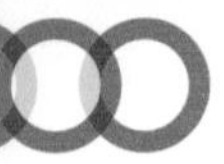

Case 55: ANSWERS

A55.i The chest x-ray shows a mass in the anterior mediastinum, which could be due to lymph nodes or may be thymic in origin. The history suggests he has developed superior vena caval obstruction.

A55.ii The blood film shows many leukaemic blast cells which are large and have relatively little cytoplasm, prominent nucleoli and convoluted nuclei. They show positivity for acid phosphatase at their poles ('polar positivity') and are likely to be T cells. The likeliest diagnosis is T-cell acute lymphoblastic leukaemia, which is often seen in this age group. Immunohistochemistry confirmed that the cells are positive for the enzyme terminal deoxynucleotidyl transferase (TdT) (Figure 55a) and have T-cell markers, for example, cluster of differentiation 3 (CD3) (Figure 55b). The cells are negative for B-cell markers, for example, CD 19 (Figure 55c). Flow cytometry should also be used to differentiate early T-cell precursor acute lymphoblastic leukaemia (ALL), which has a poorer prognosis and is positive only for cytoplasmic CD3 and CD7, from the much commoner thymic or cortical T-cell derived form of the disease. Flow cytometry is an effective way of monitoring treatment response and for detecting residual disease. These monoclonal T cells also have a discrete rearrangement of T-cell receptor genes, and this is a specific marker of the disease. It can be used to detect minimal residual disease after chemotherapy. Cytogenetic analysis should be undertaken so that a full analysis can be undertaken of the likely prognosis. Hyperdiploidy and the presence of the t(12;21) translocation indicate a good prognosis and are much rarer in adult ALL than in childhood. The presence of the Philadelphia chromosome (t(9;22)) is detected in up to 25% of adults; and its presence, or the presence of the (4;11) translocation, is associated with a poor prognosis; however, failure to clear leukaemic cells from marrow and blood for 4 weeks, and chromosome changes such as hypodiploidy would indicate a bad risk for disease.

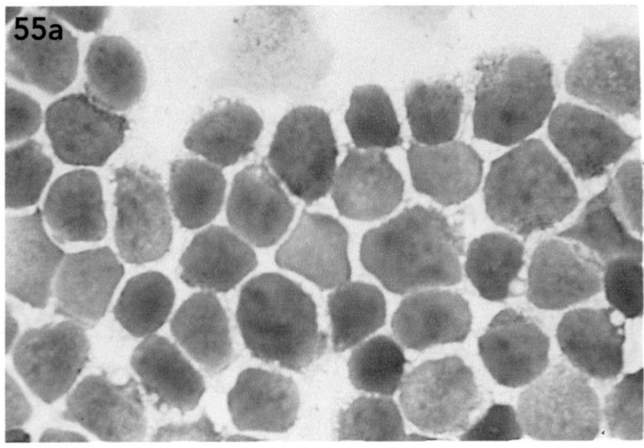

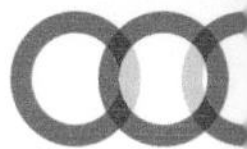

Case 55: ANSWERS (Continued)

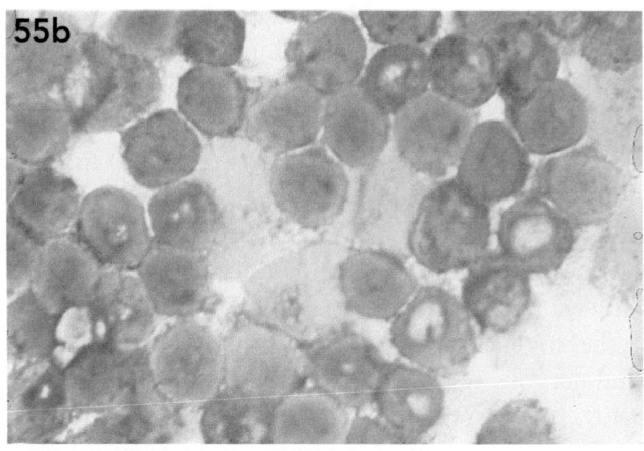

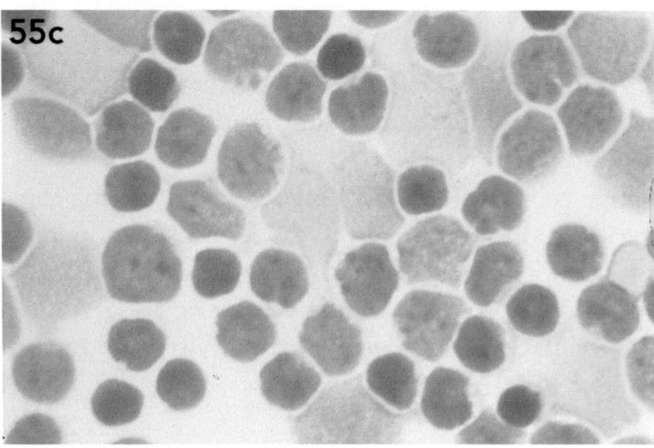

A55.iii This is an acute and rapidly proliferating tumour. Consideration should be given to preservation of fertility by storing viable sperm if feasible. A tumour lysis syndrome can occur upon commencement of chemotherapy and disseminated intravascular coagulation may supervene. Metabolic complications include acute renal failure, hyperkalaemia, hyperphospataemia, hypocalcaemia and hyperuricaemia.

He should be well hydrated with intravenous fluids and given rasburicase (after excluding the presence of glucose-6-phosphate dehydrogenase [G6PD] deficiency). This compound metabolises uric acid rapidly and is effective at preventing tumour lysis syndrome in high-risk settings. Allopurinol, which blocks the enzyme xanthine oxidase in the liver, also prevents treatment-induced gout and urate nephropathy. Urinary alkalinisation by use of intravenous sodium bicarbonate promotes excretion of harmful metabolites. A good urine output (more than 3 L daily) should be promoted during therapy.

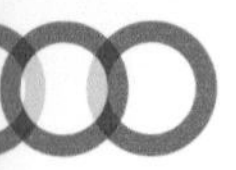

Initial chemotherapy for ALL is with a combination of pre-phase steroid therapy, induction with prednisolone, vincristine, anthracyclines (e.g. daunorubicin), L-asparaginase, cytosine arabinoside and cyclophosphamide, and intensification with high dose intravenous (IV) methotrexate to cross the blood brain barrier. A tyrosine kinase (TK) inhibitor should be added in patients with t(9;22). This is followed by consolidation with agents similar to those used at induction. Maintenance chemotherapy (e.g. daily methotrexate and 6-mercaptopurine, monthly vincristine and prednisolone, and periodic intrathecal methotrexate) should be given for 2 years. Craniospinal radiotherapy is not indicated as a prophylactic but may be needed to treat central nervous system (CNS) disease. Whereas childhood ALL is cured in >90% of cases, the outlook for adults is much more guarded and stem cell transplantation may have to be undertaken. Monoclonal antibodies are increasingly used in the treatment of relapsed ALL. Blinatumomab is used in the treatment of relapsed B-cell ALL. A part of the antibody attaches to the CD19 antigen on B cells whereas another part attaches to the CD3 antigen on T cells, allowing them to destroy the B cells.

Adoptive cell transfer (ACT) involves engineering the patient's own immune cells to recognise and treat the cancer cells; it is increasingly used in relapsed ALL. Autologous T cells can be genetically engineered to produce special receptors on their surface called 'chimeric antigen receptors' (CARs). Such CAR T cells can then be expanded in vitro and re-infused to treat the tumour.

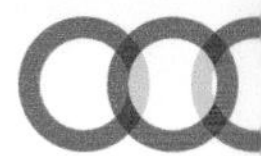

CASE 56

QUESTIONS

A 64-year-old man was noted to have an abnormal blood count at an insurance medical. He was asymptomatic, but on examination had a palpably enlarged spleen. His full blood count shows

Haemoglobin (Hb)	113 g/L
White blood cells (WBC)	73.4 × 10^9/L (blasts 1%, promyelocytes 1%, myelocytes 8%, metamyelocytes 6%, neutrophils 76%, lymphocytes 6%, monocytes 2%)
Platelets	430 × 10^9/L

His neutrophil alkaline phosphatase (NAP) score was 8 (normal range 60–120), and his liver function tests were normal.

Q56.i What is the likely diagnosis based on the history, the blood count and the blood film?

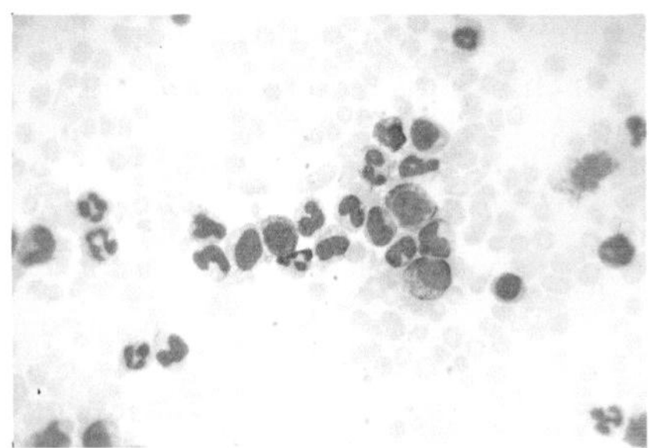

Q56.ii He is treated, and remains well for 3 years. However, he was poorly compliant with the medication. A repeat blood count at that time shows

Haemoglobin (Hb)	81 g/L
White blood cells (WBC)	96 × 10^9/L
Platelets	41 × 10^9/L

What complication has occurred based on his blood count and blood film at this time?

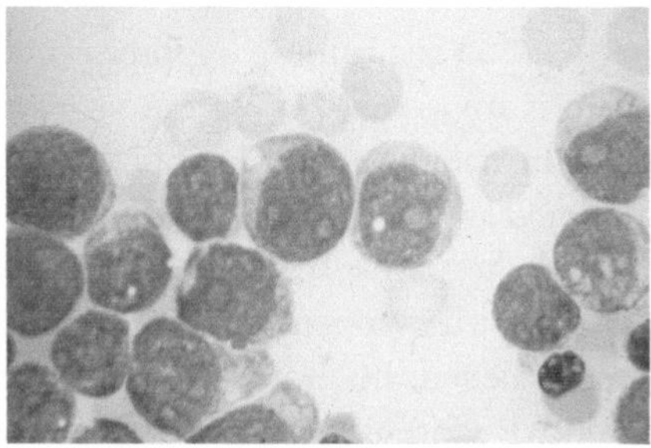

Q56.iii What further investigations are warranted?

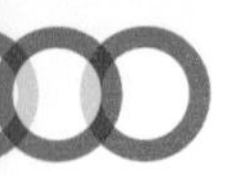

Case 56: ANSWERS

A56.i Chronic granulocytic leukaemia (CGL). The blood film shows increased numbers of granulocytic (myeloid) cells at different stages of differentiation. This patient was positive for the Philadelphia chromosome (translocation from 9 to 22). Other forms of chronic myeloid leukaemia include a Philadelphia chromosome negative form, which generally responds less well to therapy; chronic myelomonocytic leukaemia, in which there is a prominent monocytic component and other forms of myelodysplasia. He was treated with imatinib and up to 90% of compliant patients will achieve complete cytogenetic and molecular remission and remain well for 8–10 years or more.

A56.ii The blood film now shows increased numbers of immature blast cells. A bone marrow aspirate would confirm this. Flow cytometry, cytochemistry and immunocytochemistry with monoclonal antibodies will help to define the type of leukaemia that has developed. CGL usually transforms into a predominantly myeloid form of acute leukaemia (as illustrated here), but often (in approximately 10% of cases) the acute leukaemia is predominantly lymphoid. Although this tends to respond better to therapy, overall prognosis in transformed CGL is very poor, with a median survival of only 16–24 weeks. A mixed transformation is often observed.

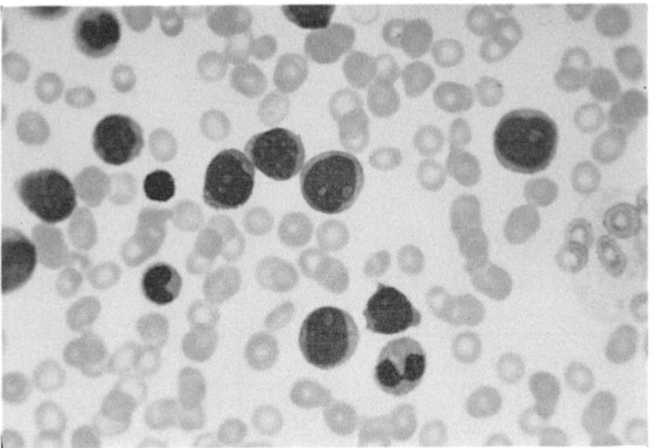

A56.iii A repeat cytogenetic investigation is appropriate, as there may be changes additional to the Philadelphia chromosome. Up to 20% of patients are found to have deletion or mutations affecting both alleles of the p53 gene at the time of transformation. p53 is a tumour suppressor gene ('anti-oncogene') and mutations within it are associated with progression of a range of haematological and non-haematological neoplasms. Treatment would be with high-dose imatinib and close monitoring. Failure to respond would indicate imatinib resistance and alternative treatment with nilotonib or dasatinib should be promptly instituted, with cytogenetic and molecular monitoring. Once complete response is achieved, he should be considered for an allogeneic stem cell transplant. The NAP score usually rises when transformation develops.

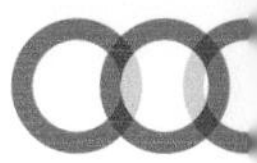

CASE 57

QUESTIONS

An 18-year-old male complains of pain in the right upper abdomen. The pain is colicky and intermittent, and it is associated with fever and jaundice. His blood count shows

Haemoglobin (Hb)	75 g/L
White blood cells (WBC)	27 $\times 10^9$/L (neutrophils 86%)
Platelets	360 $\times$ 10^9/L

Q57.i What abnormalities are seen on the blood film?

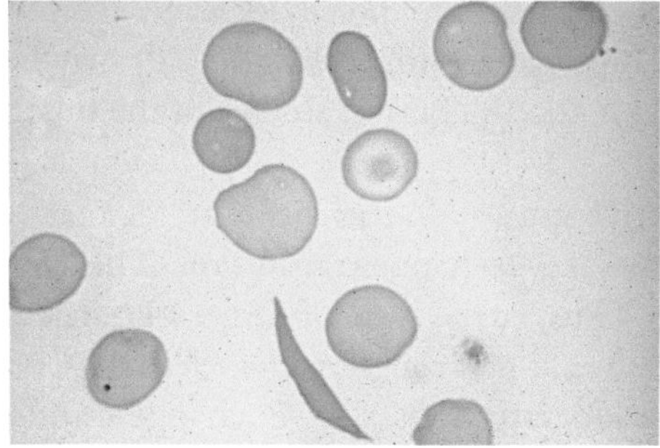

Q57.ii What is the haematological diagnosis and how would you confirm it?

Q57.iii What abnormality is shown on the abdominal ultrasound scan?

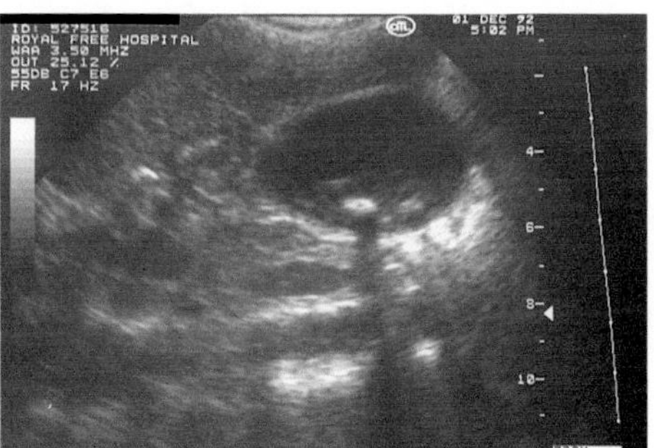

Q57.iv How should this patient be managed?

Q57.v Six months later, he presents with severe tiredness. A blood count shows

Haemoglobin (Hb)	41 g/L
Reticulocytes	0.1%

What complication has occurred?

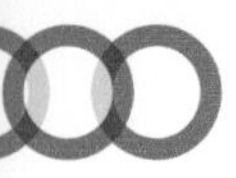

Case 57: ANSWERS

A57.i The blood film shows sickle cells, target cells and Howell–Jolly bodies.

A57.ii Homozygous sickle cell (SS) disease. Auto-infarction of the spleen leads to changes of splenic atrophy in the red blood cells. The polymorph leukocytosis suggests active infection. Confirmation of the diagnosis is by high-performance liquid chromatography (HPLC) haemoglobin electrophoresis.

A57.iii The gallbladder contains multiple gallstones.

A57.iv He should be stabilised with intravenous fluids and antibiotics. If recurrent attacks of cholecystitis occur, cholecystectomy is advised. Endoscopic retrograde cholangiopancreatography (ERCP) may help to exclude biliary obstruction, and it allows contrast studies of the biliary tract to be performed.

Any major elective surgery in patients with SS anaemia should be undertaken following exchange transfusion. This is best undertaken with a cell separator. Thus, at the time of surgery or anaesthesia the level of haemoglobin S should be brought to less than 40% of the total, to minimise the risks of a perioperative SS crisis. Exchange transfusion may occasionally also be necessary during pregnancy and during SS crisis. Red cells for transfusion should be compatible with the patient's own cells for ABO, Kell and Rh antigens, and for those other red cell antigens which can readily sensitise recipients. The use of hydroxycarbamide (with or without erythropoietin) is generally considered safe and is advocated. It increases haemoglobin F production, improves haemoglobin concentration and reduces the risk of SS crisis.

A57.v Infection with parvovirus. This leads to 'aplastic crisis' – temporary arrest of erythropoiesis, which is of little consequence to normal individuals, but causes life-threatening anaemia in individuals with hereditary haemolytic anaemia.

The common form of crisis in SS anaemia is due to deoxygenation leading to precipitation of haemoglobin S within red cells, causing shape change and thrombosis. Microvascular occlusion leads to further deoxygenation, and a cycle of sickling is promoted. Precipitating factors are usually not identified, but infection, dehydration and prolonged stasis (e.g. following a long aircraft flight) are possible precipitants. Clinical effects may include pain (abdomen, limbs, back), pulmonary sickling (dyspnoea, reduction in arterial oxygen saturation), cerebral sickling (epilepsy, stroke) and priapism. Treatment is with intravenous fluids, analgesia, oxygen and blood transfusion in selected cases.

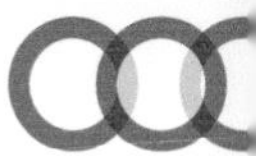

CASE 58

QUESTIONS

A 6-year-old child is assessed in the accident and emergency department, where his parents give a 1-week history of drowsiness, headache and generalised weakness. His parents concede that he has been generally unwell for 3–4 months, with tiredness and fever. On examination, he is pyrexial (38°C) and clearly drowsy, though he responds to verbal commands. He has generalised muscle weakness. There is no neck stiffness. Reflexes are normal and both plantar responses are equivocal. He has generalised lymphadenopathy and liver and spleen are both palpable. His full blood count shows

Haemoglobin (Hb)	76 g/L
White blood cells (WBC)	137 × 10^9/L
Platelets	34 × 10^9/L

Q58.i Comment on the blood film appearances (Figures 58a).

Q58.ii A lumbar puncture is performed. Comment on the appearance of the cells in the cerebrospinal fluid (Figure 58b).

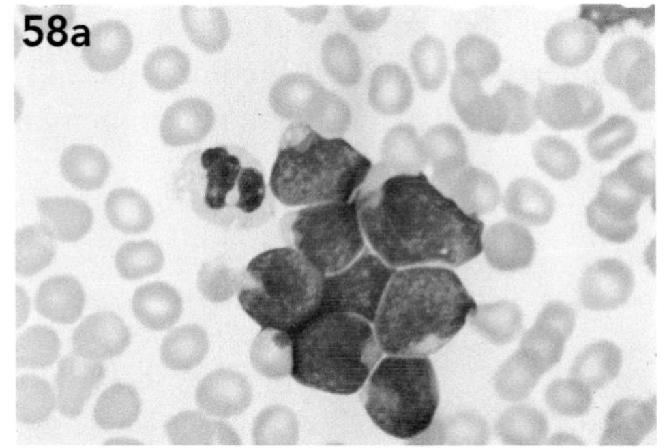
58a

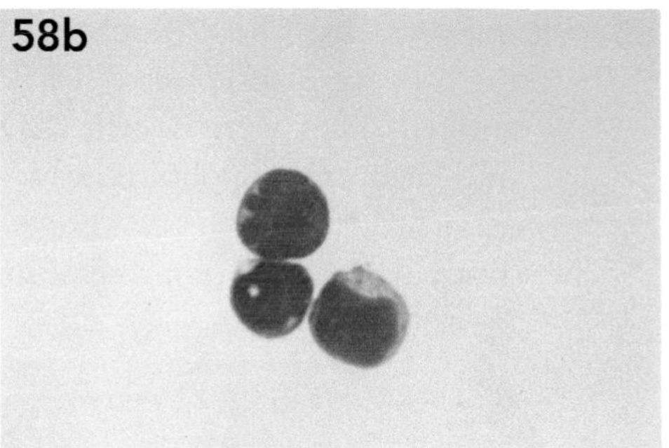
58b

Q58.iii What is the diagnosis and how would you confirm it?

Q58.iv What other tissues may be involved by this condition?

Q58.v How is this condition classified? Comment on the prognostic factors and treatment.

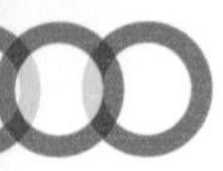

Case 58: ANSWERS

A58.i The blood film shows large numbers of primitive cells, with scanty cytoplasm, no granules and positivity for Periodic acid Schiff (PAS) reaction with blocks of positive material.

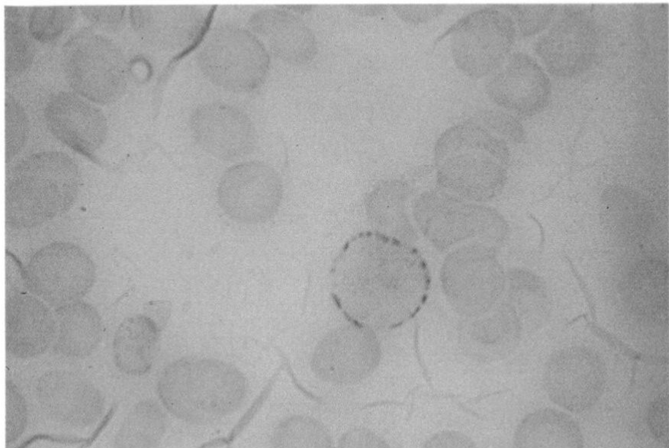

A58.ii Cells similar to the peripheral blood are seen on this cytospin preparation of cerebrospinal fluid.

A58.iii Acute lymphoblastic leukaemia (ALL) with central nervous system (CNS) involvement. The PAS reaction is important confirmatory evidence, but the cells were also positive by flow cytometry for the CD10 (common ALL) antigen. They were B-cells (CD19 positive) and had a discrete rearrangement of their immunoglobulin heavy-chain genes.

A58.iv Testicular and ovarian disease are well recognised.

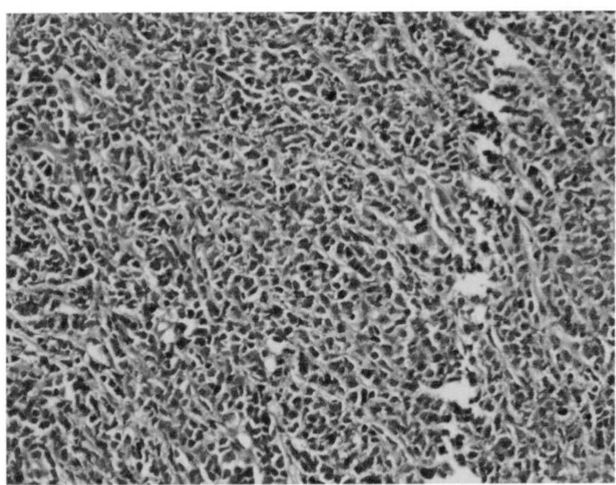

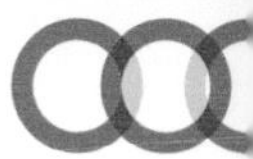

A58.v A classification based on flow cytometry is shown in the following table. The majority of tumours are of B-cell origin.

Classification of childhood ALL

B-lineage (70%)	CD 10	CD19	CD22	CD79A	Tdt	Ig
Early precursor (ProB)	–	+	+	+	+	–
Intermediate (common)	+	+	+	+	+	–
Pre B (Burkitt type)	+	+	+	+	+	+

Biphenotypic – approximately 2%–5%

T-lineage (25%)	CD1a	CD2	CD3	CD4	CD7	CD8	CD34
Pro T	–	–	Cyto	–	+	–	+/–
Pre T	–	+	Cyto	–	+	–	+/–
Cortical T	+	+	Cyto	+	+	+	–
Medullary T	–	+	Cyto surface	–	+	+	–

Risk stratification is described as follows.

Risk stratification of acute lymphoblastic leukaemia (ALL)

Good risk	Poor risk
B-cell	T-cell lineage
Age < 10 years, rapid response	Age >10 years
Hyperdiploidy	T(9:22)
T(12:21) (ETV6-RUNXI)	T(17:19)
T(1:19) (E2A-PBXI)	T(4:11) (MLL rearrangement)
	iAMP21
	Slow response

iAMP, intrachromosomal amplification of chromosome 21; MLL, mixed-lineage leukaemia.

The important phases of treatment are induction, pre-emptive central nervous system (CNS)-directed, intensification and maintenance. Induction is with a combination of vinca alkaloids, prednisolone, anthracyclines, cytarabine and L-asparaginase. All children with acute lymphoid leukaemia (ALL) are at risk of CNS disease and treatment aimed at preventing CNS disease should be offered in pre-symptomatic patients. Such treatment includes intrathecal chemotherapy and high-dose treatment with

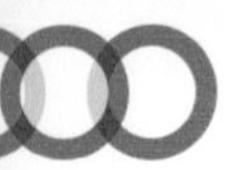

chemotherapeutic drugs that cross the blood–brain barrier (e.g. methotrexate, cytosine arabinoside). Risk stratification is applied to groups of patients, and this is based on prognostic categories and evaluation of response/assessment of minimal residual disease. The overall prognosis for childhood ALL is very good and more than 85% of patients are cured.

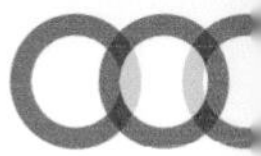

CASE 59

QUESTIONS

A 76-year-old man presented with an intensely painful and itchy rash across his lower chest. His full blood count shows

Haemoglobin (Hb)	121 g/L
White blood cells (WBC)	76 × 10^9/L (lymphocytes 91%, neutrophils 8%)
Platelets	117 × 10^9/L

Examination also revealed generalised lymphadenopathy and a palpable spleen.

Q59.i What is the dermatological diagnosis, and how should he be treated?

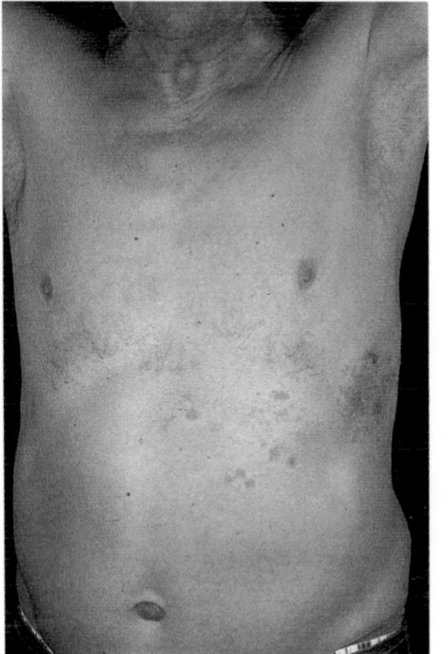

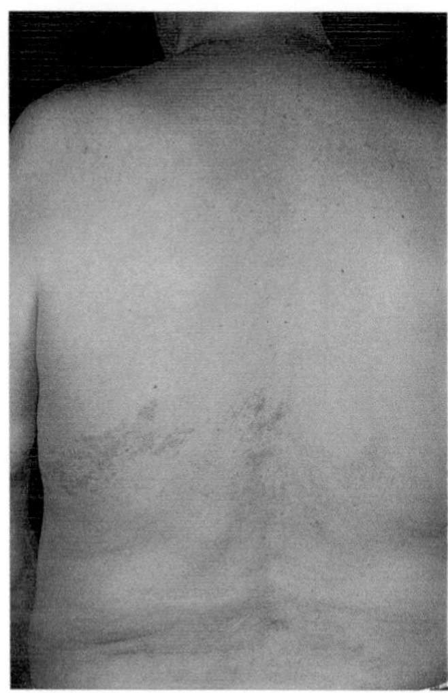

Q59.ii What abnormality is shown on the blood film, and what is the haematological diagnosis? How should this be confirmed? What important prognostic markers exist?

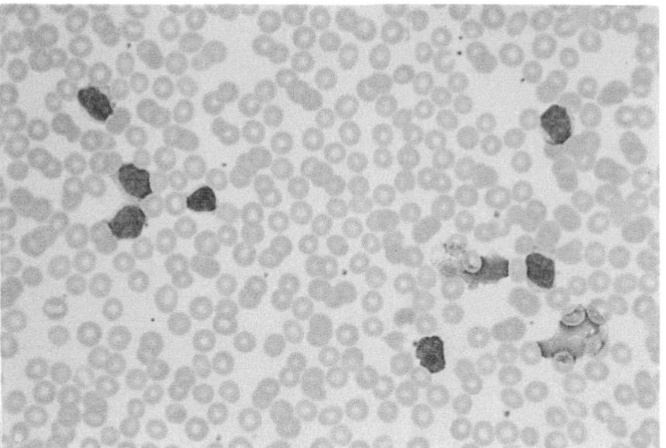

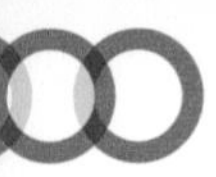

Case 59: ANSWERS

A59.i The rash is typical of shingles (herpes zoster). This condition should be treated with high doses of acyclovir, preferably intravenously.

A59.ii The blood film shows increased numbers of mature lymphoid cells and increased numbers of damaged, or smear, cells. Similar cells are seen in the marrow. These findings suggest chronic lymphocytic leukaemia (CLL). Confirmation is by flow cytometry to demonstrate positivity for the mature B lymphocyte antigens CD19, 20 and 22. The monoclonal nature of the cells is confirmed by demonstrating that the cells have only kappa or lambda light chains (but not both) on their surface. Flow cytometry of the B-cell CLL variants is shown in Table 59.1. Important determinants of prognosis in B-cell CLL are shown in Table 59.2 and in Case 10.

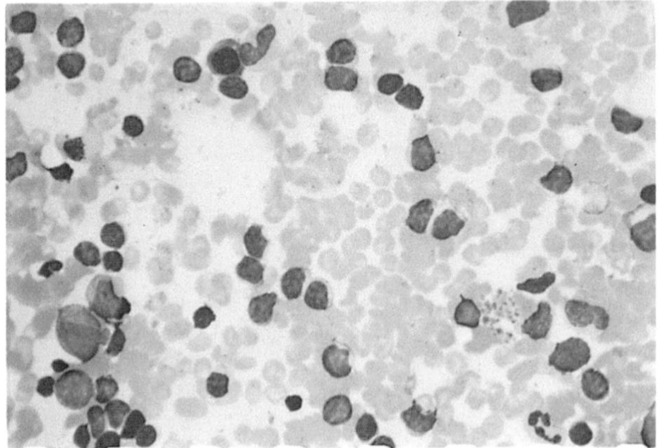

Table 59.1 Immunophenotype of B-cell chronic lymphocytic leukaemia (CLL) and variants

	Smig	CD20	CD5	CD10	CD23	CD11c	Others
CLL	−/+	−/+	+	−	+	−/+	FMC 7 Negative
B-PLL	+	+	−/+	−/+	−/+	−	c-MYC mutations
HCL	+	+	−	−	−	+	BRAF V600E mut
LPL	+	+	−	−	−	−	MYD88 mutation, CXCR4 mutation
SM2L	+	+	−/+	−	−/+	−/+	BCL-2 +
MCL	+	+	+	−	−	−	t(11;14) cyclin D1+
FL	+	+	−	+/−	−/+		t(14;18), BCL-2+

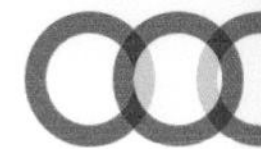

Table 59.2 Prognosis of CLL

Good	Poor
Low stage (Binet A, Rai 0,1)	Advanced stage – Binet C, Rai 4 or 5
Lymphocytic doubling time >3 years	Lymphocytic doubling time <3 years
Female	Male
Few co-morbities	Multiple co-morbidities
2AP-70 Negative	2AP-70 Positive
IGHV gene mutated	IGHV unmutated
13q deletion	P53 deletion, 11q deletion

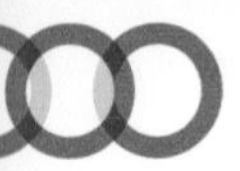

Case 59: QUESTIONS (Continued)

Q59.iii What basic therapies are available for his blood condition?

Q59.iv What variants of this haematological condition are recognised?

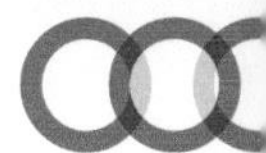

Case 59: ANSWERS (Continued)

A59.iii These patients are at increased risk of infection (because of hypogammaglobulinaemia), and they may need supportive care and treatment of complications such as immune haemolytic anaemia and immune thrombocytopenia. Many patients need no therapy at all, and stable disease should be observed and monitored. Patients with bulky or progressive disease and bone marrow failure may need combination therapy. Progressive disease is treated initially with a combination of fludarabine, cyclophosphamide and rituximab (anti-CD20 monoclonal antibody). Newer agents, such as ibrutinib and bendamustine (usually combined with rituximab) are being evaluated. In older patients, there is increasing interest in using ibrutinib as a single agent. Monoclonal antibodies other than rituximab, which can be combined with chlorambucil, include ofatumumab and obinutuzumab. Splenectomy and radiotherapy to bulky lymph nodes are other forms of therapy.

A59.iv Variants of CLL include as follows:

- B-cell CLL (as in this patient) carries a good prognosis (10 or more years).
- T-cell CLL (Figure 59a) is rare, responds less well to therapy and often affects the skin.
- Splenic marginal zone lymphoma (SMZL) and lymphoma with villous lymphocytes (SLVL) (Figure 59b), which are often accompanied by a paraprotein and responds well to splenectomy.
- B-cell prolymphocytic leukaemia is characterised by larger cells with nucleoli (Figure 59c) may evolve in patients with CLL or may appear de novo. The white cell count is usually markedly raised, splenomegaly is common, and response to therapy is often poor.
- Hairy cell leukaemia (Figure 59d) is usually B-cell but occasionally T-cell type.
- Follicular lymphoma (Figure 59e) affecting the peripheral blood, which can give rise to a similar appearance.

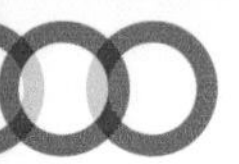

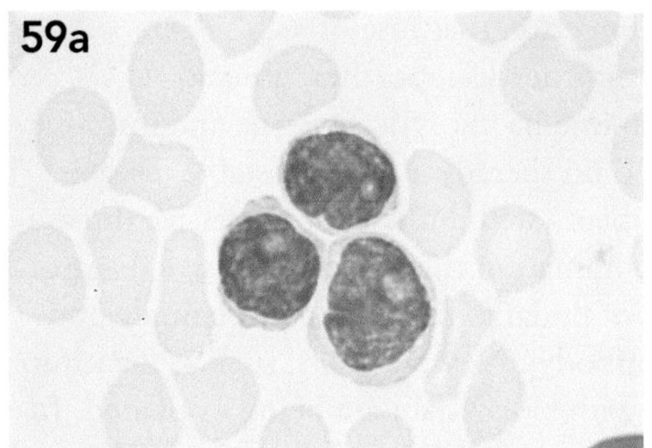

59a

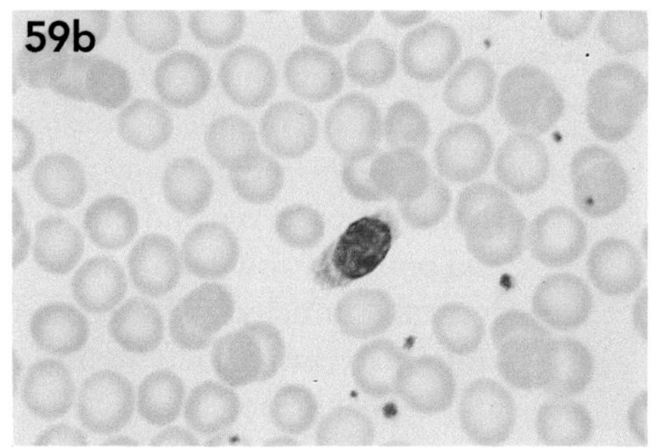

59b

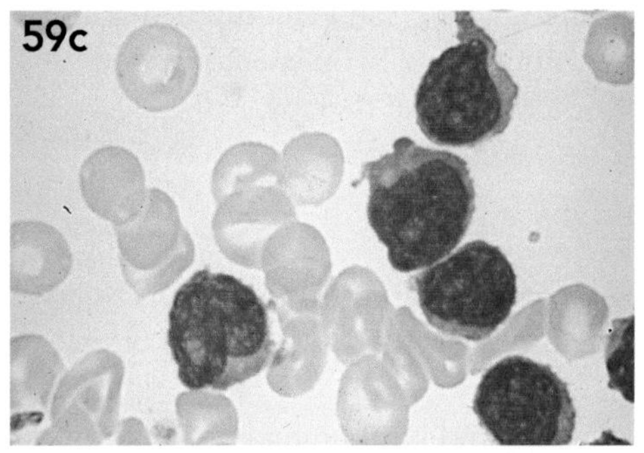

59c

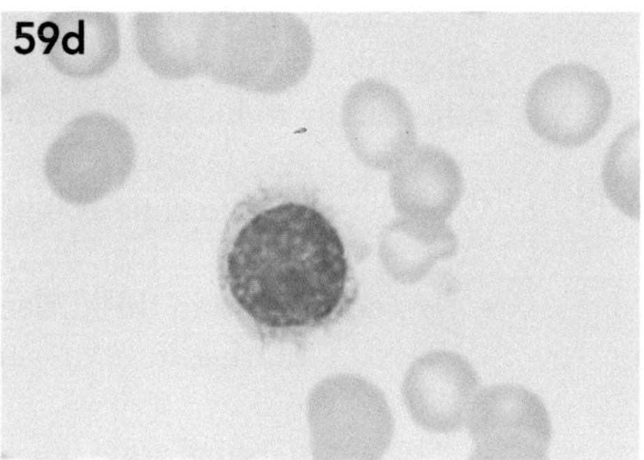

59d

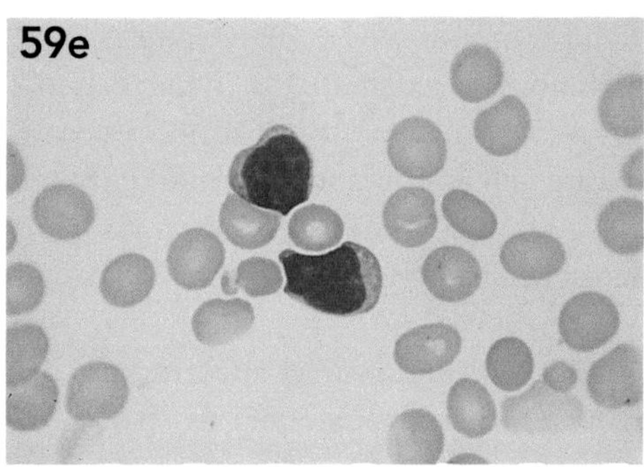

59e

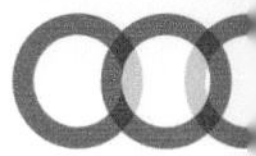

CASE 60

QUESTIONS

A 40-year-old West Indian has bilateral axillary lymphadenopathy. He has a 3- to 4-week history of gradually increasing weakness and stiffness of both legs, with lack of sensation. His full blood count shows

Haemoglobin (Hb)	111 g/L
White blood cells (WBC)	39×10^9/L
Platelets	91×10^9/L

Biochemical analysis shows

Urea	13 mmol/L
Na^+	142 mmol/L
K^+	5.5 mmol/L
Ca^{2+}	3.15 mmol/L
Albumin	38 g/L
Alkaline phosphatase	135 IU/L

Q60.i Comment on the blood film.

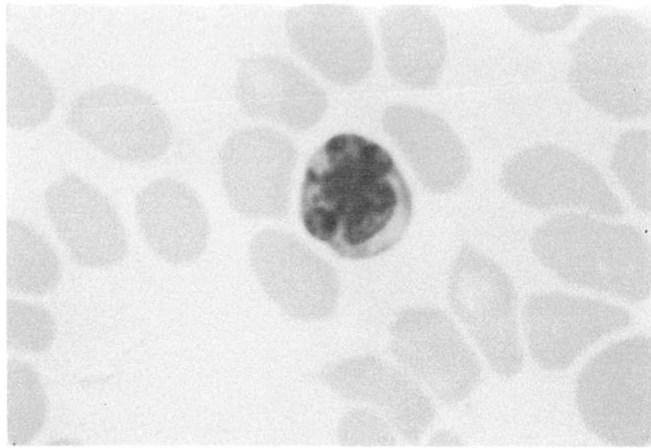

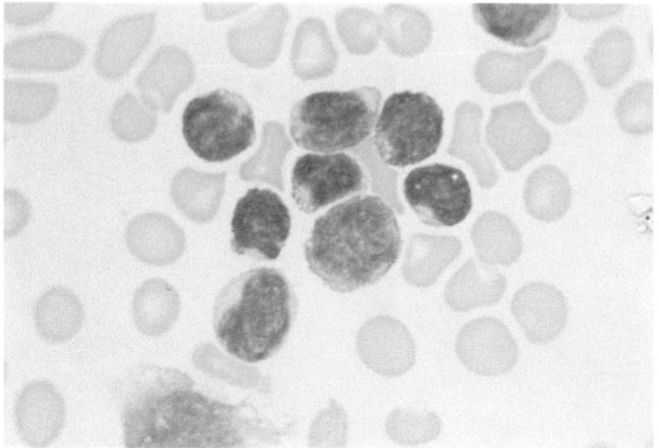

Q60.ii What further tests would you do?

Q60.iii What is the diagnosis, treatment and prognosis?

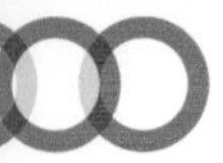

Case 60: ANSWERS

A60.i The film shows a typical lymphocytes with convoluted nuclei. He has hypercalcaemia and a history compatible with transverse myelitis.

A60.ii The following tests should be carried out:

- Serology for human T-cell lymphoma virus type 1 (HTLV-1), a retroviral infection that is endemic in the Caribbean and Japan
- A lymph node biopsy
- Staging investigations, which should include chest and abdominal computed tomography (CT) scans, bone marrow and serum lactate dehydrogenase (LDH)
- Immunophenotype analysis of peripheral blood T-cells to confirm they are T-cells

A60.iii Acute T-cell leukaemia/lymphoma. This is a high-grade lymphoma, best treated with aggressive combination chemotherapy, for example, cyclophosphamide, doxorubicin, vincristine and prednisone (CHOP).

This patient also requires hydration and steroid and/or bisphosphonate therapy (e.g. intravenous zoledronic acid) for his hypercalcaemia. This tumour is typically very aggressive and responds poorly to therapy. They are positive for the T-cell antigens CD2, CD3 (Figure 60) and CD5, and usually CD4 (helper T-cell) positive and CD8 (suppressor T-cell) negative.

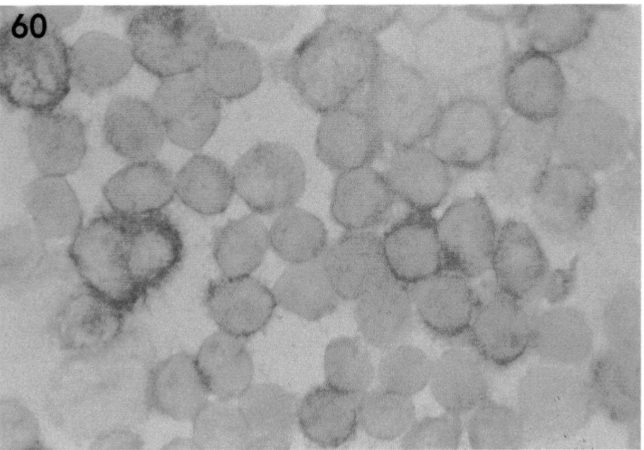

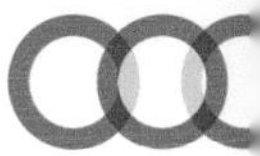

CASE 61

QUESTIONS

A 35-year-old patient has a 4- to 6-week history of fever, loss of weight, anorexia and malaise. He has no fixed abode, and also complains of an irritating cough with purulent sputum. Examination shows him to be unkempt and pyrexial (his temperature is 39°C). He has cervical lymphadenopathy. He also has bruises over his legs. Investigations show

Haemoglobin (Hb)	65 g/L
Mean corpuscular volume (MCV)	84 fL
White blood cells (WBC)	2.9×10^9/L
Platelets	34×10^9/L

Q61.i Comment on the chest x-ray findings (Figure 61a).

Q61.ii Comment on the bone marrow aspirate (Figure 61b).

Q61.iii What is the haematological diagnosis and what conditions may be associated with it?

Q61.iv What further tests should be done?

Q61.v How is this condition treated?

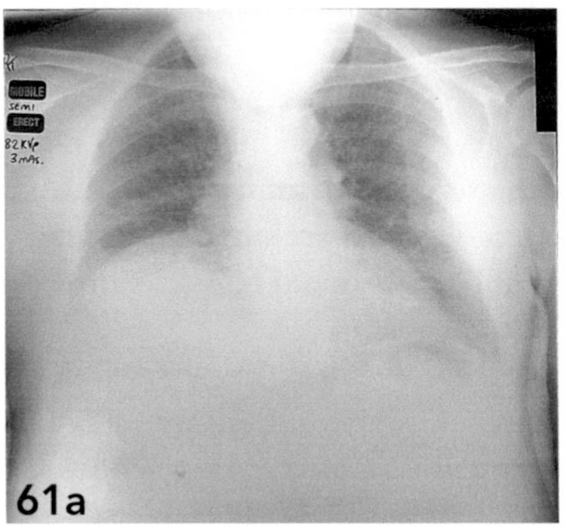

61a

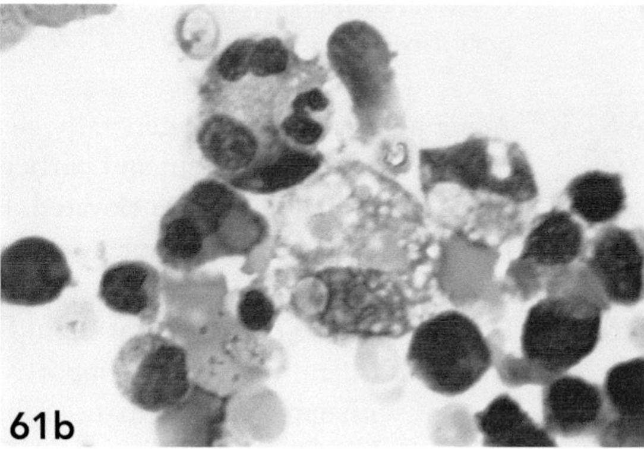
61b

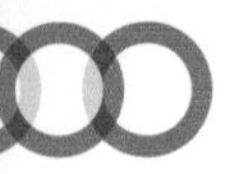

Case 61: ANSWERS

A61.i There are bilateral changes of widespread reticulonodular shadowing which, with this history, would be consistent with miliary tuberculosis.

A61.ii There are abnormal activated macrophages, which have engulfed mature red cells, white cells and platelets. The changes suggest haemophagocytic syndrome.

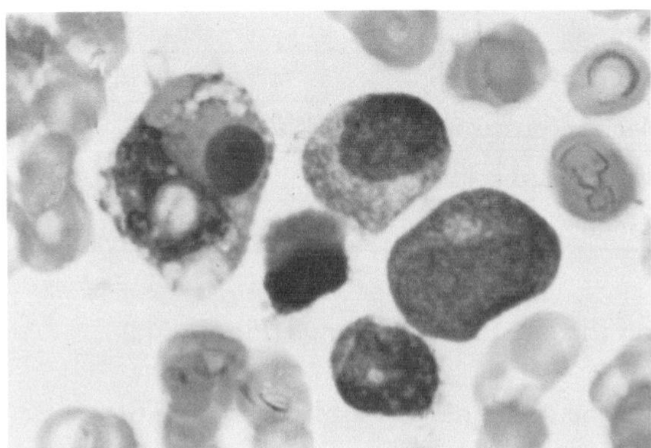

A61.iii In this context, this would be termed secondary haemophagocytic lymphohistiocytosis (HLH). This may occur in association with infection (e.g. tuberculosis or viral infections) particularly in immunosuppressed patients. It may be associated with neoplasia (e.g. malignant lymphoma) or be part of a primary histocytic neoplasm (e.g. histocytic medullary reticulosis). It is also reported in association with autoimmune conditions. Primary HLH is often familial, occurs in children and may be linked to mutations in the perforin gene.

A61.iv Acute phase markers are generally elevated – erythrocyte sedimentation rate (ESR), C-reactive protein and particularly the serum ferritin level. Plasma levels of soluble CD 25 are elevated. Liver function tests are often abnormal. Patients often have hepatosplenomegaly. An HIV test should be performed.

A61.v In secondary HLH, treatment should be aimed at the cause. There is abundant inflammation and supportive therapy, possibly cautious use of steroids with appropriate anti-microbial treatment is required. Intravenous immunoglobulin is often beneficial. In primary or familial HLH, steroids are usually combined with chemotherapy, for example, etoposide, cyclosporine, methotrexate and vincristine.

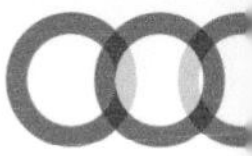

CASE 62

QUESTIONS

A 65-year-old man developed back pain over a 4-week period. He was otherwise well. Investigations show

Haemoglobin (Hb)	91 g/L
White blood cells (WBC)	12.7 × 10^9/L (neutrophils 62%, lymphocytes 31%, metamyelocytes 2%, myelocytes 1%, monocytes 2%, eosinophils 1% and basophils 1%)
Platelets	137 × 10^9/L
Nucleated red blood cells (NRBC):WBC	1:100 (ratio of nucleated red blood cells to white cells)
Erythrocyte sedimentation rate (ESR)	82 mm/h

Q62.i Comment on the differential white cell count and blood film.

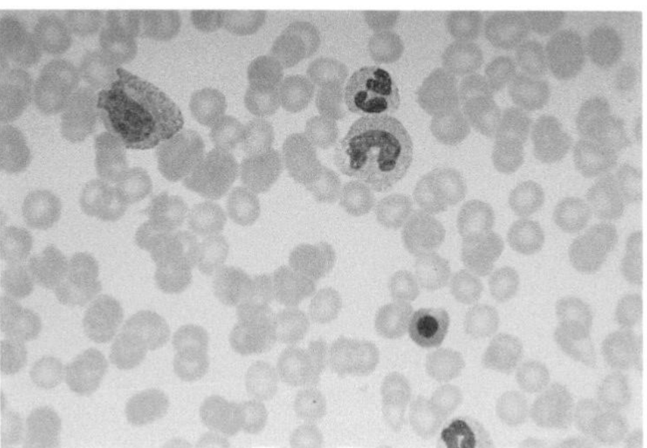

Q62.ii Comment on the bone marrow aspirate (image on the left) and the trephine biopsy (image on the right).

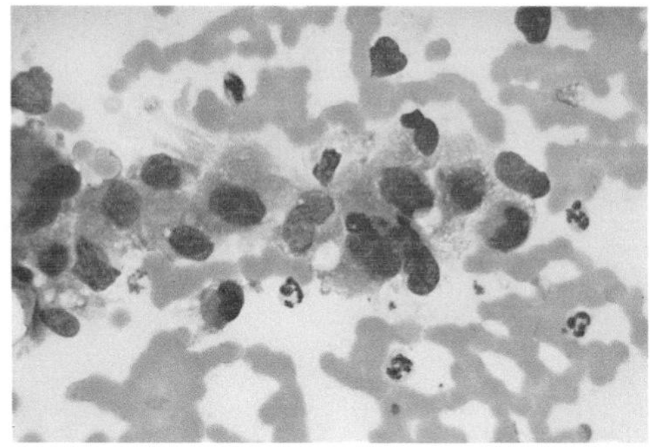

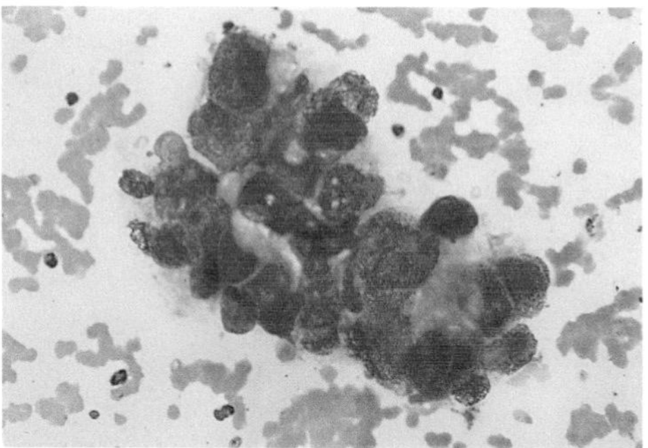

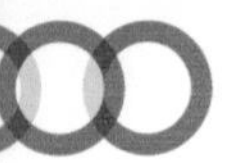

Case 62: ANSWERS

A62.i He has a leukoerythroblastic blood film, which suggests marrow infiltration by abnormal non-myeloid cells. This is an indication for bone marrow examination.

A62.ii The aspirate and trephine biopsy show infiltration by abnormal cells – glandular elements are clearly visible in the trephine biopsy. The appearance suggest secondary carcinoma. He also has back pain. The cells shown in Figure 62a are from a carcinoma of the stomach in a bone marrow aspirate, and a trephine biopsy of oat cell carcinoma of the bronchus (Figure 62b).

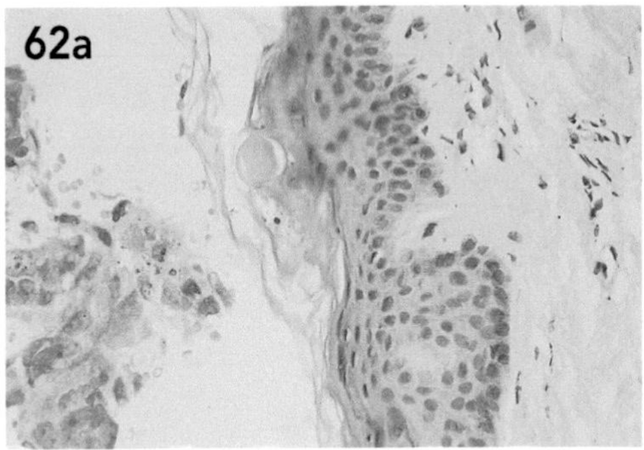

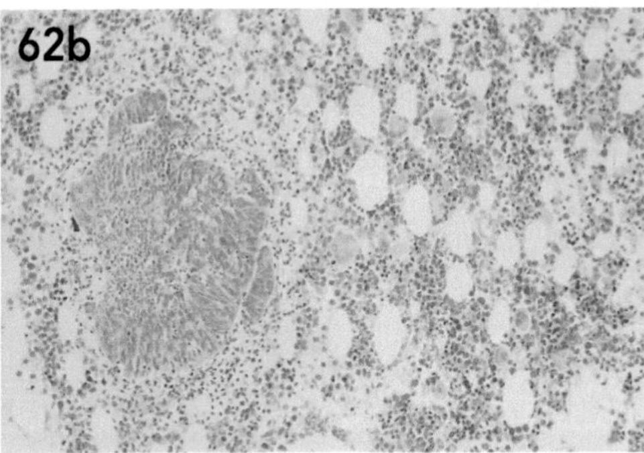

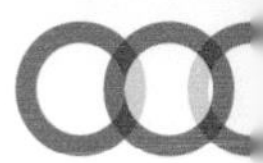

Case 62: QUESTIONS (Continued)

Q62.iii What further tests are indicated?

Q62.iv The patient underwent a retropubic prostatectomy, but post-operatively he developed severe haematuria which persisted for 12 hours despite bladder washouts.

Tests showed

Hb	61 g/L
Platelets	151×10^9/L
Prothrombin time (PT)	15 seconds (control 11–13 seconds)
Activated partial thromboplastin time (APTT)	45 seconds (control 30–40 seconds)
APTT mix with normal plasma 50:50	35 seconds
Thrombin time	40 seconds (control 15–20 seconds)
Fibrinogen	0.01 (NR 0.2–0.4 g/L)
Fibrin degradation products (FDP)	>1:160 (NR <1:10)

What complication has occurred, and how should he be treated?

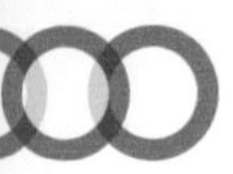

Case 62: ANSWERS (Continued)

A62.iii The prostatic specific antigen was raised. The cells in the aspirate were positive for acid phosphatase, and an isotope bone scan also showed secondary deposits. Rectal examination and prostatic biopsy confirmed the diagnosis.

A62.iv He has developed disseminated intravascular coagulation. There is a spectrum of coagulation abnormalities that occur and in this case the platelet count is relatively preserved and the effect of the consumptive coagulopathy is predominantly hyperfibrinolysis as shown by the profoundly lowered fibrinogen and markedly elevated FDPs. The prostate bed is a rich source of plasminogen activators which cause fibrin degradations; D–D dimers (formed also from fibrin degradation) would be raised.

He should have therapy with tranexamic acid not used now which is a specific inhibitor of plasminogen activators. Cryoprecipitate is also a possible option.

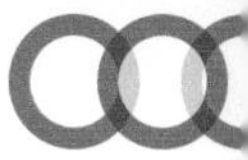

CASE 63

QUESTIONS

An 82-year-old woman has been treated for 5 months for persisting anaemia and thrombocytopenia. Her full blood count shows

Haemoglobin (Hb)	71 g/L
White blood cells (WBC)	1.3 × 10^9/L (neutrophils 40%, lymphocytes 45%, blasts 2%)
Platelets	23 × 10^9/L

Q63.i Comment on the appearance of this patient's face.

Q63.ii Comment on the appearance of the blood film.

Q63.iii What is the diagnosis?

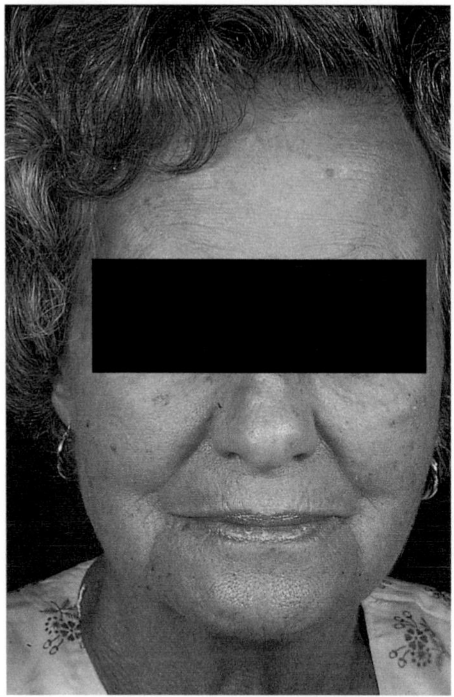

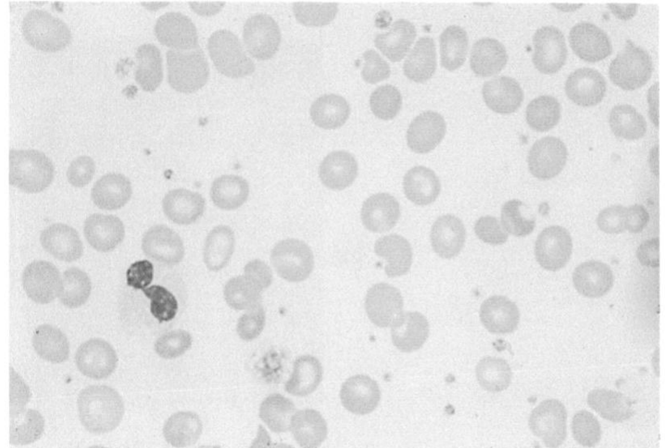

Q63.iv What is the prognosis of this condition?

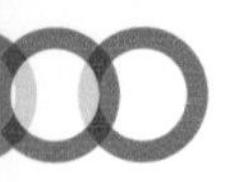

Case 63: ANSWERS

A63.i The face shows a greyish pigmentation which is due to transfusional iron overload. The bone marrow aspirate (Perl's stain) shows increased iron (Figure 63a), and the trephine biopsy shows increased haemosiderin (Figure 63b). Other complications of iron overload include endocrinopathy (e.g. diabetes), liver disease and cardiomyopathy. This patient also had extensive ecchymosis (Figure 63c) as a result of her thrombocytopenia.

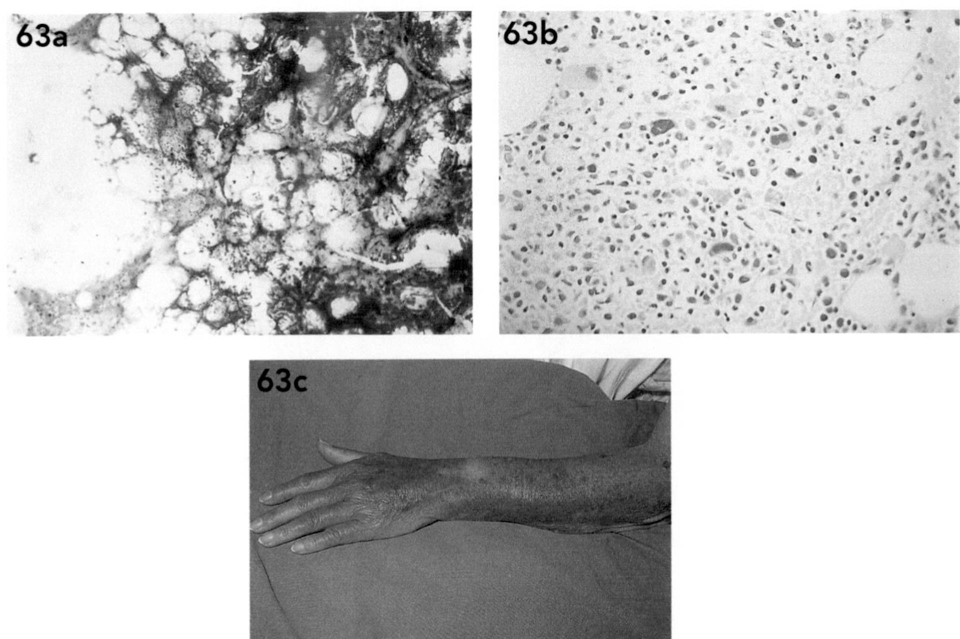

A63.ii The blood film shows hyposegmentation of neutrophil nuclei (pseudo–Pelger forms) with hypogranularity, an occasional blast and platelet/red cell anisocytosis.

A63.iii Myelodysplasia. This is characterised by cytopenias affecting more than one lineage in the face of a cellular marrow, indicating defective maturation within the marrow. Abnormal megakaryocytes and blasts are other typical features in myelodysplasia.

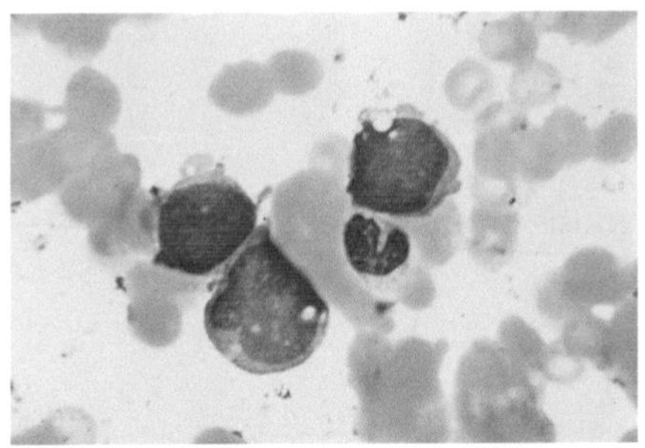

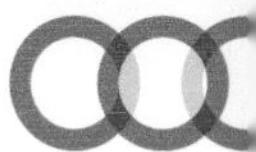

Case 63: ANSWERS (Continued)

A63.iv Myelodysplasia typically affects elderly people (but can occur at any age) and is a disorder of the haemopoietic stem cell. The below table shows a classification of myelodysplasia. Cytogenetic changes are frequently seen, and these most commonly affect chromosomes 5 and 7. Genetic mutations affecting growth and differentiation of haemopoietic stem cells are involved in the pathogenesis of these preleukaemic disorders, but the precise cause is not known. Some patients have previously received myelosuppressive chemotherapy for an unrelated neoplasm.

Classification of myelodysplasia

Myelodysplasia	IPSS Score
Refractory cytopenias with unilineage dysplasia	
Refractory anaemia	0
Refractory neutropenia	0
Refractory thrombocytopenia	0
Refractory anaemia with ring sideroblasts	0
Refractory cytopenia with mulitlineage dysplasia	1
Refractory anaemia with excess marrow blasts: Type 1 (5%–9%) Type 2 (10%–19%)	 2 3
Myelodysplastic syndromes associated with isolated del 5q	0
Myelodysplastic/myeloproliferative neoplasms	
Chronic myelomonocytic leukaemia	
Atypical chronic myeloid leukaemia, BCR-ABL1 negative	
Juvenile myelomonocytic leukaemia	
Cytogenetics • Good • Intermediate • Poor – complex (>3), chromosome 7, 11q	 0 1 2

Prognosis depends on the degree of cytopenia (which influences the risk of complications of bone marrow failure), and the proportion of blasts in blood and bone marrow and the nature and extent of cytogenetic changes (which influences the risk of leukaemic transformation). Scoring systems have been devised. Patients with early myelodysplasia (e.g. refractory anaemia with or without ringed sideroblasts) may need no therapy and have a median survival of 4–6 years. Patients with chronic myelomonocytic leukaemia and refractory anaemia with excess blasts (RAEB) have a median survival of approximately 1 year, whereas patients with more than 20% of bone marrow blasts (RAEB in transformation) or 30% blasts (acute myeloid leukemia

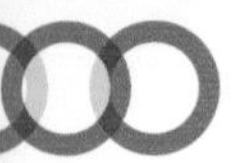

[AML]) should receive AML therapy if they are considered able to tolerate intensive therapy.

DNA methylation and histone modification are epigenetic molecular processes which alter chromatin (e.g. at the site of promoter sequences) and influence gene expression.

Treatment with 5-azacytidine (5AZT) has been shown to improve the cytopenias and reduce the blast count, as well as improve median survival, in myelodysplastic syndrome (MDS) patients who are of intermediate severity. Abnormalities of chromosome 7 seem to predict for a favourable response to 5AZT. Patients who are deemed unsuitable for intensive therapy and require blood component support may suffer iron overload and chelation therapy should be considered. Abnormalities of chromosome 5 seem to predict a favourable response to lenalidomide.

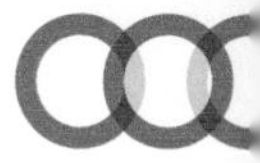

CASE 64

QUESTIONS

A 40-year-old Indian man is referred for investigation of anaemia. He has also complained recently of abdominal pain with nausea. He has had no serious illnesses in the past, and his only medications are herbal remedies. His full blood count shows

Haemoglobin (Hb)	82 g/L
Mean corpuscular volume (MCV)	95 fL
White blood cells (WBC)	Normal
Platelets	Normal

Q64.i What abnormality is seen on the blood film?

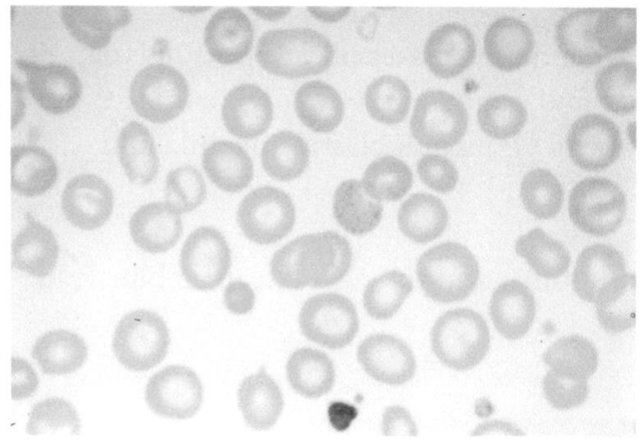

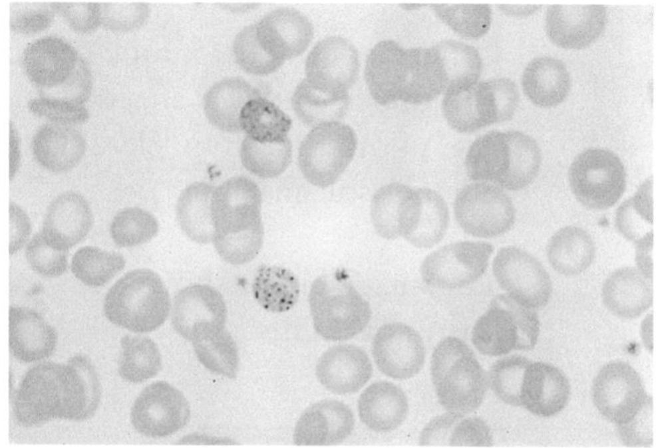

Q64.ii What is the diagnosis?

Q64.iii What further investigations/treatment would you recommend?

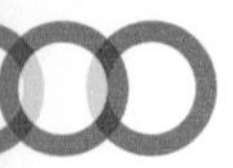

Case 64: ANSWERS

A64.i Basophilic stippling within the red cells.

A64.ii Lead poisoning, which is presumably related to a herbal remedy.

A64.iii The herbal preparation should be sent for analysis, and other users and the manufacturers should be alerted. A serum lead level should be performed.

Lead poisoning may also explain the abdominal pain, and it can cause encephalopathy, circulatory collapse and muscle cramps. Lead interferes with the haem biosynthetic pathway, and the level of urinary delta aminolaevulinic acid is elevated. Treatment in acute stages of lead poisoning, if excessive ingestion is recent and particularly if there is encephalopathy, should include gastric lavage and instillation of a chelating agent in the stomach, for example, D-penicillamine. Oral D-penicillamine can be repeated three times daily and is particularly suitable in children.

Other causes of basophilic stippling include thalassaemia, myelodysplasia, immune haemolytic anaemia, alcohol and congenital enzymyopathies (e.g. pyrimidine-5′-nucleotidase deficiency), megaloblastic anaemia and sideroblastic anaemia.

The image below shows his teeth and gums, and the characteristic blue lead line in his gums.

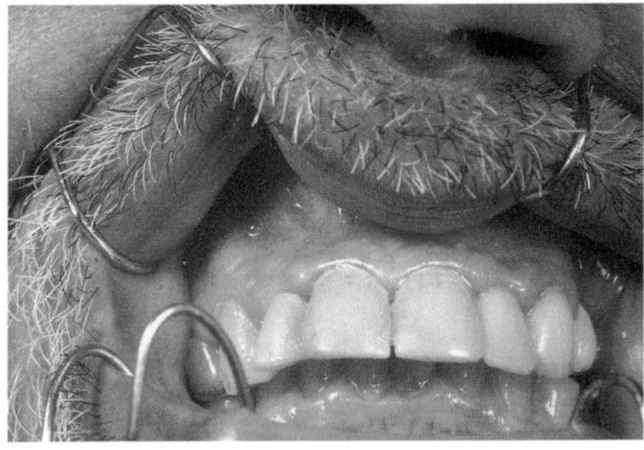

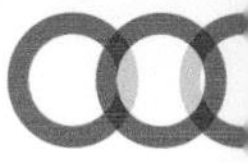

CASE 65

QUESTIONS

Q65.i What abnormality is shown in this blood film?

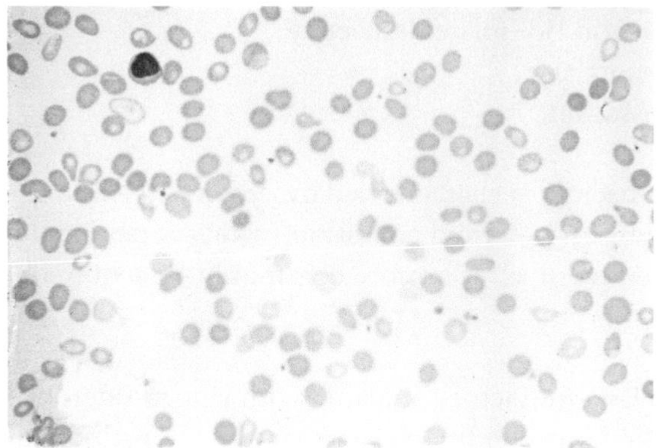

Q65.ii What are the possible causes?

Q65.iii What abnormality is shown in the bone marrow aspirate?

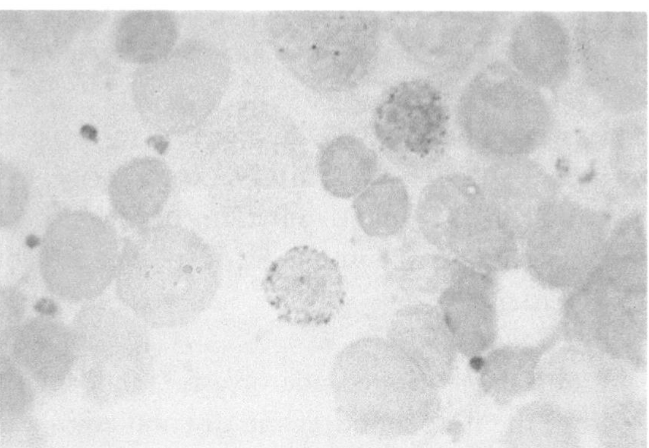

Q65.iv What is the treatment?

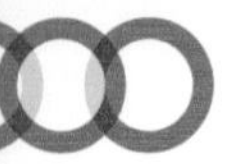

Case 65: ANSWERS

A65.i The blood film shows a dimorphic population of red blood cells, and is from a patient with sideroblastic anaemia. One population of red cells is hypochromic while the other has a normal haemoglobin content. Other causes of two red cell populations include

- Mixed iron and B_{12}–folate deficiency.
- Acute haemorrhage.
- Blood transfusion.

A65.ii Sideroblastic anaemia is characterised by defective synthesis of haem. This can be caused by an inherited condition (which is rare, and is typically seen as a sex-linked recessive). It is more commonly an acquired condition; causes include

- Myelodysplasia (refractory anaemia with ringed sideroblasts [RARS], probably the same condition as primary or idiopathic acquired sideroblastic anaemia)
- Drugs (alcohol, chloramphenicol, isoniazid)
- Lead poisoning
- Vitamin B_6 (pyridoxine) deficiency

(Note that RARS, as part of myelodysplasia, is often associated with thrombocytopenia or leukopenia, and is a clonal, pre-leukaemic condition.)

The spliceosome is a complex intracellular structure which is critically important in processing the primary mRNA tyranscript, to form the mature mRNA that is transcribed. Somatic mutations of the genes encoding the protein components of the spliceosome occur in over 50% of myelodysplastic syndrome (MDS) patients.

A65.iii The iron (Perl's) stain shows ringed sideroblasts – abnormal accumulation of iron granules within the mitochondria and distributed in a circular fashion around the nucleus.

A65.iv Treatment depends on the cause, and persistent symptomatic anaemia usually requires blood transfusion.

Vitamin B_6 is the co-factor for the enzyme delta-amino-laevulinic acid synthetase, which is an important step in haem synthesis. Isoniazid therapy should be combined with vitamin B_6 supplements to prevent sideroblastic anaemia.

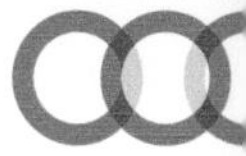

CASE 66

QUESTIONS

A 76-year-old man has a 2- to 3-week history of headache and lethargy. He smokes 15 cigarettes daily but does not have a history of chronic lung disease. His appetite is good and his weight is steady. He has also noticed generalised pruritus after a hot shower. Examination reveals a palpable spleen. Investigations show

Haemoglobin (Hb)	196 g/L
Mean corpuscular volume (MCV)	76 fL
Red blood cells (RBC)	7.4×10^9/L
Packed cell volume (PCV)	0.59 fL
White blood cells (WBC)	16.1×10^9/L (neutrophils 66%)
Platelets	452×10^9/L

Q66.i Comment on this patient's facial appearance.

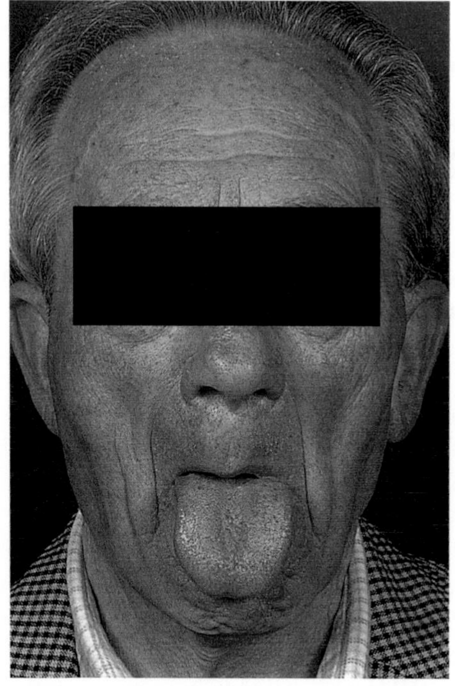

Q66.ii What are the causes of a raised haemoglobin?

Q66.iii What further tests are indicated?

Q66.iv What is the diagnosis? Is this condition familial?

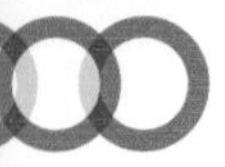

Case 66: ANSWERS

A66.i He has plethora.

A66.ii A raised haemoglobin may be due to a true erythrocytosis (or polycythaemia) or it may be spurious (or relative).

Spurious polycythaemia occurs as a concentration effect in people with reduced plasma volume ('stress polycythaemia'). This is seen in hypertension, during diuretic therapy and in association with smoking.

True polycythaemia may be appropriate (or physiological), for example, at high altitude, in people with chronic lung disease or cyanotic congenital heart disease, or in association with a high oxygen affinity haemoglobin variant. Inappropriate polycythaemia occurs in response to an erythropoietin-secreting tumour (e.g. renal cysts, hypernephroma, uterine and hepatic tumours) or in polycythaemia rubra vera (PRV) or primary proliferative polycythaemia (PPP), which is a myeloproliferative disorder.

A66.iii The presence of splenomegaly strongly suggests PPP, but an abdominal ultrasound should be performed to confirm that the abdominal mass is not an enlarged kidney. The *JAK2 V617F* mutation is present in >95% of patients with PRV. Patients with homozygous mutations are typically more severely affected. A urate level should be documented, as these patients are at increased risk of developing gout. The neutrophil alkaline phosphatase score is usually raised in PPP.

Pulmonary function tests will exclude long-standing lung disease as a contributory cause for the raised haemoglobin.

More than 50% of patients with PPP have raised white cell and platelet counts as part of their myeloproliferative disorder. A red cell mass and plasma volume estimation is useful to document the presence of a true polycythaemia but is only rarely required with the advent of *JAK2* testing.

A66.iv PRV or PPP. Familial polycythaemia can arise due to mutations in the erythropoietin receptor. Mutations in genes which result in increased activity of hypoxia inducible factors (HIFs) will increase erythropoietin production. Familial polycythaemia can result from a mutation in the von Hippel-Lindau gene (VHL) (so called 'Chuvash polycythaemia') and mutations in the *PHD2* gene have a similar effect. Mutations of HIF2 alpha can increase erythropoietin production to cause familial polycythaemia.

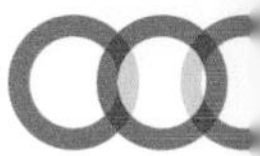

Case 66: QUESTIONS (Continued)

Q66.v How should he be treated?

The patient subsequently went on to develop a generalised, intensely pruritic skin rash over his trunk (Figure 66a), associated with abdominal pain and diarrhoea. A repeat bone marrow examination (Figure 66b) was carried out at this stage.

Q66.vi What condition has now developed?

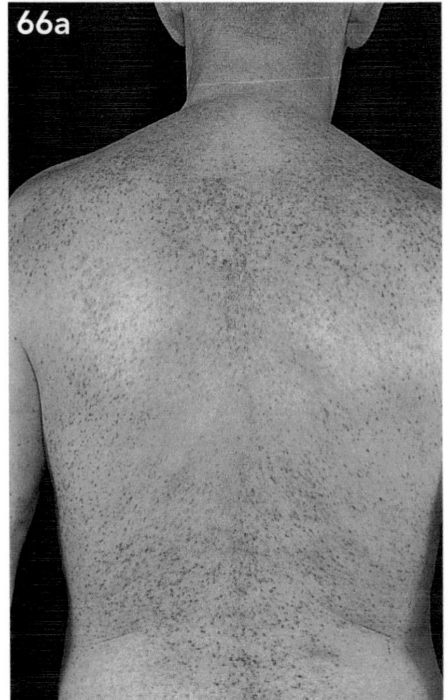

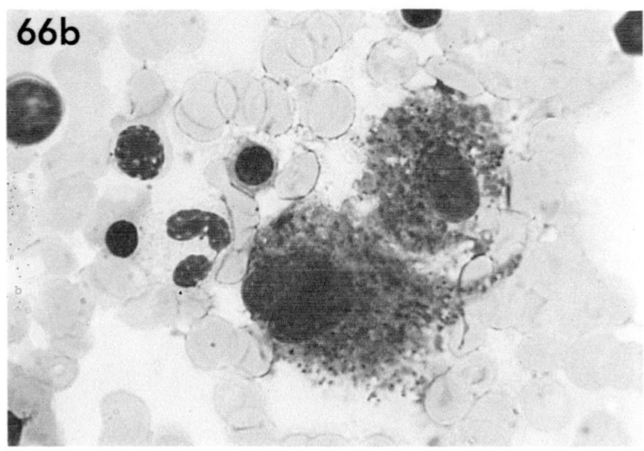

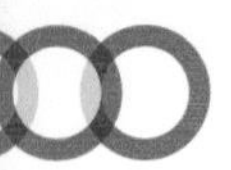

Case 66: ANSWERS (Continued)

A66.v The aim in PPP is to maintain the packed cell volume (PCV) at less than 0.45, as this reduces the risk of thrombosis. This is most easily achieved with regular venesection, but chemotherapy (e.g. oral hydroxycarbamide) may be required. Iron therapy should be avoided.

Patients with myeloproliferative disorder have an increased risk of developing leukaemia, and some therapies (e.g. chlorambucil and other alkylating agents, and 32P) have been shown to increase the risk further. A bone marrow aspirate is shown below from a patient with PPP, treated with long term 32P, who has developed acute myelomonocytic leukaemia.

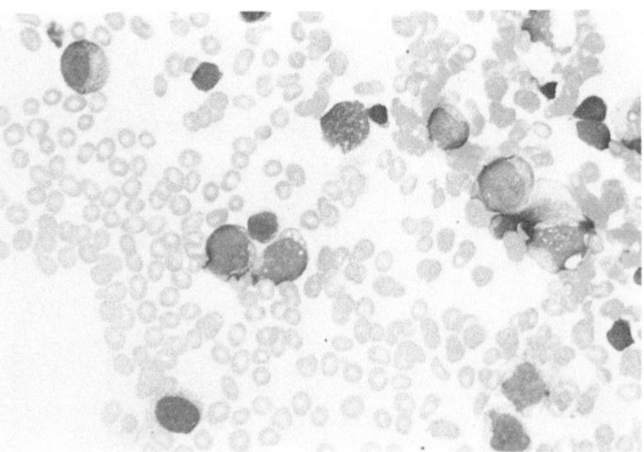

Low-dose anti-platelet therapy (e.g. aspirin 150 mg on alternate days) will reduce the thrombotic tendency.

A66.vi The bone marrow shows infiltration by mast cells. This, together with the skin rash, suggests he has developed systemic mastocytosis, which is associated with the myeloproliferative disorders.

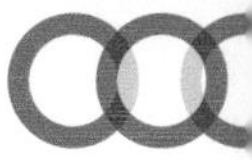

CASE 67

QUESTIONS

A 50-year-old woman has excessive bleeding following tooth extraction. She has never had excessive bleeding before, and there is no relevant family history. She has had two normal vaginal deliveries in the past. Physical examination is normal.

Investigations show

Haemoglobin (Hb)	135 g/L
White blood cells (WBC)	6.7×10^9/L
Platelets	80×10^9/L
Prothrombin time (PT)	12 seconds (control 11–13 seconds)
Activated partial thromboplastin time (APTT)	39 seconds (control 30–40 seconds)
Ivy template bleeding time	4 minutes (normal range up to 10 minutes)

Q67.i Comment on her blood film appearance and on the above results.

Q67.ii Discuss the differential diagnosis.

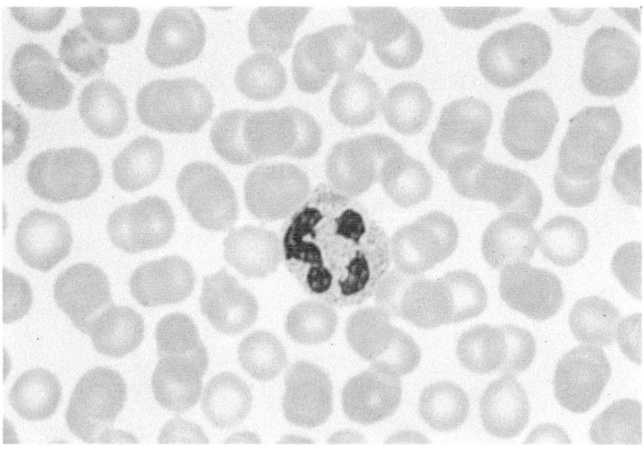

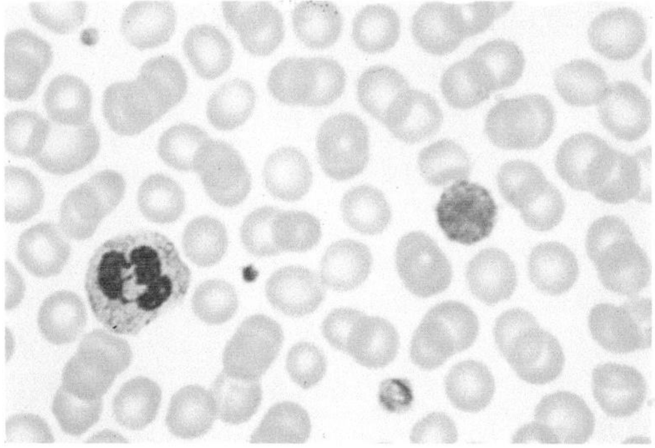

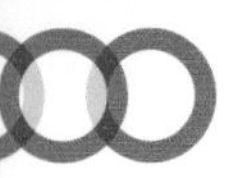

Case 67: ANSWERS

A67.i The blood film shows giant platelets. The neutrophil has an abnormal inclusion which is similar to the Dohle body, found as a feature of neutrophils responding to severe infection. There is a mild thrombocytopenia. The clinical history suggests that she may have a mild bleeding disorder, but the coagulation tests and bleeding time are normal.

A67.ii This patient suffers from the May–Hegglin anomaly, a rare, dominantly inherited disorder which runs a benign course. Bleeding manifestations are rare and platelet function studies are essentially normal. Bernard–Soulier syndrome is an autosomal recessive or codominant trait also associated with giant platelets and thrombocytopenia; but there are no neutrophil inclusions, bleeding manifestations are common and platelet membranes lack glycoprotein Ib and fail to aggregate in response to ristocetin.

Giant platelets may be confused with red cells by automatic cell counters to lead to a spurious thrombocytopenia. They also occur in myelodysplasia, myelofibrosis and as part of thrombocytosis in essential thrombocythaemia and iron deficiency. Giant platelets with thrombocytopenia appear as a benign abnormality in certain Mediterranean populations and is reported in Down's syndrome and with autosomal dominant nephritis and deafness (Epstein's syndrome).

Chediak–Higashi syndrome is a rare autosomal recessive condition wherein partial ocular and cutaneous albinism are associated with a bleeding tendency, severe granulocyte functional abnormalities and abnormal inclusions in developing and mature myeloid cells.

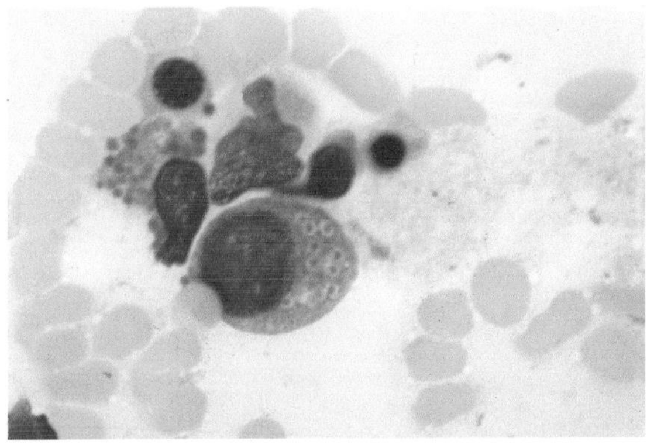

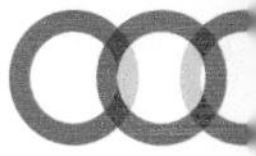

CASE 68

QUESTIONS

A 58-year-old female gives a 4-week history of being generally unwell. She has had intermittent fever, loss of appetite and has lost almost 4 kg (8 pounds) in weight over 2 months. She has had joint pains affecting hands, wrists and ankles which have persisted despite treatment with diclofenac. She developed a generalised skin rash 3 days after commencing a course of amoxycillin. Some 6 months previously she had developed hypothyroidism.

Examination reveals a pale woman who appears ill. She has generalised lymphadenopathy in the cervical, axillary and inguinal regions, and both liver and spleen are palpable. She has swelling of the proximal interphalangeal joints and wrists and a faint macular rash affecting her trunk and upper part of her thighs. Investigation shows

Haemoglobin (Hb)	86 g/L
Mean corpuscular volume (MCV)	81 fL
White blood cells (WBC)	$11.6 \times 10^9/L$
Platelets	$65 \times 10^9/L$
Urea	9.8 mmol/L
Aspartate transaminase (AST)	320 (normal 5–40 units/L)
Alanine transaminase (ALT)	170 (normal 5–40 units/L)
Alkaline phosphatase	275 (normal 35–130 units/L)
Erythrocyte sedimentation rate (ESR)	110 mm/h

Protein electrophoresis shows a faint paraprotein band (later characterised as IgG kappa, 6 g/L) with remaining immunoglobulins at the lower limit of normal.

A bone marrow aspirate is performed.

Q68.i Comment on the appearance of the blood film (Figure 68a) and bone marrow (Figure 68b).

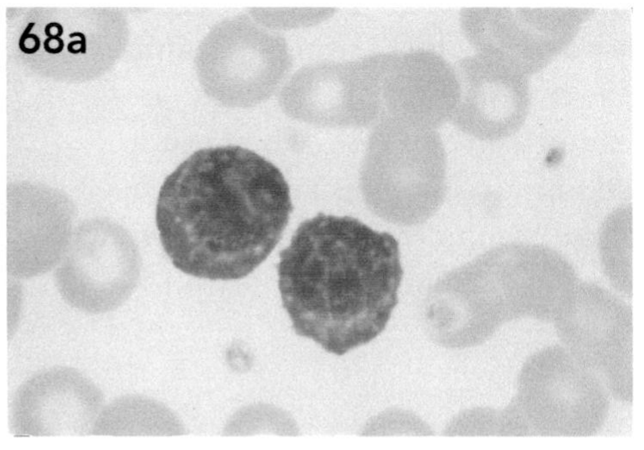
68a

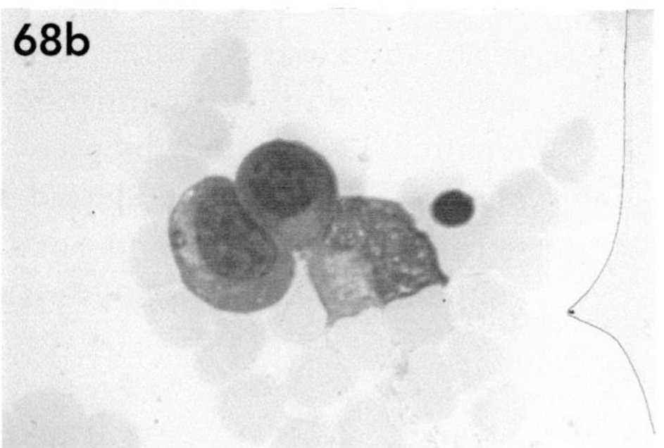
68b

Q68.ii What is the differential diagnosis?

Q68.iii What further management would you suggest?

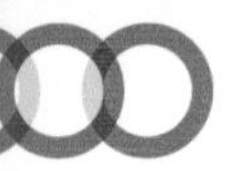

Case 68: ANSWERS

A68.i The peripheral blood film (Figure 68a) shows circulating differentiated B lymphocytes which are plasma cells. Figure 68b shows similar cells (plasma cells or immunoblasts) in the marrow.

A68.ii The clinical history, with skin rash, arthralgia, drug sensitivity, lymphadenopathy, fever, organomegaly and past history of endocrinopathy, is classical for angioimmunoblastic lymphadenopathy with dysproteinaemia (AILD). Autoimmune thrombocytopenia and haemolytic anaemia frequently occur. Lymph node biopsy (Figure 68c) characteristically shows effacement of architecture with arborisation of blood vessels (the angio-component of AILD) and a higher-power view of the node (Figure 68d) shows a polymorphous infiltrate with numerous immunoblasts. A high proportion of patients have clonal rearrangements of T-cell receptor and/or immunoglobulin genes and the condition progresses to overt lymphoma in about a third of cases. Differential diagnosis is wide and includes connective tissue disease, drug hypersensitivity, infection (e.g. viral hepatitis, bacterial endocarditis), lymphoma and myeloma.

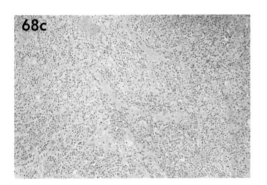

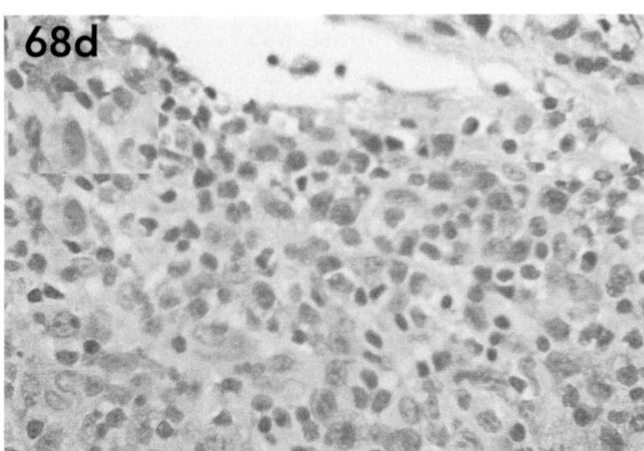

A68.iii Further diagnostic procedures (e.g. lymph node biopsy, liver biopsy if coagulation tests permit, computed tomography [CT] scan, autoimmune serology and urine examination for paraprotein, protein and casts) are required. Lymph node biopsy was diagnostic in this case. Therapeutic options for AILD are wide and include immunosuppressive therapy (e.g. steroids, cyclophosphamide) and intensive combination chemotherapy with a lymphoma regime. Prognosis is poor and 2-year survival is only 30%

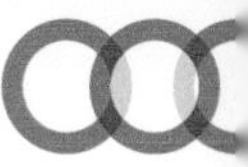

CASE 69

QUESTIONS

Q69.i What abnormality is seen on this blood film?

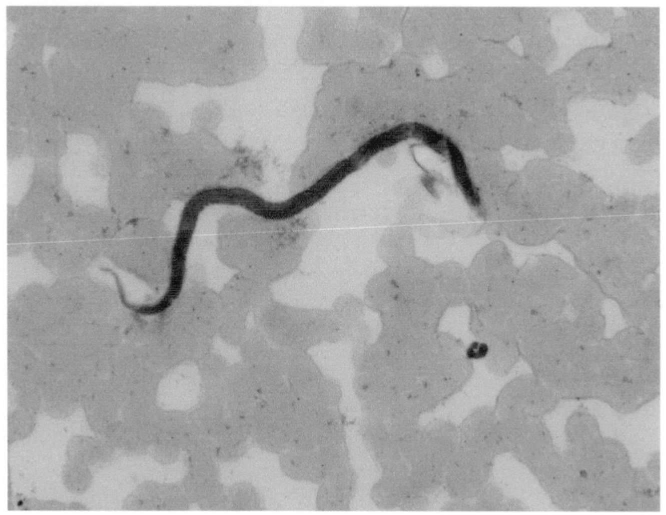

Q69.ii What haematological changes commonly accompany this abnormality?

Q69.iii How is this condition treated?

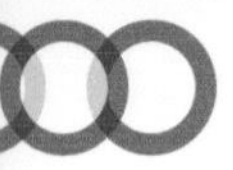

Case 69: ANSWERS

A69.i Filariasis, probably due to *Wuchereria bancrofti*. The larvae are transmitted by mosquito bites, adult worms then develop in the lymphatics and mature females release microfilariae into the blood stream. These microfilariae are ingested by biting mosquitoes.

A69.ii Eosinophilia ($1–30 \times 10^9$/L) and lymphocytosis are frequently seen. Tropical eosinophilia is associated with dyspepsia, wheezing, chest pain and pyrexia, and is frequently due to occult filariasis with pulmonary and lymphatic involvement.

A69.iii Treatment is with oral diethylcarbamazine which is usually given for 21 days.

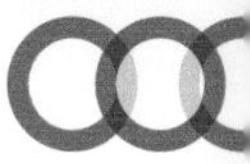

CASE 70

QUESTIONS

A 27-year-old male has recently returned from southern Africa. He complains of intermittent fever. His full blood count shows

Haemoglobin (Hb)	71 g/L
White blood cells (WBC)	17.5×10^9/L (eosinophils 4×10^9/L, lymphocytes 9×10^9/L)
Platelets	56×10^9/L

Q70.i What is the diagnosis?

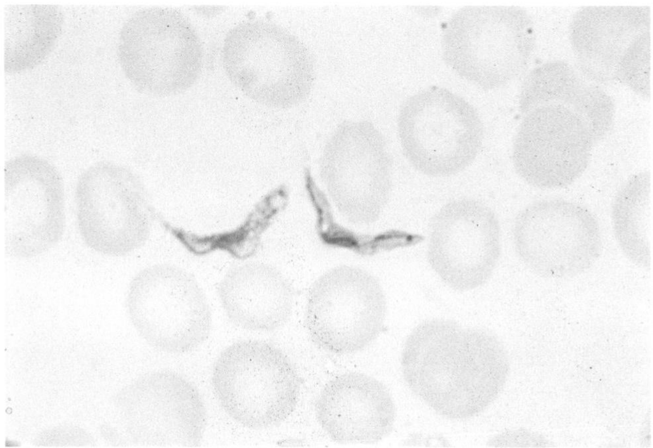

Q70.ii What other haematological complications may occur?

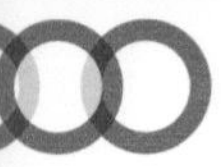

Case 70: ANSWERS

A70.i Trypanosomiasis, probably due to *Trypanosoma rhodesiense.*

A70.ii Splenomegaly is frequently seen. Anaemia is due to haemolysis, caused by release of haemolysins by trypanosomes, erythrophagocytosis within the reticuloendothelial system and splenomegaly with pooling. Thrombocytopenia arises through splenic pooling and disseminated intravascular coagulation (DIC).

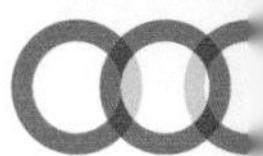

CASE 71

QUESTIONS

A 53-year-old male visits his general practitioner (GP) for a blood pressure check. The GP decides to perform a series of screening blood tests which show the following.

His full blood count shows

Haemoglobin (Hb)	138 g/L
White blood cells count and differential	Normal
Platelets	Normal
Urea and electrolytes	Normal
Vitamin B_{12}	Normal
Folic acid	Normal
Serum iron	33.4 μmol/L (NR 11–36)
Total iron binding capacity	38 μmol/L (NR 53–85)
Percentage transferrin saturation	88% (NR 20–40)
Ferritin	1031 μg/L (NR 30–340)

Q71.i He is referred to you in clinic. What further history would you obtain?

Q71.ii What further tests would you do and why?

Q71.iii How would you manage him?

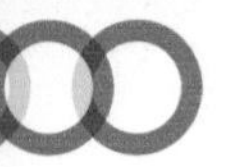

Case 71: ANSWERS

A71.i A full history is mandatory. The additional history required is his alcohol intake (alcohol can raise the serum ferritin) and whether there is a relevant family history. Hereditary haemochromatosis is due to mutations in the high Fe (HFE) gene and is inherited in an autosomal recessive fashion. In the United Kingdom, it is often seen in individuals of Irish heritage. Hepcidin is a protein synthesized by the liver which lowers the levels of ferroportin present on the portal vein border of intestinal cells. It therefore serves to reduce iron absorption. Hepcidin also reduces release of iron from macrophages to transferrin. HFE, hemojuvelin (HJV) and the minor transferrin receptor 2 TFR2 all control hepcidin synthesis; mutations in any of the corresponding genes can lower hepcidin secretion and lead to iron overload.

A71.ii Important additional tests are liver function, blood glucose level to exclude diabetes. The iron (transferrin) saturation is elevated indicating true increase in iron stores and this mandates DNA testing of the HFE gene locus. Particular mutations that may indicate haemochromatosis are homozygosity at *C282Y* and *H63D*, and are found in >90% of subjects with haemochromatosis. Heterozygosity is not associated with iron overload. The absence of mutations at HFE may warrant analysis of mutations at other genetic loci. Many subjects have homozygous mutations but no biochemical or clinical evidence of iron overload. Referral for specialist liver evaluation should be considered if liver function is abnormal.

A71.iii The aim of treatment is to reduce iron stores with regular venesection. The aim is to reduce transferrin saturation and the serum ferritin into the normal range and to maintain it there. Regular attendance and review is mandatory and subjects should be advised to have family members screened.

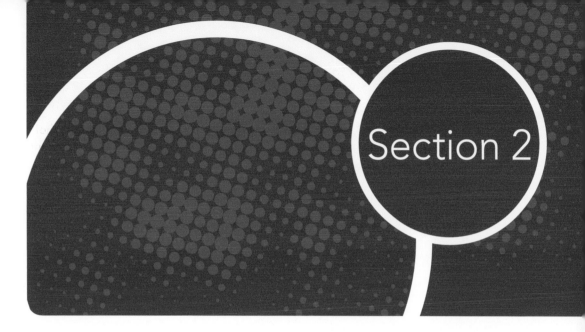

COAGULATION

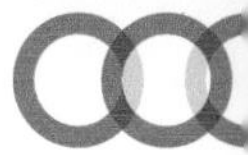

CASE 72

QUESTIONS

A 4-year-old boy presents with excessive bleeding following a fall while riding his bicycle. He has not had surgery previously, but his mother reveals that he does bleed easily and that he bleeds excessively following cuts and abrasions. There is no relevant family history. Physical examination is normal. His investigations show

Haemoglobin (Hb)	9.7 g/dL
White blood cells (WBC)	12.9 × 10^9/L (neutrophils 67%)
Platelets	310 × 10^9/L
Prothrombin time (PT)	11 seconds (control 11–13 seconds)
Activated partial thromboplastin time (APTT)	>120 seconds (control 30–40 seconds)
Thrombin time	18 seconds (control 18–20 seconds)
PTTK with 50:50 mix with normal plasma	55 seconds (control 30–40 seconds)

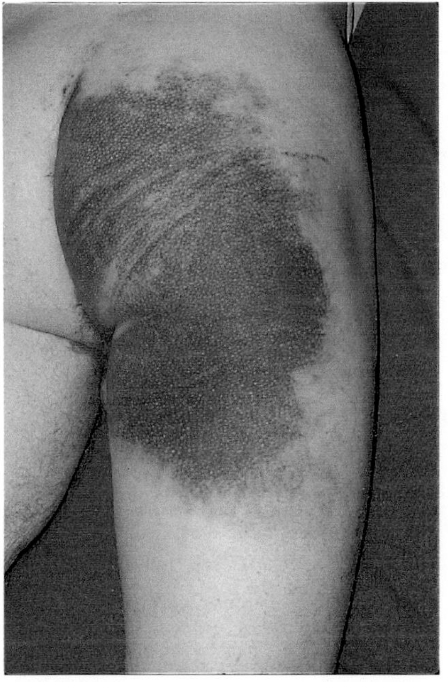

Q72.i What is the likely diagnosis?

Q72.ii What further investigations are required?

Q72.iii How should this condition be treated?

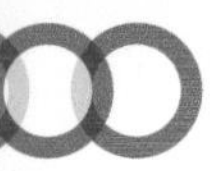

Case 72: ANSWERS

A72.i The history and finding of a prolonged activated partial thromboplastin time (APTT) which shows partial correction by addition of normal plasma suggests an inherited bleeding tendency within the intrinsic pathway of the coagulation cascade. These findings would be compatible with

- Haemophilia A (Factor VIII deficiency)
- Haemophilia B (Christmas disease, Factor IX deficiency)
- von Willebrand's disease
- Factor XI deficiency

An acquired deficiency is much less common in children and the near full correction of the prolonged APTT is against an acquired abnormality. A contact factor deficiency could explain the prolonged but would not be associated with bleeding.

A72.ii Essential further investigations are: assays of Factors VIII, IX, XI and von Willebrand factor. In this case the results showed Factor VIII:C 1.5 IU/dL with normal levels of the other factors and so the diagnosis is moderate Haemophilia A. About half of new presentations have no family history. Both haemophilia A and B are X-linked (i.e. the genes for Factors VIII and IX are encoded on the X chromosome) and family members should be screened, because the mother and sisters may be carriers and male siblings may have the disease. Screening of potential carriers generally requires identification of the genetic abnormality in the index case first. Plasma should be routinely screened for the presence of a Factor VIII inhibitor, though such inhibitors are usually present only after treatment with clotting factor concentrates.

A72.iii Treatment is best conducted at a haemophilia centre with full laboratory, clinical and community services. Current guidelines favour the use of *recombinant* Factor VIII concentrate for treatment of bleeding episodes and prophylaxis at times of surgery. An important complication of earlier therapy with plasma-derived concentrates that had not been heat-treated was transmission of viral infections such as HIV and hepatitis C.

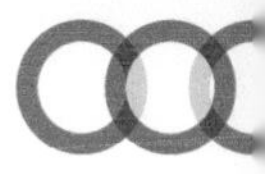

CASE 73

An 18-year-old girl presents with an antepartum haemorrhage 20 weeks into her first pregnancy. She requires a blood transfusion. In her past history, she reports heavy bleeding after a tonsillectomy. She was returned to theatre for cauterisation to achieve haemostasis and required a post-operative blood transfusion. She has had no other procedures and reports normal menstrual blood loss. Her father similarly required blood transfusion after tonsillectomy and she believes that he received treatment during subsequent surgeries to prevent bleeding.

Investigations prior to transfusion

	Test Results	Normal Range
Prothrombin time	14 s	[12–16]
APTT	50 s	[26–36]
APTT 50:50 mix	38:34	
Factor VIII:C one stage	34 IU/dL	[50–150]
Factor IX:C	75 IU/dL	[50–150]
Factor XI:C	81 IU/dL	[70–150]
VWF:Ag	93 IU/dL	[50–150]
VWF:CB	90 IU/dL	[50–150]
VWF:RCo	55 IU/dL	[50–150]
Hb	65 g/dL	[11–16]
WBC	8.3 × 10^9/L	
Platelets	320 × 10^9/L	[150–400]

QUESTIONS

Q73.i Comment on the history and results, list a differential diagnosis and outline further investigation.

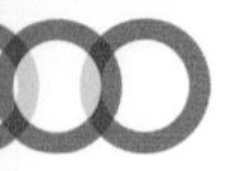

Case 73: ANSWERS

A73.i The main abnormalities are the reduced Factor VIII level and VWF:RCo which are disproportionately low compared with the VWF:Ag. Although both are in their respective normal ranges this may reflect pregnancy-induced elevations. There is a history of unexpected bleeding following surgery in both the patient and her father raising the possibility of an inherited disorder of coagulation. The commonest cause of a low Factor VIII in a female with this history is VWD. The discrepancy between one of the functional assays and the antigen and the fact that the Factor VIII level is lower than the VWF levels suggests type 2 disease. Carriership of haemophilia A is also a possibility but would not be associated with discrepancy in the VWF assays. Acquired haemophilia is much rarer and the mixing studies do not indicate the presence of an inhibitor. These are all possibilities that should be addressed with subsequent investigations which should include

- FVIII chromogenic assay
- FVIII inhibitor screen
- VWF multimer analysis
- VWF FVIII binding assay

Further investigations

	Test Results	Normal Range
FVIII chromogenic	28 IU/dL	[50–150]
FVIII inhibitor screen	Negative	

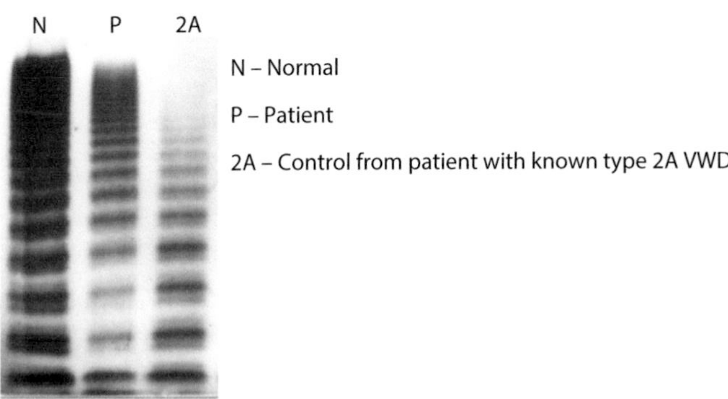

Figure 73a Von Willebrand factor multimers.

Factor VIII (FVIII) binding assay (normal control FVIII bound to von Willebrand factor (VWF) from normal control, case of known homozygous type 2N and patient).

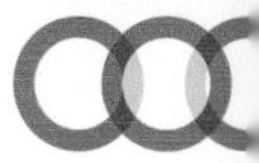

Case 73: ANSWERS (Continued)

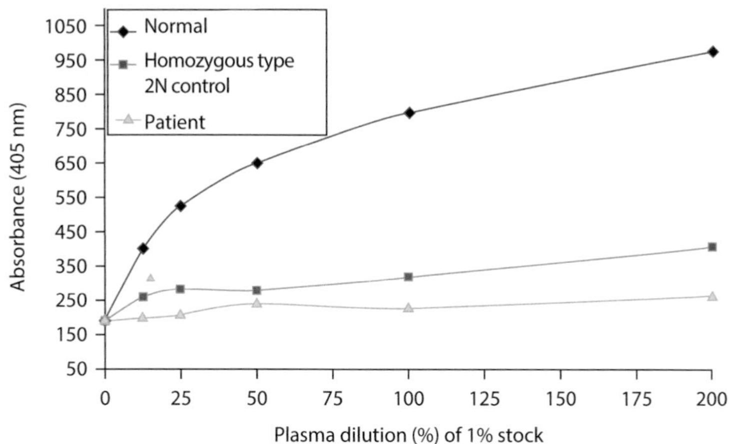

Figure 73b Factor VIII binding assay.

Case 73: QUESTIONS (Continued)

Q73.ii Report these results. What is the diagnosis? Are there any additional tests that can be done to confirm the diagnosis?

Q73.iii Outline a management plan for the patient to cover pregnancy, labour and the post-partum period.

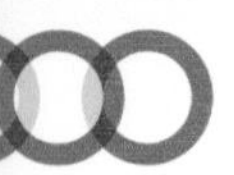

Case 73: ANSWERS (Continued)

A73.ii The diagnosis is type 2N VWD. The mutimer gel shows a normal electrophoretic pattern but the diagnosis is clinched by the FVIII binding assay which shows severely reduced binding of normal FVIII by the patient's VWF.

A73.iii The risk of bleeding in type 2N is most closely linked to the FVIII, rather than the VWF level. In this case, the FVIII level is mildly reduced and so it is unlikely that this is the sole cause of the antepartum haemorrhage. There may be an obstetric abnormality that requires management as well as treatment of the low FVIII level. Mild deficiencies of FVIII can be treated by concentrate to elevate the level in combination with adjunctive therapies such as the anti-fibrinolytic agent: tranexamic acid. It is generally necessary to keep a level well into the normal range for 1–2 weeks. Plasma-derived intermediate purity VWF-containing concentrate is likely to be more effective than recombinant FVIII concentrate in this condition. Desmopressin may also be effective but as this elevates endogenous abnormal VWF, the effect may be short-lived. Prophylactic rather than on demand therapy is likely to be adequate for the rest of the antenatal period but delivery is likely to require replacement therapy with correction of the FVIII level until the risk of post-partum haemorrhage is negligible. Patients with mild bleeding disorders generally require post-partum tranexamic acid for a minimum of 4 weeks or until the lochia is no longer bloody.

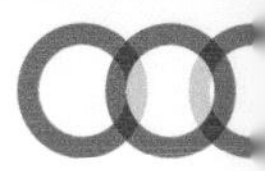

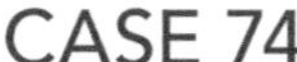

CASE 74

A 56-year-old man is referred for anti-coagulation with warfarin as he has atrial fibrillation. His only other medication is frusemide. However, it proves very difficult to increase the international normalised ratio (INR) above 1.5 and 4 months after commencing warfarin his INR is 1.4 despite being prescribed 25 mg of warfarin daily for the last fortnight. The patient insists that he is compliant with his medication and religiously takes the correct dose at the same time each day.

QUESTIONS

Q74.i What further investigations would you carry out?

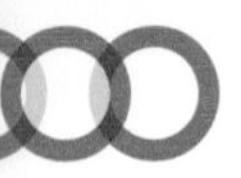

Case 74: ANSWERS

A74.i The most common cause of an apparent unresponsiveness to warfarin is lack of patient compliance. This is difficult to monitor in the community but a direct assay for warfarin will demonstrate whether or not the drug is actually being taken. Malabsorption might result in low warfarin levels after ingestion but as warfarin is very easily absorbed there would be very obvious symptoms of a malabsorption syndrome if this was the explanation. Although the INR measures the effect of warfarin, it is not specific for this drug. Warfarin acts as a competitive inhibitor of vitamin K in the pathway responsible for γ-carboxylation of coagulation factors. Thus in correctly anti-coagulated patients, there will be elevated levels of factors that are not γ-carboxylated. These are referred to as proteins induced by vitamin K absence (PIVKA) and can be directly measured. Thus, measurement of serum warfarin and PIVKA levels will indicate whether the drug is being taken and if it is, whether it is having a therapeutic effect.

Additional investigations

	Test Results	Normal Range
Prothrombin time	16 s	[12–16]
INR	1.4	[therapeutic range 2.0–3.0]
Serum warfarin	2.48 mg/L	[therapeutic range 0.7–2.3 mg/L]
PIVKA	0.1 AU/mL	[<0.2]

Case 74: QUESTIONS (Continued)

Q74ii Comment on these results. What is the likely explanation for the sub-therapeutic INR?

Q74iii How would you manage this patient?

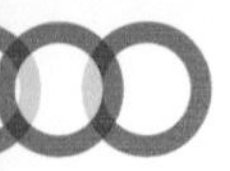

A74.ii The serum warfarin level is elevated indicating that the drug is being taken and getting absorbed. However, the PIVKA levels are not elevated (the result is within the normal range seen in individuals not on warfarin) indicating that there is no effective inhibition of γ-carboxylation by warfarin. The most likely explanation for this is that there is an abnormality in the Vitamin K Epoxide Reductase Complex (VKORC1) that makes it insensitive to inhibition by warfarin. Alternatively, there may be abnormal metabolism of warfarin due to variants in the cytochrome P450 pathway. Genetic testing demonstrated a likely pathogenic variant in *VKORC1* in this case.

A74.iii Of the main anti-coagulant drugs, only warfarin is affected by mutations in VKORC1 or cytochrome P450. Therefore, a direct thrombin or Factor Xa inhibitor would be effective in this case.

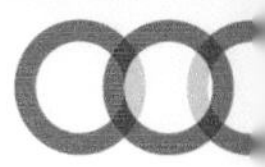

CASE 75

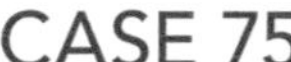

An 8-year-old boy from Iran presents with easy bruising and recurrent nosebleeds. His elder sister is in Iran and suffers from severe menorrhagia for which she has required blood transfusion. His parents are first cousins.

Initial investigations

	Test Result	Normal Range
Prothrombin time	14 s	[12–16]
APTT	30 s	[26–36]
Factor VIII:C one stage	114 IU/dL	[50–150]
Factor IX:C	85 IU/dL	[50–150]
Factor XI:C	75 IU/dL	[70–150]
VWF:Ag	98 IU/dL	[50–150]
VWF:CB	90 IU/dL	[50–150]
VWF:RCo	103 IU/dL	[50–150]
Hb	125 g/dL	[11–16]
WBC	$5.2 \times 10^9/L$	
Platelets	$245 \times 10^9/L$	[150–40]

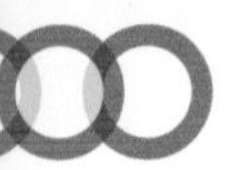

Figure 75a Platelet aggregometry tracings.

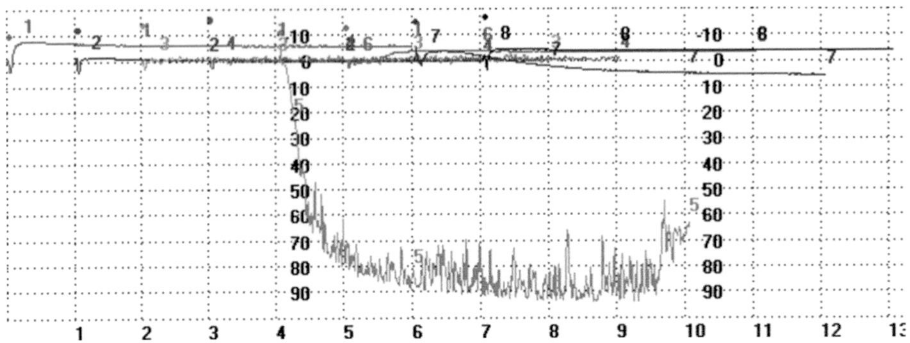

Lane	Agonist	% Aggregation at 5 Minutes
1	ADP	0
2	ADP 10 µM	0
3	Adrenaline 10 µM	0
4	Ristocetin 0.5 g/L	0
5	Ristocetin 1.5 g/L	67
6	Collagen 2 µg/L	0
7	Arachidonic acid 1 mM	6
8	U46619 1 µM	0

QUESTIONS

Q75.i How would you report these results? What is the likely diagnosis?

Q75.ii What is the molecular basis of this disorder? What confirmatory tests would you do?

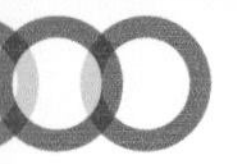

Case 75: ANSWER

A75.i The history is suggestive of an inherited bleeding disorder but there are no abnormalities in the clotting tests or factor assays. The aggregometry shows an absent response to all agonists with the exception of ristocetin to which there is a normal response. This indicates a severe platelet dysfunction and the most likely diagnosis is Glanzmann's thrombasthenia. Although aggregometry is almost absent in this case the bleeding history is suggestive of a milder form of the disease.

A75.ii This disorder is caused by abnormalities in the glycoprotein (Gp) IIb/IIIa complex. This receptor is involved in the binding or signalling of many platelet agonists but not ristocetin, which binds and signals exclusively through the Gp Ib/IXa complex. It is extremely rare except in communities where consanguinity is more common. The diagnosis should be confirmed by measurement of levels of the receptor which is easily done by flow cytometry. Analysis of the genes encoding the proteins of the receptor complex is also useful.

The family returns to Iran and 10 years later, the patient returns to the United Kingdom to attend university. He has had recurrent tonsillitis and the ENT surgeons have recommended tonsillectomy. While in Iran, he received several platelet transfusions during his teenage years following severe epistaxis and bleeding after dental extraction. He reports that after the last extraction a year ago, he suffered extensive haemorrhage despite receiving several pools of platelets both before and after the procedure.

Case 75: QUESTIONS (Continued)

Q75.iii What further investigations would you carry out? How would you cover the surgery?

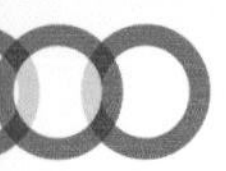

A75.iii Generally, first-line therapy is with platelet transfusion in this condition. Tranexamic acid is a useful adjunct but desmopressin rarely has any benefit. Patients should receive human leukocyte antigen (HLA)-matched platelets but it is unlikely that this would have been achievable in Iran. The history is suggestive of platelet refractoriness which is most likely to be due to the presence of HLA antibodies and so a test for these should be carried out. There should then be a discussion with the blood transfusion service to determine whether appropriately matched platelets can be provided. If not, recombinant Factor VIIa can be an effective haemostatic agent in this condition. However, the therapeutic response is generally poorer than with platelets and the treatment has to be given frequently, perhaps as often as 3–6 hourly in the immediate peri-operative period. In this particular case, the frequency was reduced to 8 hourly after 24 hours and treatment continued for a total of 72 hours. Monitoring of bypassing agents is difficult but can be achieved with global tests of haemostasis such as thromboelastometry or thrombin generation.

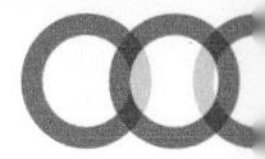

CASE 76

A 40-year-old woman is scheduled for elective thyroid surgery for Hashimoto's disease. She has no other medical problems. She tells the surgeons that she was diagnosed with a 'blood disorder' during childhood but cannot remember any specific details.

The results of pre-operative blood tests are shown below and the surgeons refer her to haematology for further assessment and investigation.

Initial tests

	Test Results	Normal Range
Prothrombin time	34 s	[12–16]
APTT	28 s	[26–36]
Thrombin time	14 s	[11–15]
PT 50:50 mix	16:14	

QUESTIONS

Q76.i How would you investigate this case?

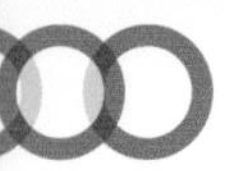

Case 76: ANSWERS

A76.i The initial tests show an isolated prolongation of the prothrombin time suggesting a defect in the extrinsic pathway. Possible causes at this stage would be a coagulation factor deficiency or an inhibitor. Lupus anti-coagulant is by far the most common cause of an inhibitor that affects the prothrombin time and although most lupus anti-coagulants would affect the activated partial thromboplastin time (APTT) this is dependent on the specificity of the anti-phospholipid antibody. As the thromboplastin reagent used in the prothrombin time contains phospholipid it is not at all uncommon for some prolongation to be seen in the presence of lupus anti-coagulant. Although mixing studies do not suggest an inhibitor, correction does not exclude a lupus anti-coagulant and so this possibility needs to be excluded with a more specific assay.

Additional investigations

	Test Results	Normal Range
Factor II:C	94 U/dL	[50–150]
Factor V:C	101 U/dL	[50–150]
Factor VII:C	23 U/dL	[50–150]
Factor X:C	88 U/dL	[50–150]
DRVVT	1.10	[0.8–1.2]

On taking a more detailed history, she reports two normal vaginal deliveries without any post-partum bleeding and three dental extractions without any bleeding. She also underwent removal of a meningioma 5 years ago without any bleeding problems.

Case 76: QUESTIONS (Continued)

Q76.ii How would you manage the surgery?

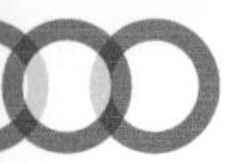

Case 76: ANSWERS (Continued)

A76.ii Second-line investigations should test for lupus anti-coagulant and deficiencies of the coagulation factors that might cause prolongation of the prothrombin time. The normal dilute Russell viper venom time (DRVVT) makes a lupus anti-coagulant highly unlikely although guidelines recommend the use of two specific tests to exclude it.

The factor assays indicate a marked Factor VII deficiency. Deficiencies of Factors II, V and X would be expected to cause prolongation of the APTT as well.

Factor VII deficiency is a mild bleeding disorder unless there is complete absence of Factor VII protein. In the most severe cases, life-threatening bleeding can be seen from infancy. As levels of above 15 U/dL are generally adequate for normal haemostatic function, milder forms of the disease are often asymptomatic.

As previous haemostatic challenges have not been associated with any bleeding it is likely that thyroid surgery would also not be associated with bleeding. However, the consequences of bleeding at this site would be serious and so it would be safer to provide some form of haemostatic cover. In this situation, tranexamic acid alone would be a reasonable first-line treatment. Replacement therapy with plasma-derived products such as fresh-frozen plasma (FFP) or Factor VII concentrate, or recombinant Factor VIIa is not required in mild cases.

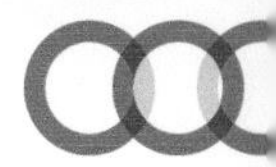

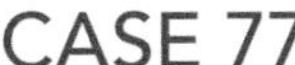

CASE 77

An 18-year-old girl is referred for investigation of a possible clotting factor deficiency. When she was 5, she had recurrent epistaxis and required cauterisation. At the time, she was found to have a Factor VII level of 8 U/dL and given a diagnosis of Factor VII deficiency. The epistaxis settled after the cauterisation and she had no further bleeding symptoms.

She has recently consulted her general practitioner (GP) with symptoms of menorrhagia. Because of the history of Factor VII deficiency, the GP refers her to the haematology clinic.

Initial tests

	Test Result	Normal Range
Prothrombin time	14 s	[12–16]
APTT	28 s	[26–36]
Thrombin time	14 s	[11–15]
Factor VII:C	43 U/dL	[50–150]

QUESTIONS

Q77.i How do you explain these findings?

Q77.ii What other tests would be useful in this situation?

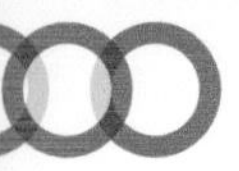

Case 77: ANSWERS

A77.i Factor VII deficiency does not improve spontaneously over time. The most likely explanation is that the deficiency is due to a mutation in *F7* that affects the binding of the Factor VII protein with tissue factor. The measured activity of the mutant Factor VII then varies depending upon the thromboplastin used as this is the source of the tissue factor used in the Factor VII assay.

Previously, animal thromboplastins were commonly used in prothrombin times and Factor VII assays as they are cheaper and were more easily produced than human thromboplastin which is now generally made by recombinant methods. Rabbit and bovine thromboplastins were the most common and there are subtle differences in the tissue factors from different species. This makes little difference with wild-type human Factor VII but rabbit tissue factor binds poorly to some mutant human Factor VIIs. Well-known mutations in the Factor VII protein causing this effect are p.Arg139Gln and p.Arg364Gln (FVII Padua). In this case, the historical value was obtained using a rabbit thromboplastin and a near normal level is now obtained with a human thromboplastin.

A77.ii Genetic analysis will be useful to demonstrate the mutation. A Factor VII antigen measurement will generally produce a level similar to that obtained with human thromboplastin confirming that this is a protein where the dysfunctionality is specific to the type of thromboplastin used.

From a practical perspective, a Factor VII level of 43 U/dL would not cause any bleeding symptoms and cannot be responsible for the menorrhagia.

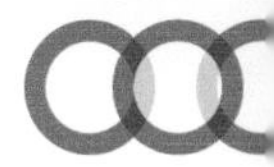

CASE 78

A 19-year-old male is referred to the outpatient clinic for investigation of thrombocytopenia. He is generally fit and well and has not had any surgery or invasive procedures. He does report that he often has nosebleeds and sometimes, these can last for up to 1 hour. He has recently noticed unexplained oral bleeding and often wakes up with a blood-stained pillow. He consulted his general practitioner (GP) who carried out a full blood count, the results of which are shown below. He has also been to see his dentist who has advised that a tooth extraction is required.

He has no other relevant past medical history and is not on any medication.

He has one younger brother who also has nosebleeds but has not been investigated. His mother reports no bleeding symptoms. His father died when he was a young child while undergoing surgery on his neck.

Initial investigations

	Test Results	Normal Range
Hb	145 g/L	[110–160]
WBC	7.1 × 10^9/L	[3.5–11]
Platelets	45 × 10^9/L	[150–400]
Prothrombin time	13 s	[12–16]
APTT	32 s	[26–36]
Factor VIII:C one stage	50 IU/dL	[50–150]
VWF:Ag	25 IU/dL	[45–175]
VWF:CB	8 U/dL	[45–175]
VWF:RCo	<10 IU/dL	[45–175]

QUESTIONS

Q78.i What is the differential diagnosis?

Q78.ii What further tests should be carried out?

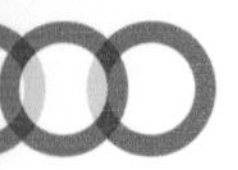

Case 78: ANSWERS

A78.i There is a significant deficiency of von Willebrand factor (VWF) and the functional assays (ristocetin co-factor [RCo] and collagen binding [CB]) are much lower than the antigen value with Ag:RCo and Ag:CB ratios well below 0.7. There is also a significant thrombocytopenia and so the most likely diagnosis that accounts for all these findings is type 2B von Willebrand disease (VWD). Less common is pseudo- or platelet-type VWD. Another type of VWD with thrombocytopenia due to an unrelated cause is also a possibility.

Type 2B VWD is caused by a gain of function mutation in the Gp1b binding region of the A1 domain of VWF. This results in the formation of VWF-platelet complexes which are removed from the circulation to prevent thrombosis. Clearance of VWF and platelets leads to a deficiency of both. In pseudo-VWD the gain of function mutation is in the Gp1b receptor on the platelet surface.

A78.ii The important investigations are VWF multimer analysis and a low-dose ristocetin-induced platelet aggregation (RIPA). The multimer analysis shows a relative loss of high-molecular weight multimers (HMWM) on a background of an overall reduction in VWF protein. In normal platelet-rich plasma aggregation is caused by ristocetin at 1.5 g/L but not at 0.5 g/L. In type 2B and pseudo-VWD the low dose of ristocetin does cause aggregation.

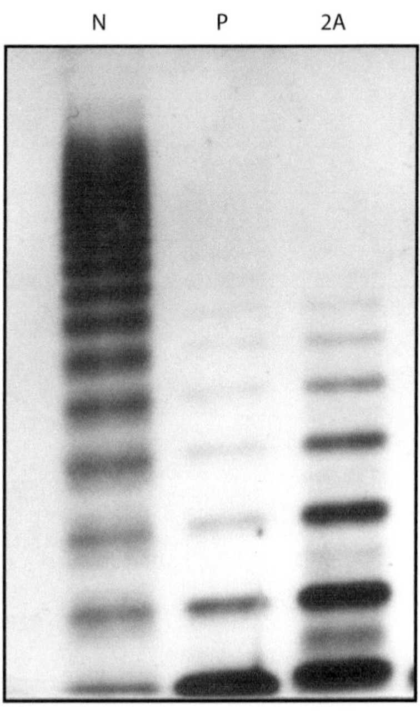

Figure 78a Von Willebrand factor (VWF) multimer analysis. N = normal plasma, P = patient, 2A = known case of type 2A.

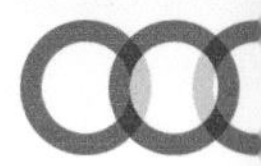

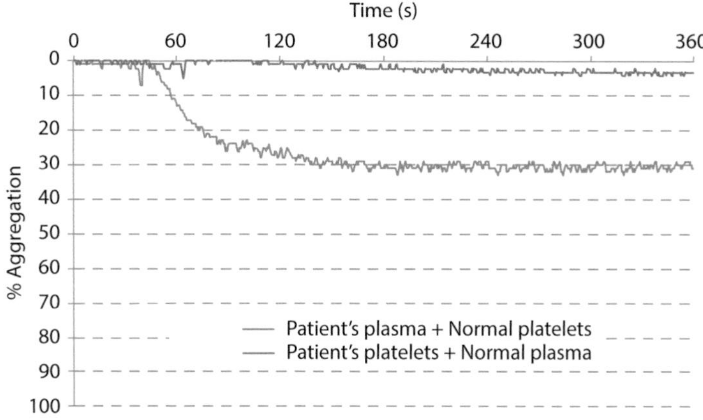

Figure 78b Platelet aggregation using low-dose ristocetin 0.5 g/L.

Case 78: QUESTIONS (Continued)

Q78.iii Report these additional results.

Q78.iv How would you manage the tooth extraction?

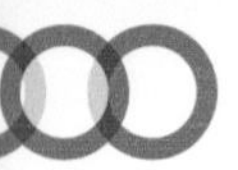

Case 78: ANSWERS (Continued)

A78.iii The way to differentiate these diagnoses is by mixing studies as shown in Figure 78b. As one would expect the combination of the patient's platelets and normal plasma, does not cause aggregation, but the patient's plasma is able to aggregate normal platelets. This shows that the defect is in the patient's plasma. In pseudo-VWD, the patient's platelet would aggregate even when mixed with normal plasma. The diagnosis is therefore type 2B VWD.

The diagnosis can be confirmed by genetic analysis of the *VWF* gene which will show a mutation affecting the A1 domain. This is inheritable as an autosomal dominant trait and will facilitate screening of the younger brother.

A78.iv There is an increased risk of bleeding during tooth extraction. Desmopressin is relatively contraindicated in type 2B VWD as the increase in endogenous VWF levels worsens the thrombocytopenia. Replacement therapy with VWF-containing concentrate is the treatment of choice with adjunctive therapy with tranexamic acid which can be given as a mouthwash. Platelets are also an effective treatment.

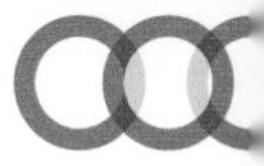

CASE 79

A 60-year-old man is admitted from the haematology clinic with gum bleeding. He has noticed a sudden onset of spontaneous bruising that started about a week previously. On examination, he has extensive bruising covering most of his leg (see the image below). The calf is tender and swollen.

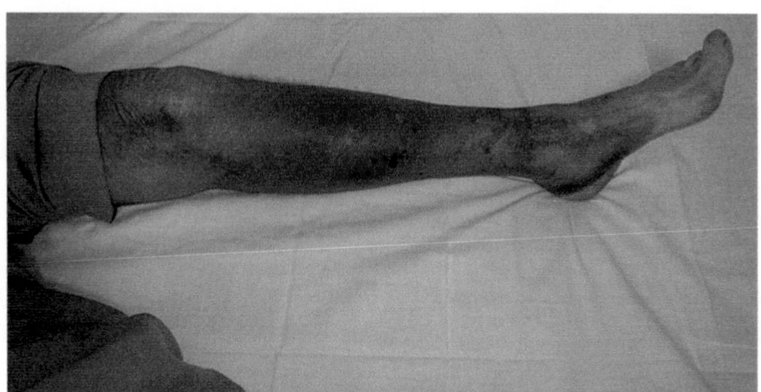

He has no significant past medical history and is not on any medication. Prior to the bruising, starting a week beforehand he was feeling fit and well. An ultrasound scan shows a large calf haematoma with no evidence of thrombosis. There is no family history of note.

Initial investigations

	Test Results	Normal Range
Hb	85 g/L	[110–160]
WBC	13.1×10^9/L	[3.5–11]
Platelets	325×10^9/L	[150–400]
Prothrombin time	13 s	[12–16]
APTT	82 s	[26–36]
APTT 50/50 mix	34/30	

QUESTIONS

Q79.i Discuss these results and list the most relevant subsequent investigations.

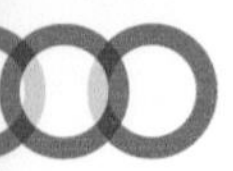

Case 79: ANSWERS

A79.i The sudden onset of bleeding symptoms with a marked prolongation of the activated partial thromboplastin time (APTT) in a man with no previous history of bleeding symptoms is very suggestive of an acquired inhibitor. The most likely diagnosis is, therefore, acquired haemophilia A. Although mixing studies are designed to screen for these, they may be time dependant and so can be unreliable if the standard incubation time for the APTT of 2–5 minutes is used. In order to allow for a time-dependant inhibitor to manifest, a 2-hour incubation is recommended prior to carrying out further investigations which should include a Factor VIII level and Bethesda assay for Factor VIII inhibitor. Acquired von Willebrand disease is a much less likely possibility.

The results of subsequent investigations performed with 2-hour incubation are shown below:

Further investigations

	Test Results	Normal Range
Factor VIII:C one stage	7 IU/dL	[50–150]
Bethesda assay	16 BU/mL	[<0.6]
VWF:Ag	65 IU/dL	[45–175]
VWF:CB	72 U/dL	[45–175]
VWF:RCo	67 IU/dL	[45–175]

Case 79: QUESTIONS (Continued)

Q79.ii What is the diagnosis? How would you treat the immediate bleeding symptoms? How can treatment be monitored in this setting?

Q79.iii What would be your long-term treatment strategy?

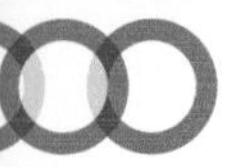

Case 79: ANSWERS (Continued)

A79.ii These results confirm the diagnosis of acquired haemophilia A. Unlike congenital haemophilia, the factor level does not correlate well with the risk of bleeding and in a symptomatic patient with drop in haemoglobin this should be treated as a severe bleeding disorder. Immediate bypassing therapy is the most effective way of stopping the bleeding and currently the preferred options are recombinant Factor VIIa or FEIBA (Factor VIII inhibitor bypassing agent). Newer therapies on the horizon include recombinant porcine Factor VIII and other bypassing agents. Prothrombin complex concentrate may also have some benefit but fresh frozen plasma (FFP) or Factor VIII concentrate are unlikely to be of benefit. There is no value in monitoring the Factor VIII level or the inhibitor in the early stages and if need be the bypassing therapy may be monitored by global haemostatic assays such as thromboelastography or thrombin generation.

Compartment syndrome is a not infrequent consequence of limb bleeding in this condition and the left leg should be monitored closely for any signs of this.

A79.iii In the longer term, immunosuppression will be required to clear the inhibitor. A variety of agents can be used in this condition with steroids alone or in combination with cyclophosphamide being most popular. Remission rates are 50%–80% with first-line therapy and on average it takes about 5 weeks before the Factor VIII level normalises and the inhibitor becomes undetectable.

About half of the cases of acquired haemophilia A are idiopathic. Additional investigations to rule out underlying causes such as malignancy and autoimmune disease should be considered.

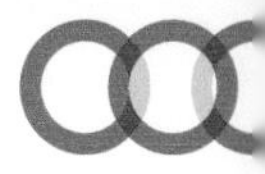

CASE 80

You are asked to see a 62-year-old man on the ward by the urologists. Since he underwent an uncomplicated transurethral resection of the prostate (TURP) the previous day, he has had continuous haematuria. On further questioning, he reports that he bled profusely after a tonsillectomy in his 20s and required a blood transfusion. At school, he was a promising footballer but had to give up because he would develop haematomas after playing. Last year, he underwent a tooth extraction and had to return to the dentist after 2 days because of ongoing bleeding. This settled after the dentist restitched the wound.

Initial investigations

	Test Results	Normal Range
Prothrombin time	10 s	[12–16]
APTT	37 s	[26–36]
Factor VIII:C one stage	47 IU/dL	[50–150]
Factor IX:C	105 IU/dL	[50–150]
Factor XI:C	85 IU/dL	[70–150]
DRVVT ratio	1.0	[0.8–1.1]
VWF:Ag	124 IU/dL	[45–175]
VWF:CB	115 U/dL	[45–175]
VWF:RCo	118 IU/dL	[45–175]

Platelet count and function testing showed no abnormalities.

QUESTIONS

Q80.i Comment on these results. What further tests would you do?

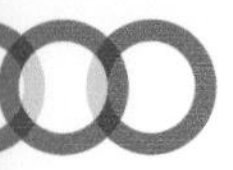

Case 80: ANSWERS

A80.i The initial tests show a slight prolongation of the activated partial thromboplastin time (APTT) and a very slight deficiency of Factor VIII. Note that the Factor VIII level is much lower than the von Willebrand factor levels and normally these two proteins tend to have similar levels as they circulate together in the plasma. Although a very mild haemophilia A could explain these bleeding symptoms the extent of the bleeding is out of keeping with the level of the deficiency. Therefore, the Factor VIII level should be rechecked using a two-stage or chromogenic assay.

Additional investigations

	Test Results	Normal Range
Factor VIII:C chromogenic assay	7 IU/dL	[50–150]

Case 80: QUESTIONS (Continued)

Q80.ii What is the explanation for these results?

Q80.iii What are the treatment options for the bleeding?

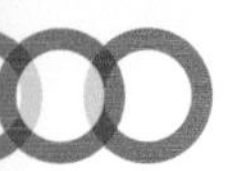

A80.ii The chromogenic assay gives a much lower level than the one stage and this value, although still within the range for classification as a mild haemophilia, is much more consistent with the bleeding history.

Both the chromogenic and two-stage assays have two endpoints. First, the contribution of Factor VIII to the formation of Factor Xa is allowed to go to completion. In the second part of the test, the amount of Factor Xa formed is measured using either a chromogenic substrate or in a clot-based assay that measures the amount of fibrin clot formed (two stage). In comparison, the one-stage assay measures the direct contribution of Factor VIII to the formation of fibrin clot.

In some cases of haemophilia A, the mutation leads to a molecule that has reduced stability and becomes inactivated more rapidly. In the one-stage assay, the relatively short incubation time does not allow this defect to become apparent and so the Factor VIII function appears relatively normal. In the other assays which allow the formation of Factor Xa to go to completion, the increased susceptibility to inactivation reveals the defect and gives a true, lower level that better reflects physiological function.

A80.iii With a factor level in single figures, replacement therapy with Factor VIII concentrate is required to stop the bleeding. In the future, it may be useful to assess the response to desmopressin as this may be a therapeutic option for minor bleeding. However, desmopressin tends to result in a three- to fivefold increase in levels that would barely take the level into the normal range in this case. In addition, desmopressin should be used with caution in patients over the age of 65 because of cardiovascular risk factors. Anti-fibrinolytics are a useful adjunct in these cases.

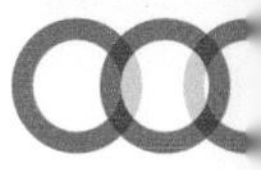

CASE 81

A 28-year-old woman requests screening for haemophilia A. She has a maternal male cousin who has haemophilia A. She is not sure what the severity is but knows that at the age of 35, he has already got chronic hip disease and has undergone several hip operations. He attends a haemophilia centre in another part of the United Kingdom. She recently got married and wishes to start a family. She has no bleeding symptoms herself and has no other significant medical problems. The aforementioned cousin is the only affected individual in the family.

Initial investigations

	Test Results	Normal Range
Prothrombin time	13 s	[12–16]
APTT	35 s	[26–36]
Factor VIII:C one stage	78 IU/dL	[50–150]
Factor IX:C	75 IU/dL	[50–150]
VWF:Ag	135 IU/dL	[45–175]
VWF:CB	125 U/dL	[45–175]
VWF:RCo	128 IU/dL	[45–175]

QUESTIONS

Q81.i Comment on these results. Are there any additional steps to be taken in determining her carrier status?

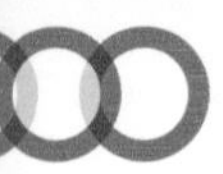

Case 81: ANSWERS

A81.i A normal factor level does not exclude carriership of haemophilia A or B. The only definitive way of establishing whether or not a woman is a carrier is through genetic analysis to look for the mutation that has previously been identified in the family. If the mutation has not been identified it is not possible to exclude carriership.

Having said that, measurement of factor levels is of some value. In a minority of carriers, the factor level will be reduced and females may have bleeding symptoms similar to that of a male with mild haemophilia. Normally, factor VIII (FVIII) and von Willebrand factor (VWF) should have similar levels and a FVIII:VWF ratio of <0.7 suggests that the patient is a carrier.

In the United Kingdom, the majority of haemophilia A patients has undergone genetic analysis and part of the consent process for this test is to ask patients if they are willing for their results to be used for the screening of relatives. It is normal practice in the United Kingdom to ask for further information about the index case in a pedigree from the haemophilia centre where the case is registered. In this case, the cousin's doctors stated that he had mild disease but that he also had a congenital abnormality of his hip that was unrelated to the haemophilia but required surgical intervention.

Correspondence with her cousin's haemophilia centre confirms that he is registered with mild haemophilia A and a Factor VIII: C level of 17 IU/dL. He has undergone genetic analysis and his report states

Hemizygous for c.541G>A, p.Val181Met. This mutation has been reported multiple times in association with mild haemophilia A and is consistent with the reported phenotype.

With this information, the patient undergoes genetic testing and is found to be heterozygous for c.541G>A, p.Val181Met.

She is reviewed in the clinic and is anxious because she has read about haemophilia and is aware that joint damage is a feature of the severe form of the disease. She wishes to avoid having a son with severe haemophilia A.

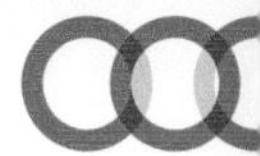

Case 81: QUESTIONS (Continued)

Q81.ii What would you say to her about her carrier status? What are the chances of any sons that she has having severe haemophilia A?

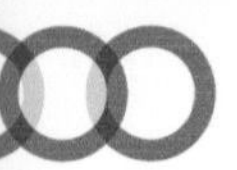

Case 81: ANSWERS (Continued)

A81.ii Genetic analysis confirms that she is a carrier of haemophilia A. However, she can be reassured that her cousin, and indeed all other previously reported cases with the same mutation, have had mild, and not severe, disease. Although any sons that she has will have a 50% chance of having haemophilia A and this will be of the mild type.

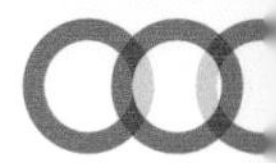

CASE 82

Two sisters (III.2 and III.3, as shown below) attend to be screened for haemophilia B. Their brother (III.1) and uncle (II.1) are known to have severe haemophilia B. Genetic analysis of the brother showed complete failure of amplification by polymerase chain reaction (PCR) of all *F9* exons indicating that the defect is a deletion of the whole *F9* gene. As large deletions cannot be directly detected by conventional sequencing techniques, a linkage analysis is carried out to detect a restriction fragment length polymorphism (RFLP) in intron 3 of *F9* that affects cleavage by the restriction endonuclease *XmnI*. Depending on whether the polymorphism is present or not, the band sizes amplified by PCR are 124 or 163 bp.

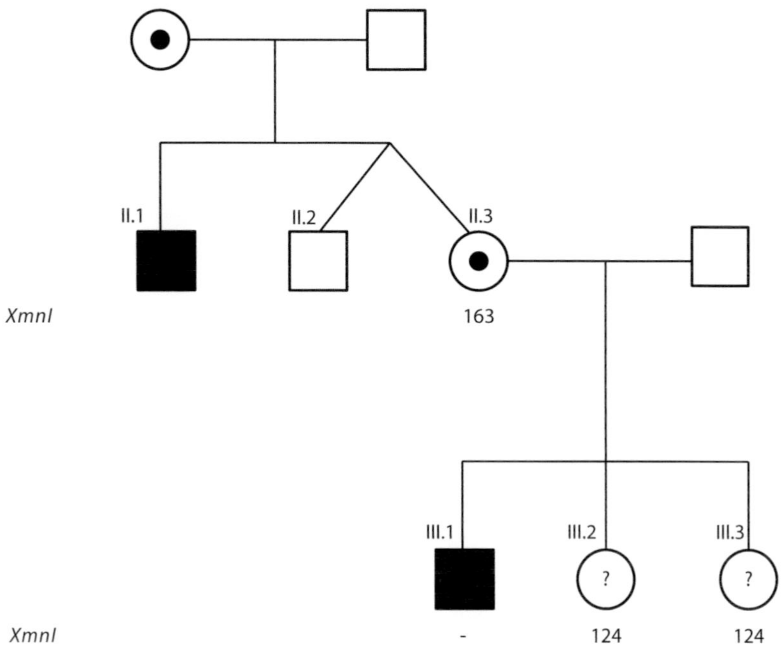

Pedigree with restriction fragment length polymorphism (RFLP) sizes on tested family members.

QUESTIONS

Q82.i Work out the sister's carrier status. How would you counsel them regarding the risk of having an affected child?

Q82.ii Regardless of your answer to Q82.i, assume that the sisters are both carriers and wish to avoid having a son with haemophilia. What are their options?

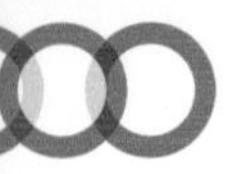

Case 82: ANSWERS

A82.i Both sisters are carriers. Their mother (II.3) is an obligate carrier as she has a son with haemophilia and a male relative in her generation with haemophilia. Therefore, she must carry the whole *F9* gene deletion. As this does not amplify her *XmnI* 163-bp band must be on the normal allele. Her daughters have not inherited this allele because they have a 124-bp band that must mark their normal paternal allele. Therefore, their maternal allele must have the whole gene deletion.

Note that a non-carrier daughter in this pedigree would have inherited normal alleles from both mother and father and would therefore have both bands (163/124).

The probability of a male foetus being affected is 0.5. The probability of a female foetus being a carrier is 0.5.

A82.ii Carriers of severe haemophilia are entitled to treatment on the National Health Services (NHS) if they wish to avoid having a son with haemophilia. This is provided through specialist fertility clinics. The main options are prenatal diagnosis by amniocentesis or chorionic-villous biopsy which may then be followed by termination of an affected foetus, or pre-implantation genetic diagnosis. The latter requires in vitro fertilization and embryos are then tested genetically to ascertain whether they carry the abnormal gene. This allows normal embryos to be selected for implantation.

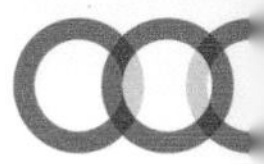

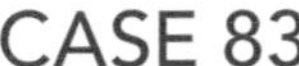

CASE 83

A 28-year-old man known to have mild haemophilia A is admitted following a road traffic accident. He has an expanding intra-abdominal haematoma and requires emergency laparotomy. He has a bleeding disorder registration card that gives his baseline Factor VIII levels as 20 by both the one-stage and chromogenic assays. He is able to tell you that he bleeds infrequently and has previously only received treatment for procedures or trauma-related bleeding. His last treatment was an infusion of desmopressin 3 years before for a dental extraction. Prior to that, he has received Factor VIII concentrate on a few occasions.

QUESTIONS

Q83.i Discuss how you would manage the haemophilia during the surgery.

At laparotomy, a hepatic tear is found and is repaired. Three days later, a post-treatment sample is taken and shows Factor VIII:C 23 IU/dL.

Q83.ii What investigations would you carry out?

Q83.iii What would your initial management be?

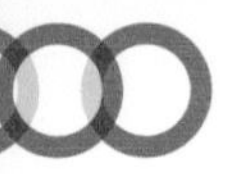

Case 83: ANSWERS

A83.i In most patients with mild haemophilia A, desmopressin induces an approximate threefold rise in factor levels. While this might be sufficient for a minor procedure, it would not provide adequate cover here. The Factor VIII level should be elevated to 100 IU/dL prior to surgery by means of an infusion of Factor VIII concentrate. Subsequently, the trough level should be maintained in the normal range until there is adequate wound healing. This is likely to be 7–14 days. This can be achieved by means of repeated bolus injections or a continuous infusion with regular monitoring of levels. This would require at least daily factor levels for the first few days.

A83.ii A lack of response to treatment suggests that a Factor VIII inhibitor has developed. The standard test for detection is a Bethesda assay.

A83.iii There is still a significant risk of bleeding and the factor level is likely to fall further as the inhibitor develops. Further replacement therapy will have no effect and so bypassing therapy with either recombinant Factor VIIa or Factor VIII inhibitor bypassing agent (FEIBA) is required. Prothrombin complex concentrate is a less effective alternative.

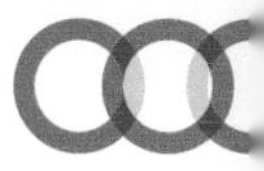

CASE 84

A 46-year-old man is seen in the accident and emergency (A&E) department with central chest pain. The pain settles spontaneously but there are ischaemic changes on the ECG and he is started on aspirin. The cardiologists wish to carry out an angiogram but have noticed some abnormalities on the coagulation screen. The patient is a heavy smoker but has no other medical history. He is aware that his sister has some sort of blood disorder that was diagnosed following a pulmonary embolism (PE) when she was aged 32. She is on lifelong warfarin.

Initial investigations

	Test Results	Normal Range
Prothrombin time	13 s	[12–16]
APTT	32 s	[26–36]
Thrombin time	34 s	[10–14]
Reptilase time	31 s	[10–14]

QUESTIONS

Q84.i What further investigations would you carry out?

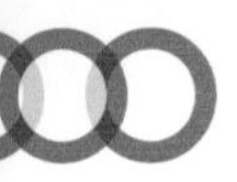

Case 84: ANSWERS

A84.i Common causes of a prolonged thrombin time (TT) are heparin contamination and a deficiency of fibrinogen. As the TT is very sensitive to heparin, it is quite possible for it to be prolonged without a rise in activated partial thromboplastin time (APTT). The reptilase time is insensitive to heparin and so this possibility is excluded because the reptilase time is also prolonged. Other causes include an inhibitor of fibrinogen cleavage, such as fibrinogen degradation products, or a low albumin that causes an artificial prolongation.

Measurement of fibrinogen function, which is most commonly done by a Clauss assay, and protein level with an antigen assay are required.

Further investigations

	Test results	Normal Range
Fibrinogen Clauss	0.6 g/L	[1.5–4.0]
Fibrinogen antigen	2.8 g/L	[1.5–4.0]

Case 84: QUESTIONS (Continued)

Q84.ii What is the diagnosis and what advice would you give the cardiologists?

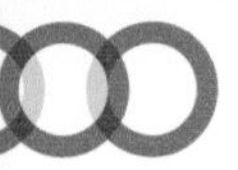

Case 84: ANSWERS (Continued)

A84.ii These results are indicative of a dysfibrinogenaemia as the activity level is markedly reduced while the protein level is normal. Dysfibrinogenaemias may be associated with bleeding or thrombotic complications and very rarely both in the same family. The family history warrants further investigation. In this case, it transpired that the sister had genetic analysis which showed a mutation in the *FGA* gene that had previously been described in association with thrombosis. This is consistent with the decision to place her on lifelong warfarin after a single thrombotic episode. Therefore, the risk for the angiogram was primarily one of thrombosis rather than bleeding. Heparin was used at a therapeutic dose and there were no complications. As the patient does not himself have a history of venous thrombosis, he does not require anti-coagulation at the moment. However, he should stop smoking and one would need to consider using thromboprophylaxis during periods of increased risk in the future.

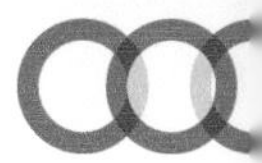

CASE 85

A 25-year-old man from Poland is referred following a routine blood test that shows an abnormality on the clotting screen. He is fit and well and on no medication. He has had three dental extractions which have all been uneventful. He recalls that his sister was diagnosed with haemophilia some years ago in Poland. The sister is now in her late 20s and has had two children without any bleeding complications. As far as he knows, the sister has not had any bleeding symptoms.

Initial investigations

	Test Results	Normal Range
Prothrombin time	11 s	[12–16]
APTT	172 s	[26–36]
APTT 50/50 mix	33/32	
Thrombin time	14 s	[12–16]
Factor VIII:C one stage	106 IU/dL	[50–150]
Factor VIII:C chromogenic	116 IU/dL	[50–150]
Factor IX:C	100 IU/dL	[50–150]
Factor XI:C	84 IU/dL	[70–150]
DRVVT ratio	0.9	[0.8–1.1]
Normalised SCT ratio	1.1	[<1.16]
Lupus interpretation	Lupus negative	
VWF:Ag	102 IU/dL	[45–175]
VWF:CB	100 U/dL	[45–175]
VWF:RCo	108 IU/dL	[45–175]

QUESTIONS

Q85.i Comment on these results. Consider the most likely diagnosis and what advice would you give to this man if he needed to have major surgery.

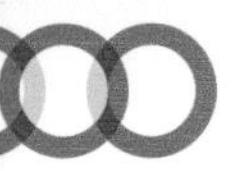

Case 85: ANSWERS

A85.i There is a marked prolongation of the activated partial thromboplastin time (APTT) that fully corrects on mixing studies. This suggests a deficiency in the intrinsic pathway. However, he has normal levels of all the clinically relevant intrinsic factors and there is no history of bleeding either in himself or his sister. Therefore, the most likely diagnosis is a clinically insignificant abnormality in the contact system. Although further investigation is not essential in this case, the Factor XII level was found to be <1 U/dL. The patient had mistakenly assumed that because his sister had been found to have an abnormality after testing in a haemophilia centre that was the diagnosis.

The patient can be reassured that there is no risk of bleeding with a contact factor deficiency and indeed, these are of no proven clinical significance. No specific treatment is required prior to surgery. Note that the extent of the prolongation of the APTT does not correlate with the risk of bleeding. Thus, a patient with a very high APTT is not necessarily more likely to bleed than a patient with a slightly high APTT.

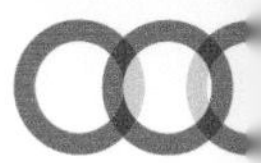

CASE 86

A 65-year-old man presents with a 4-month history of unexplained bruising, gum bleeding and prolonged bleeding after minor trauma. This has been getting progressively worse and he is admitted in A&E with a nosebleed that lasted for 2 hours.

He also reports severe back pain and tenderness over his chest wall on the right side. He is very tired and finds that he becomes short of breath after walking upstairs. Prior to this illness, he was fit and well and had undergone surgery on three occasions without any bleeding problems. He is not on any medication.

Initial investigations

	Test Results	Normal Range
Prothrombin time	30 s	[12–16]
APTT	85 s	[26–36]
Prothrombin time 50/50 mix	25/14	
APTT 50/50 mix	62/32	
Thrombin time	14 s	[12–16]
Fibrinogen Clauss	2.6 g/L	[1.5–4.0]
DRVVT ratio	1.0	[0.8–1.1]
Normalised SCT ratio	1.0	[<1.16]
Lupus interpretation	Lupus negative	
Hb	75 g/L	[110–160]
MCV	87 fL	[80–100]
WBC	7.1×10^9/L	[3.5–11]
Platelets	110×10^9/L	[150–400

QUESTIONS

Q86.i Provide a differential diagnosis.

Q86.ii Outline a plan of investigation focusing on those most useful in making the diagnosis.

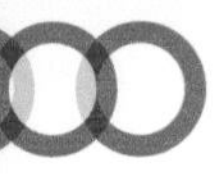

Case 86: ANSWERS

A86.i The history is that of an acquired coagulopathy. There are marked prolongations of clotting times which do not correct on mixing. This suggests an acquired inhibitor. Two tests for lupus are negative and so an anti-phospholipid antibody is effectively excluded. A consumptive coagulopathy is unlikely as the fibrinogen is normal and the platelet count is only mildly reduced. There is, however, a marked normocytic anaemia and along with symptoms of bone pain, this makes myeloma the likely diagnosis. Metastatic cancer with disseminated intravascular coagulation (DIC) or a specific factor inhibitor is a less likely possibility.

A86.ii A myeloma screen is the key investigation and in this case confirmed the diagnosis.

Subsequently, protein electrophoresis showed an IgM paraprotein with immunoparesis. Chest x-ray shows lytic lesions in the ribs on the right side and a spine x-ray shows vertebral collapse.

Despite packing of the nose, there is recurrent nosebleeds and fresh bruising the day after admission.

Case 86: QUESTIONS (Continued)

Q86.iii How would you manage the bleeding symptoms?

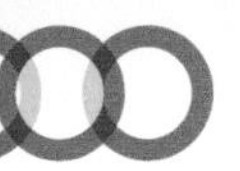

A86.iii Paraproteins often have a non-specific inhibitory effect on coagulation factors that leads to clinically significant bleeding. Usually, these symptoms do not require specific treatment and standard treatment of the myeloma with subsequent reduction in paraprotein levels is sufficient to alleviate the bleeding symptoms. In this case, however, the bleeding symptoms require specific treatment. Replacement therapy with fresh-frozen plasma (FFP) is ineffective because the paraprotein simply swamps any exogenous factor. Bypassing therapy with, for example, prothrombin complex concentrate or Factor VIII inhibitor bypassing agent (FEIBA), will have some effect but carries a risk of thrombosis in cancer patients. The most effective treatment is often removal of the paraprotein with plasma exchange.

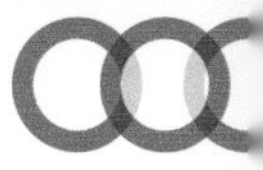

CASE 87

A 24-year-old woman presents with excessive per vaginal (PV) bleeding a week after giving birth to her first child. She has no significant past medical history and is not on any medication. Antenatally, she had normal blood tests and the pregnancy was uneventful. She had a normal, non-instrumental vaginal delivery and was discharged on the first post-partum day with little lochia.

Shortly after admission, she has a fit and requires treatment with anti-convulsants.

Initial investigations

	Test Results	Normal Range
Prothrombin time	12 s	[12–16]
APTT	26 s	[26–36]
Thrombin time	14 s	[12–16]
Fibrinogen Clauss	2.6 g/L	[1.5–4.0]
Hb	75 g/L	[110–160]
MCV	87 fL	[80–100]
WBC	7.1×10^9/L	[3.5–11]
Platelets	11×10^9/L	[150–400]

QUESTIONS

Q87.i What is the most likely diagnosis? List the key investigations.

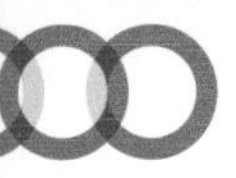

Case 87: ANSWERS

A87.i The main abnormalities are anaemia and severe thrombocytopenia with a normal coagulation screen. As we know that the platelet count was normal prior to delivery, the most likely diagnosis is thrombotic thrombocytopenic purpura. This condition has an increased incidence in the peri-partum and would explain the neurological symptoms. Other acquired causes of thrombocytopenia would generally be associated with abnormal coagulation as part of a consumptive coagulopathy.

Additional investigations

	Test Results	Normal Range
ADAMTS13 activity level	<5%	[60–123]
IgG anti-ADAMTS13 level	44%	[<6%]

The key investigations should look for other features of the condition. Micro-angiopathic haemolytic anaemia can be demonstrated by the presence of red cell fragments on blood film examination and raised bilirubin levels. The pentad of features classically seen in full-blown forms of the disease include renal impairment and so measurement of U&E is essential. The diagnosis can be confirmed by measurement of ADAMTS13 levels and antibody levels.

Case 87: QUESTIONS (Continued)

Q87.ii How is ADAMTS13 (a disintegrin and metalloproteinase with a thrombospondin type 1 motif, member 13) measured (i.e. what are the principles of the assay)?

Q87.iii How would you manage this case?

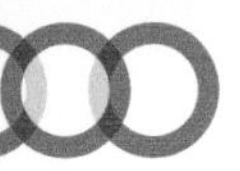

Case 87: ANSWERS (Continued)

A87.ii ADAMTS13 cleaves the high-molecular weight forms of von Willebrand factor (VWF) which are primarily responsible for its collagen binding function. Activity assays measure the residual amount of collagen binding function using an enzyme-linked immunosorbent assay (ELISA). Alternatively, activity can be assessed by measuring the ability of the patient sample to cleave a short peptide containing the residues around the VWF cleavage site. Antigen measurements can be used to measure the enzyme concentration. Inhibitory antibodies can differentiate between the congenital and acquired forms of the disease. Congenital deficiency can present in adulthood and be unmasked by pregnancy.

A87.iii The cornerstone of treatment is plasma exchange. Solvent detergent plasma is preferred to reduce the risk of transmission of transfusion associated infections and allergic reactions, but if not available then fresh-frozen plasma (FFP) or cryosupernatant may be used. Daily plasma exchanges should be continued until a minimum of 2 days after normalisation of the platelet count.

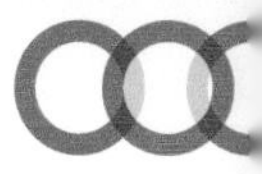

CASE 88

An 85-year-old woman with Alzheimer's disease is referred to the haematology clinic for investigation of unexplained bruising and oral bleeding of recent onset. She has been looked after in the same nursing home for the last 5 years. In the last 6 months, her family had noticed on numerous occasions unexplained bruises up to 20 cm across and suspected the staff in the home of physical abuse. She is unable to give a coherent history. According to the general practitioner (GP) records, there is no history of unexpected bleeding prior to 6 months ago and she had five deliveries without any abnormal bleeding.

Initial investigations

	Test Results	Normal Range
Prothrombin time	12 s	[12–16]
APTT	26 s	[26–36]
Thrombin time	14 s	[12–16]
Fibrinogen Clauss	4.6 g/L	[1.5–4.0]
Hb	115 g/L	[110–160]
MCV	87 fL	[80–100]
WBC	7.1×10^9/L	[3.5–11]
Platelets	350×10^9/L	[150–400

QUESTIONS

Q88.i What additional investigations would you request?

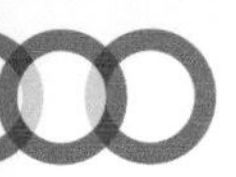

Case 88: ANSWERS

A88.i The history is suggestive of an acquired bleeding disorder. Although physical abuse might account for the bruising, it would not explain the oral bleeding. The normal clotting screen effectively excludes acquired haemophilia. Acquired von Willebrand disease is a very unlikely possibility as it is very uncommon and would normally be associated with a low Factor VIII level and a prolonged activate partial thromboplastin time (APTT). Nevertheless, von Willebrand factor levels should be checked. The most likely diagnosis is an acquired platelet dysfunction and so tests of platelet function such as platelet aggregometry and platelet nucleotide assays are required.

Additional investigations

	Test Results	Normal Range
Factor VIII:C one stage	185 IU/dL	[50–150]
VWF:Ag	155 IU/dL	[45–175]
VWF:CB	168 IU/dL	[45–175]
VWF:RCo	172 IU/dL	[45–175]

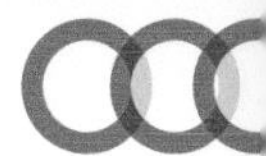

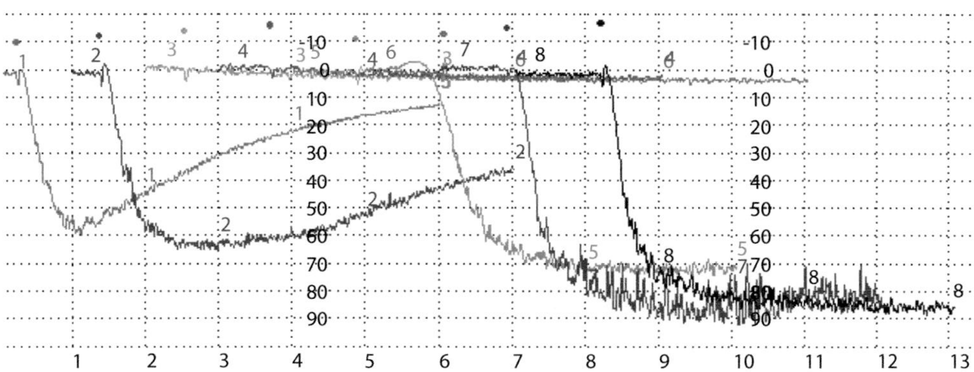

Platelet aggregometry.

Lane	Agonist	% Aggregation at 5 Minutes
1	ADP 2 μM	0
2	ADP 5 μM	0
3	Adrenaline 3 μM	0
4	Adrenaline 10 μM	0
5	Collagen 2 μg/L	67
6	Arachidonic acid 1 mM	0
7	Ristocetin 1.5 g/L	6
8	U46619 1 μM	0

Case 88: QUESTIONS (Continued)

Q88.ii Report the additional investigations. What is the most likely explanation for the bruising?

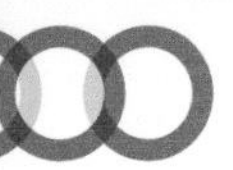

Case 88: ANSWERS (Continued)

A88.ii Acquired von Willebrand disease is excluded by the normal levels. The aggregometry traces are abnormal with an absence of the response to arachidonic acid being the most significant abnormality. There is also a reduced response to adenosine diphosphate (ADP) and adrenaline. The most likely explanation is that the patient is taking aspirin or a similar medication. In this case, it subsequently became clear that another resident in the care home had been administering aspirin to treat low back pain.

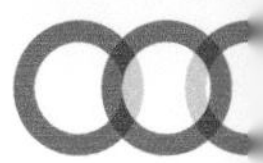

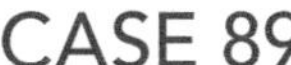

CASE 89

A 22-year-old girl presents with a sudden onset of pain and swelling in her left leg that has been getting gradually worse over the previous 5 days. There is no significant past medical history or family history and her only medication is a combined oral contraceptive that she has been taking for 3 years. She has been smoking 10 cigarettes a day for 5 years.

The D-dimer is elevated at 2647 ng/mL [<130] and a Doppler ultrasound scan shows an extensive deep vein thrombosis (DVT) involving several deep veins in the thigh and the internal and external iliac veins.

QUESTIONS

Q89.i How would you treat this patient? What is the value of thrombophilia testing in this situation?

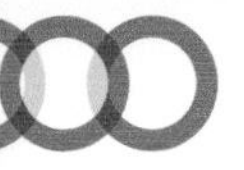

Case 89: ANSWERS

A89.i Oestrogen-containing contraceptives are a risk factor for venous thrombosis. There is some evidence that smoking may also be a minor risk factor. In this case, the thrombosis is most likely to be provoked by these factors.

The standard treatment for this patient would be 3–6 months of anti-coagulation. Iliofemoral DVT has a particularly poor prognosis with high rates of recurrence and post-thrombotic syndrome. Studies have shown that these outcomes can be improved by catheter-directed thrombolysis using low dose of thrombolytics such as tissue plasminogen activator (tPA) over a couple of days. However, the bleeding risk is significantly higher on thrombolysis and this needs to be carefully monitored, so safety may prevent its use in a non-specialist setting.

Assuming that she is able to stop smoking and the oral contraceptive is discontinued, anti-coagulation could be discontinued after 3–6 months. Elevated D-dimer levels after the discontinuation of anti-coagulation are associated with an increased risk of recurrence. There is little value in repeating the ultrasound scan after completing treatment as many patients have residual abnormalities and this does not add anything further to estimating the risk of recurrence. There is a reasonable argument for long-term anti-coagulation in patients with extensive initial thrombus if the bleeding risk with anti-coagulation is low, as it would be in this case.

Thrombophilia testing is most likely to reveal pertinent findings in patients with a first episode of unprovoked thrombosis below the age of 40 or those with a positive family history. Although this patient is under 40, there are provoking factor(s) and so thrombophilia testing is unlikely to be of value in this setting.

She consults a doctor who carries out a thrombophilia screen from which the only result of interest is that she is heterozygous for Factor V Leiden. She is placed on indefinite anti-coagulation using warfarin with a target international normalised ratio (INR) range of 2.0–3.0, and the oral contraceptive is stopped.

Five years later, she is complaining of intermittent pain and swelling in her left leg such that by the end of the day she finds it difficult to stand. Data from the anti-coagulant clinic shows that her time in therapeutic range was 45% in the first year of anti-coagulation and has been 65% since. The D-dimer level is now 450 ng/mL and a further scan shows chronic residual thrombus with recanalization and some varicosities in the proximal veins.

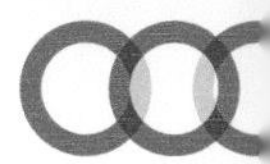

Q89.ii What is the significance of heterozygosity for Factor V Leiden in this case? How would you manage the symptoms of pain and swelling in the leg?

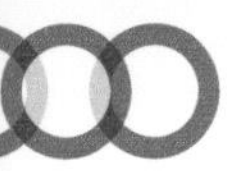

Case 89: ANSWERS

A89.ii Heterozygosity for Factor V Leiden has no influence on the risk of recurrence after a first thrombosis. In some cases, where it is likely to have been a significant causative factor there might be value in screening of family relatives. In this case, it is unlikely to have been a major causative factor and so the risk of thrombosis in first degree relatives of the index case is increased whether or not they have Factor V Leiden.

Post-thrombotic syndrome occurs (PTS) in about 25% of patients after a first episode of DVT. Although anti-coagulation reduces the risk of this complication, the use of graduated compression stockings is of more value in treating the symptoms. However, there is conflicting data on whether graduated compression stockings reduce the incidence of PTS after the initial episode.

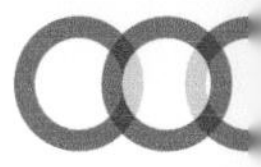

CASE 90

A 28-year-old male presents with a 1-week history of gradually increasing pain and swelling of his left leg as shown in the below image. Over the previous 24 hours he has coughed up blood-stained sputum on 2 occasions. His father died suddenly of unknown causes at the age of 46 and his 27-year-old sister suffered a deep vein thrombosis during pregnancy.

Initial investigations

(Hb)	134 g/L
(WBC)	7.9 × 10^9/L
Platelets	313 × 10^9/L
(PT)	12 seconds (control 11–13 seconds)
(APTT)	34 seconds (control 30–40 seconds)

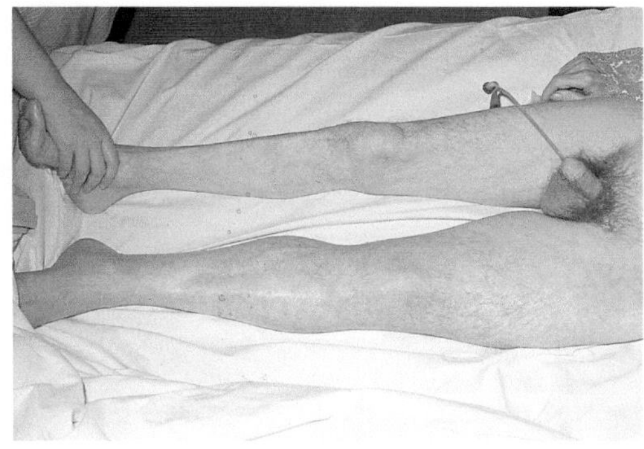

QUESTIONS

Q90.i What is the diagnosis and how would you confirm it?

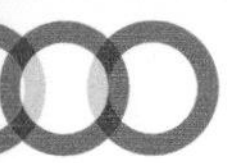

Case 90: ANSWERS (Continued)

A90.i He has marked swelling of the whole of the left leg suggesting a deep vein thrombosis. As the clinical suspicion is high a D-dimer is not of diagnostic value and a Doppler ultrasound should be done to confirm this. A venogram is an alternative more invasive test. The illustration shows the presence of thrombus in the deep veins of the calf and popliteal region with extensive collaterals. The history of haemoptysis suggests a pulmonary embolism. This may be confirmed by a ventilation/perfusion isotope scan but pulmonary angiography should be considered as he may be a candidate for surgery

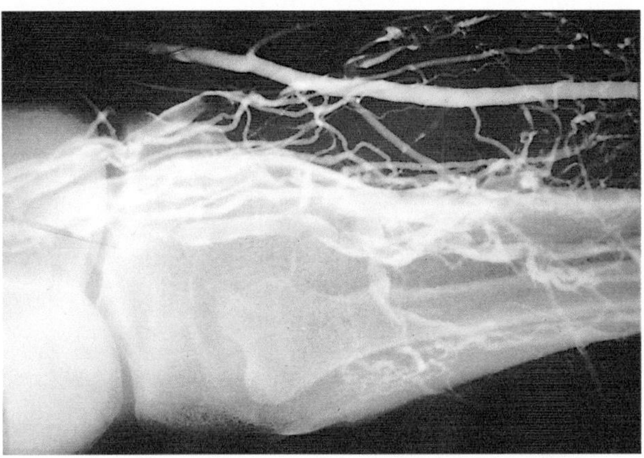

Case 90: QUESTIONS (Continued)

Q90.ii What additional investigations should be performed?

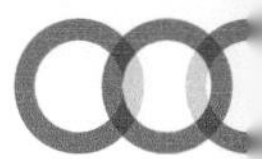

Case 90: ANSWERS (Continued)

A90.ii The family history is suggestive of an inheritable thrombophilia. He should be screened for the presence of a familial or acquired hypercoagulable state after the initial course of anti-coagulation is completed. Thrombophilia screening in the acute setting does not give reliable results.

He is treated with rivaroxaban for 3 months and makes a good recovery. A thrombophilia screen is carried out off anti-coagulation.

Results from thrombophilia screen

Prothrombin time	13 s	[11-13]
APTT	36 s	[30-40]
Thrombin time	14 s	[12-16]
Factor VIII:C one stage	165 iu/dL	[50-150]
Protein C:Ac	131 iu/dL	[70-140]
Antithrombin:Ac	95 iu/dL	[79-121]
Protein S:Free bioassay	105 iu/dL	[70-150]
Protein S:Free antigen	122 iu/dL	[60-140]
Protein S:Total antigen	140 iu/dL	[70-140]
DRVVT ratio	1.1	[0.8-1.1]
DRVVT correction	5%	[<10%]
Normalised SCT ratio	1.0	[<1.16]
APCr ratio	0.7	>2.0
Factor V Leiden	Homozygous Q/Q	
Prothrombin 3'UTR variant	Normal G/G	

Case 90: QUESTIONS (Continued)

Q90.iii What is the diagnosis? How would you manage this case? Is there any advice you would offer to his sister?

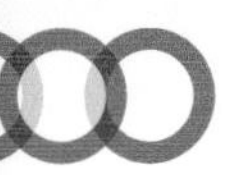

A90.iii He is homozygous for the Factor V Leiden (FVL) variant. This also explains the very low activated protein C resistance ratio (APCr).

Heterozygosity for FVL occurs in about 3% of the population and is a low risk factor for venous thrombosis (approximately 4-fold increased risk) it does not have a significant effect on the risk of recurrence as the hazard ratio for recurrence of thrombosis is 1.4. Homozygosity occurs in about 1 in 5000 and carries a much greater risk of thrombosis (approximately 20-fold increased risk). The risk of recurrence does appear to be increased with severe thrombophilias and so long-term anti-coagulation would be recommended in this case.

There is a 0.25 probability of his sister also being homozygous for Factor V Leiden and so she should be offered screening. Should she turn out to be homozygous then long-term anti-coagulation would need to be considered. However, if she is heterozygous then thromboprophylaxis during periods of increased risk, rather than on-going anti-coagulation, would be appropriate.

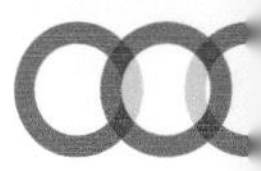

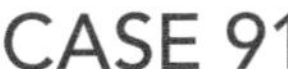

CASE 91

A 55-year-old woman is referred to the haematology clinic for advice regarding the use of hormone replacement therapy (HRT). She developed a pulmonary embolism aged 35 after internal fixation of a fracture of femur and was anti-coagulated for 6 months. She made a full recovery and has no residual respiratory symptoms.

She has severe post-menopausal symptoms that are preventing her from working.

QUESTIONS

Q91.i What advice would you give regarding the use of HRT in this case?

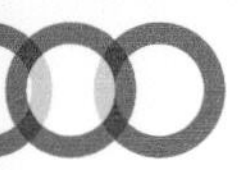

Case 91: ANSWERS

A91.i As with other oestrogen-containing medications, HRT is associated with an increased risk of thrombosis. However, this risk may be outweighed by other benefits such as a reduction in the risk of osteoporosis. In younger women, in particular, all-cause mortality may be reduced in those on HRT. In this case, the absolute risk of recurrence is low as the single thrombotic episode was associated with a transient provoking factor.

The thrombotic risk with HRT is affected by the dose of oestrogen and route of administration. In this case, a preparation with a low dose of oestrogen or a transdermal preparation would be preferable. However, if these do not provide adequate symptom relief then the use of higher strength HRT could be considered after a frank explanation of the risks and benefits.

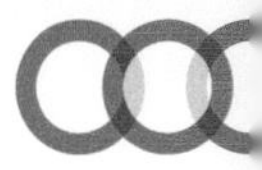

CASE 92

A 31-year-old woman is referred from the obstetrician following a miscarriage at 25 weeks. There is a history of two previous miscarriages at 10 and 22 weeks of gestation and one normal vaginal delivery. There is no personal or family history of thrombosis and there is no other past medical history of note. A thrombophilia screen was carried out 6 months after the miscarriage and is shown below

Thrombophilia screen

	Test Results	Normal Range
Prothrombin time	11 s	[12–16]
APTT	31 s	[26–36]
Thrombin time	15 s	[12–16]
Factor VIII:C one stage	65 IU/dL	[50–150]
Protein C:Ac	85 IU/dL	[70–140]
Anti-thrombin:Ac	92 IU/dL	[79–121]
Protein S:Free bioassay	40 IU/dL	[70–150]
Protein S:Free antigen	78 IU/dL	[60–140]
Protein S:Total antigen	85 IU/dL	[70–140]
DRVVT ratio	0.9	[0.8–1.1]
Normalised SCT ratio	1.1	[<1.16]
Lupus interpretation	Lupus negative	
Factor V Leiden	Heterozygous for Arg506Gln	
Prothrombin 3′UTR variant	Normal G/G	

QUESTIONS

Q92.i How would you interpret these results? What additional tests would you do?

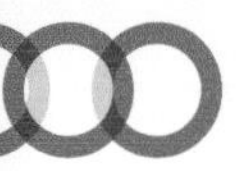

Case 92: ANSWERS

A92.i Protein S levels are reduced during pregnancy and so in this case, testing has been correctly deferred until well after the initial event.

Protein S is bound by C4b-binding protein and it is the free (non-bound) fraction that is functionally active. Total protein S levels are measured by an antigen assay while the free fraction can be measured by both coagulation-based bioassay and antigen assays using an antibody specific for the free fraction. Functional assays are the most sensitive and are able to detect all types of protein S deficiency particularly type II deficiency which may have normal levels with the antigen-based assays. However, functional assays can give falsely reduced levels in the presence of Factor V Leiden. There are two ways around this. Increased plasma dilution may be used to negate the effect of Factor V Leiden or molecular analysis of the *PROS1* gene can be carried out as this will demonstrate a missense mutation in nearly all cases of type II deficiency.

In this case, only the functional protein S assay is reduced and the patient is heterozygous for Factor V Leiden which is the most likely explanation for the low level.

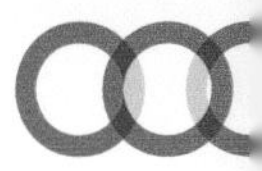

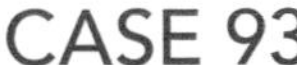

CASE 93

A 30-year-old woman is referred from the antenatal clinic as she is 8 weeks into her first pregnancy. She has a history of unprovoked proximal deep vein thrombosis (DVT) occurring 6 years previously. She was anti-coagulated for 6 months and subsequently diagnosed with anti-thrombin deficiency. Her only treatment since then has been prophylactic doses of low-molecular weight heparin prior to flying.

Initial investigations

	Test Results	Normal Range
Anti-thrombin:Ac	45 IU/dL	[80–120]
Anti-thrombin:Ag	55 IU/dL	[85–130]

QUESTIONS

Q93.i How would you manage the risk of thrombosis in this case?

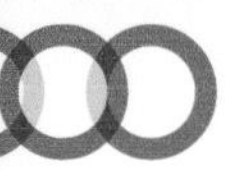

Case 93: ANSWERS

A93.i These results are indicative of a type 1 anti-thrombin deficiency. The risk of thrombosis rises steadily during pregnancy although there is normally no change in antithrombin levels. This patient requires thromboprophylaxis during pregnancy and the main issue is whether this should be for the whole or part of the pregnancy. During early pregnancy, the use of anti-coagulants is associated with an increased risk of bleeding and so this decision needs to be made in conjunction with the obstetricians. If there are obstetric concerns regarding the risk of bleeding a reasonable compromise here is to initiate a prophylactic dose of low-molecular weight heparin in the third trimester. The medication can be discontinued when labour commences and restarted after delivery. If there is no post-partum bleeding, the thromboprophylaxis should be continued for a minimum of 6 weeks after delivery.

There is considerable debate regarding the value of anti-Xa monitoring with no clear evidence indicating what anti-Xa level to aim for. Antithrombin deficiency might be associated with resistance to heparins and so monitoring is generally advocated in these cases.

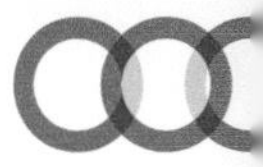

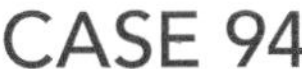

CASE 94

A 16-year-old boy is referred for screening. He has no significant personal history but there is a strong family history of thrombosis. His father experienced an unprovoked pulmonary embolism (PE) in age 12 and suffered a recurrence in age 23. He was diagnosed with anti-thrombin deficiency and is now on lifelong anti-coagulation with warfarin. His paternal grandfather had a fatal PE at the age of 30.

Initial investigations

	Test Results	Normal Range
Anti-thrombin:Ac	55 IU/dL	[80–120]
Anti-thrombin:Ag	125 IU/dL	[85–130]

QUESTIONS

Q94.i Are there any further tests that you would carry out? How would you treat this case?

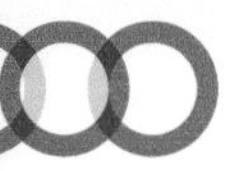

Case 94: ANSWERS

A94.i The marked discrepancy between the anti-thrombin activity and antigen levels indicates a type II deficiency. In this case, molecular analysis confirmed heterozygosity for a mutation in the anti-thrombin gene that had previously been described in a family with thrombosis at an early age. With type II deficiency, the risk of thrombosis at an early age can be very high and this is one of the few indications for initiation of anti-coagulation before the first thrombotic event. Anti-coagulation with warfarin to the standard target International Normalised Ratio (INR) range of 2–3 is effective.

Following confirmation of type II anti-thrombin deficiency by molecular analysis prophylactic anti-coagulation was recommended. The patient refused and developed a deep vein thrombosis (DVT), aged 20, following which he was maintained on lifelong anti-coagulation.

Five years later, he suffered a compound fracture of his tibia that required internal fixation.

Case 94: QUESTIONS (Continued)

Q94.ii How would you cover the surgery?

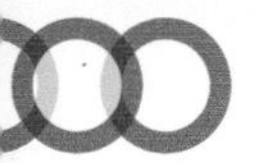

A94.ii The risk of further thrombosis is high and bridging is required. However, heparin in any form may be ineffective in type II deficiency because it is an indirect anti-coagulant acting via anti-thrombin. In type I anti-thrombin deficiency, this may be overcome by using high doses of heparin but in type II disease anti-thrombin concentrate is required in combination with heparin or low-molecular weight heparin.

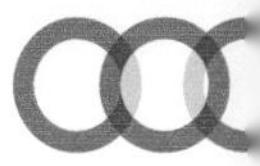

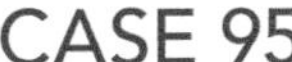

CASE 95

A 32-year-old woman is referred from the gynaecology clinic having had a miscarriage at 18 weeks. There is no other past medical history and no significant family history. A thrombophilia screen carried out in the gynaecology clinic gives the following results.

Results from thrombophilia screen

	Test Results	Normal Range
Prothrombin time	15 s	[12–16]
APTT	31 s	[26–36]
Thrombin time	14 s	[12–16]
Factor VIII:C one stage	105 IU/dL	[50–150]
Protein C:Ac	135 IU/dL	[70–140]
Anti-thrombin:Ac	102 IU/dL	[79–121]
Protein S:Free bioassay	120 IU/dL	[70–150]
Protein S:Free antigen	124 IU/dL	[60–140]
Protein S:Total antigen	135 IU/dL	[70–140]
DRVVT ratio	1.4	[0.8–1.1]
DRVVT correction	12%	[<10%]
Normalised SCT ratio	1.1	[<1.16]
Lupus interpretation	Lupus positive	
Factor V Leiden	Normal R/R	
Prothrombin 3′UTR variant	Normal G/G	

QUESTIONS

Q95.i What advice would you offer? Are there any additional investigations that you would carry out?

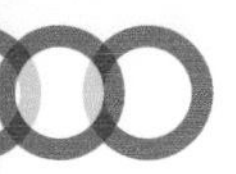

Case 95: ANSWERS

A95.i The finding of a weakly positive lupus anti-coagulant in isolation is of doubtful significance and not diagnostic of anti-phospholipid antibody syndrome (APLS), although the history is consistent with this condition. The tests should be repeated after 12 weeks with measurement of anti-phospholipid antibodies.

The blood tests are repeated after 3 months with some additional investigations.

Repeated anti-phospholipid tests

	Test Results	Normal Range
DRVVT ratio	1.5	[0.8–1.1]
DRVVT correction	25%	[<10%]
Normalised SCT ratio	1.1	[<1.16]
Lupus interpretation	Lupus positive	
Cardiolipin IgG	35 GPLU/mL	[0–10]
β2 glycoprotein 1 antibodies	Strong positive	

Case 95: QUESTIONS (Continued)

Q95.ii What advice would you now give regarding future pregnancies?

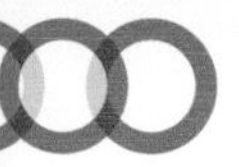

Case 95: ANSWERS (Continued)

A95.ii These tests are now diagnostic of APLS. Although this patient has only had a single miscarriage, patients who are triple positive have the highest rate of APLS-related complications. Additionally, the anti-phospholipid antibodies are of high titre. This patient should be offered heparin or low-molecular weight heparin and low-dose aspirin as soon as she falls pregnant.

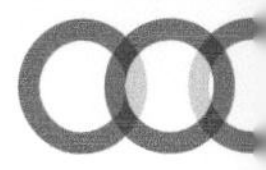

CASE 96

A 76-year-old man is diagnosed with an acute myocardial infarction and treated with coronary angioplasty and insertion of a bare metal stent. There is a past history of a hip replacement 6 months previously. He is treated with unfractionated heparin and started on dual anti-platelet therapy.

Three days later, he develops a painful leg and a Doppler ultrasound scan shows thrombus in the femoral vein. A full blood count at admission was normal and repeat blood tests are carried out.

Tests carried out after the deep vein thrombosis (DVT) is diagnosed

	Test Results	Normal Range
Hb	135 g/L	[110–160]
MCV	97 fL	[80–100]
WBC	5.1×10^9/L	[3.5–11]
Platelets	55×10^9/L	[150–400]
Prothrombin time	12 s	[12–16]
APTT	62 s	[26–36]
APTT heparin ratio	2.2	[1.5–2.5]
Anti-platelet Factor IV screen OD	1.2	[<0.4]
Anti-platelet Factor IV screen interpretation	Positive	

QUESTIONS

Q96.i What is the most likely diagnosis?

Q96.ii How would you treat this patient?

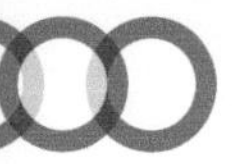

Case 96: ANSWERS

A96.i There has been a significant drop in the platelet count and anti-platelet Factor 4 antibodies have been detected. These results are indicative of heparin-induced thrombocytopenia. The development of a new thrombosis despite having a heparin ratio in the target range is typical of this condition. Generally, the platelet count starts to fall 7–14 days after starting heparin but can fall earlier if there has been relatively recent previous exposure to heparin. In this case, thromboprophylaxis would have been given during the recent orthopaedic surgery.

A96.ii The key to treatment is replacement of heparin with an alternative anti-coagulant. There may be cross-reactivity with low-molecular weight heparin (LMWH) and so better choices are direct Factor Xa inhibitors such as danaparoid or argatroban. At a later stage, oral anti-coagulation can be introduced. There is relatively little bleeding risk with a thrombocytopenia of this level and platelet transfusions should not be given. The co-administration of anti-platelet drugs does increase the risk of bleeding significantly and so discussion with the cardiologists is required to see if the anti-platelet regimen can be reduced. Often, some form of anti-platelet therapy is required in this situation and so careful monitoring of the anti-coagulation is required to reduce the risk of bleeding.

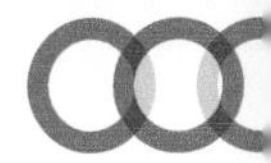

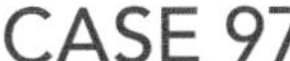

CASE 97

A 42-year-old man is diagnosed with an unprovoked proximal deep vein thrombosis. He is adopted and so there is no family history. He is started on warfarin and a thrombophilia screen is requested shortly afterwards.

Thrombophilia screen

	Test Results	Normal Range
Prothrombin time	25 s	[12–16]
INR	2.3	[0.9–1.2]
APTT	39 s	[26–36]
Thrombin time	27 s	[12–16]
Reptilase time	23 s	[12–16]
Fibrinogen (Clauss)	0.7 g/L	[1.5–4.0]
Fibrinogen:Ag	3.1	[1.8–4.0]
Factor VII:C	26 IU/dL	[50–150]
Factor VIII:C (one stage)	120 IU/dL	[50–160]
Protein C:Ac	62 IU/dL	[70–140]
Antithrombin:Ac	114 IU/dL	[79–121]
Protein S:Free antigen	46 IU/dL	[60–140]
DRVVT ratio	1.6	[0.8–1.1]
DRVVT correction	5%	[<10%]
Normalised SCT ratio	1.0	[<1.16]
Lupus interpretation	Lupus negative	
Factor V Leiden	Heterozygous for Arg506Gln	
Prothrombin 3′UTR variant	Normal G/G	

QUESTIONS

Q97.i Report these results and comment on whether there are any significant abnormalities that might have contributed to the thrombosis.

Q97.ii How long would you anti-coagulate for?

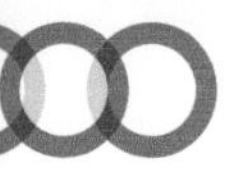

Case 97: ANSWERS

A97.i Many of the abnormalities are due to the effect of warfarin. This would explain the international normalised ratio (INR), prolonged activated partial thromboplastin time (APTT) and reduced levels of Factor VII, protein C and protein S. The raised Dilute Russell viper venom time (DRVVT) ratio is also due to the warfarin as the lack of correction shows that it is not phospholipid dependant.

This man is heterozygous for Factor V Leiden which is a weak thrombophilic defect. There is a dysfibrinogenaemia as shown by the abnormal thrombin and reptilase times and the discrepant fibrinogen activity and protein levels. Some dysfibrinogenaemias are thrombotic rather than bleeding disorders and identification of the underlying molecular defect may help to elucidate this in the absence of a family history.

A97.ii The standard duration would be 6 months. Heterozygosity for Factor V Leiden in isolation would not alter this. If the dysfibrinogenaemia turned out to be due to a strongly prothrombotic variant then indefinite anti-coagulation should be considered.

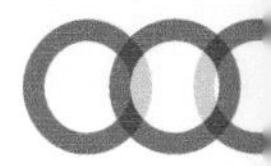

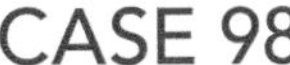

CASE 98

A 32-year-old woman is admitted with severe headache and vomiting that has gradually been getting worse over the previous week. She has no significant past medical history and she is otherwise fit and well. A magnetic resonance imaging (MRI) scan shows cerebral venous sinus thrombosis. There is no family history of thrombosis and there are no obvious provoking factors. She completes 6 months of anti-coagulation with warfarin. She is now asymptomatic and a repeat MRI scan shows residual thrombus although the overall size has reduced. A thrombophilia screen is carried out and shows a weakly positive dilute Russell viper venom time (DRVVT). Three months later, the DRVVT is still weakly positive and tests for anti-cardiolipin and anti-β2 glycoprotein 1 antibodies are negative.

QUESTIONS

Q98.i How would you manage this case?

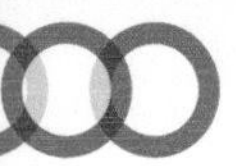

Case 98: ANSWERS

A98.i The combination of thrombosis and a positive test for anti-phospholipid antibodies leads to a diagnosis of anti-phospholipid syndrome. Note that the absence of positivity in the immunological tests does not exclude the diagnosis and the risk of thrombosis is most closely correlated with positivity for lupus anti-coagulant. The risk of further thrombotic events is relatively high in this situation and this is an indication for long-term anti-coagulation which should be restarted in this case unless there is evidence of an increased bleeding risk.

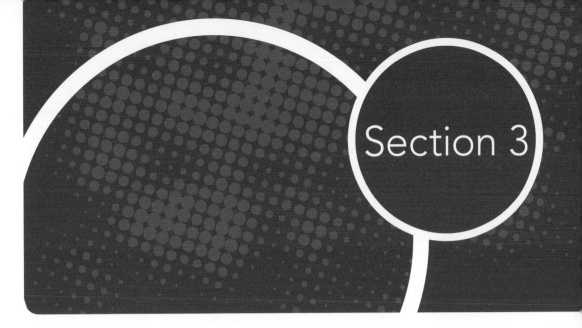

QUALITY CONTROL

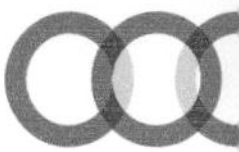

CASE 99

QUESTIONS

The results shown in the images below are your laboratory's performance in an external quality control (QC) exercise.

Q99.i Please comment on the results. What action would you take?

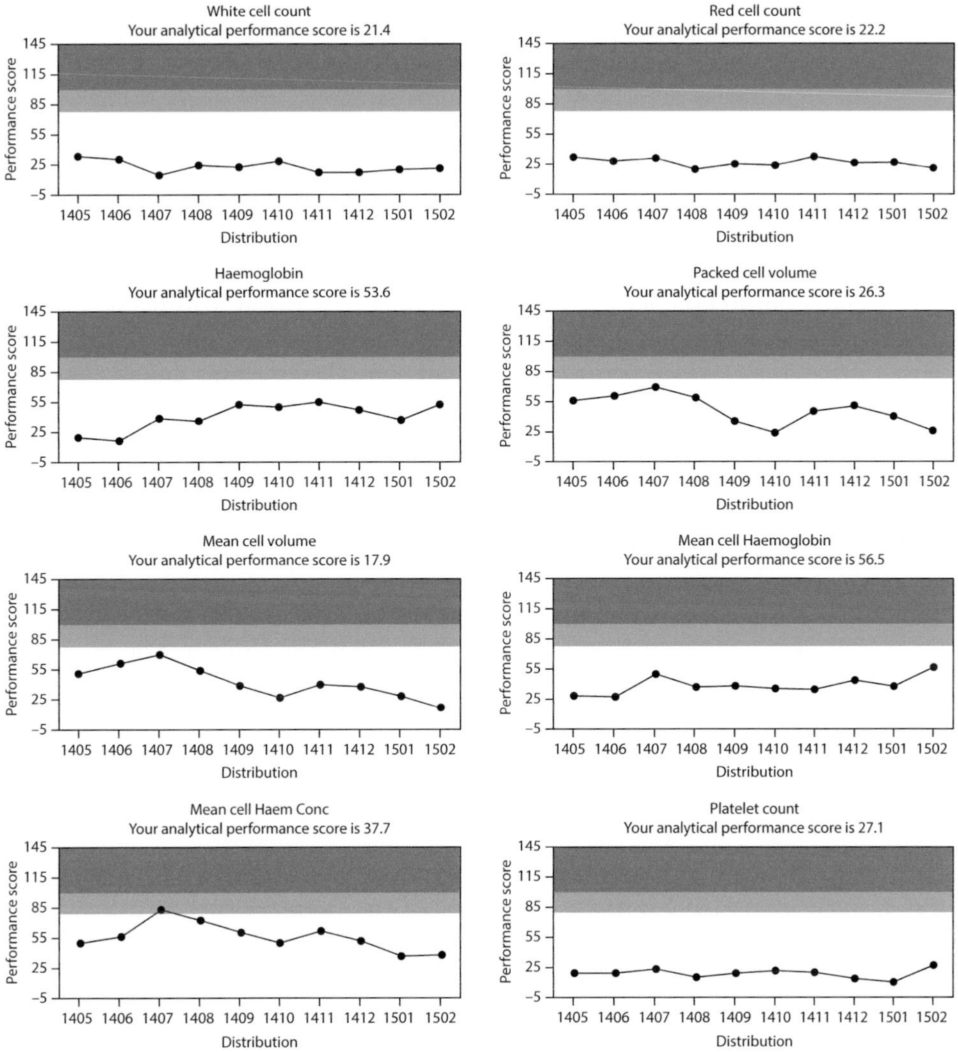

White cell count
Your analytical performance score is 21.4

Red cell count
Your analytical performance score is 22.2

Haemoglobin
Your analytical performance score is 53.6

Packed cell volume
Your analytical performance score is 26.3

Mean cell volume
Your analytical performance score is 17.9

Mean cell Haemoglobin
Your analytical performance score is 56.5

Mean cell Haem Conc
Your analytical performance score is 37.7

Platelet count
Your analytical performance score is 27.1

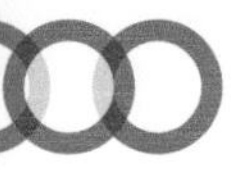

Case 99: ANSWERS

A99.i QC procedures are a central element of haematology laboratory practice. Each laboratory will have a range of protocols and standard operating procedures (SOPs) in place to ensure a high quality of service. External QC schemes play an important part in these QC procedures and are essential to gain accreditation and also to demonstrate the validity of the results produced by the laboratory. Specimens are distributed from a central source to all participating laboratories in the United Kingdom. Specialised schemes will cover the full spectrum of laboratory practice and laboratories will register for the basic schemes and the specialised ones relevant to their practice. Specimen quality can be an issue and participants are asked to comment on this. Specimens must be processed in the same way and by the same staff members as the routine samples.

Results are distributed 1–2 months after the exercise and they document the performance of the individual laboratory by expressing the results obtained for the exercise alongside the results obtained in other laboratories. The aim is not to produce a 'correct' answer but to perform 'within consensus' and are grouped according to the technical platform or test kit in use. Laboratories which perform consistently outside consensus should critically examine their procedures and will be contacted by the scheme organisers to review their performance. For specialised tests, an incorrect result will be given a red score and the laboratory will be asked to perform an investigation and provide evidence of the investigation with corrective actions to prevent further failures.

The performance score reflects the extent to which results from your laboratory deviate from the consensus for your technical platform. The greater the performance score, the greater the deviation.

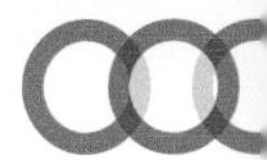

Case 99: ANSWERS (Continued)

These results show that there are several parameters – Haemoglobin concentration, mean corpuscular haemoglobin (MCH), mean corpuscular haemoglobin concentration (MCHC) – where your laboratory's results deviate significantly from median values obtained by other participants. The results for the white cell count and the platelet count are acceptable. The performance scores indicate a trend over the last 2–3 exercises of worsening performance.

You should approach the section lead biomedical scientist (BMS) and together review the QC samples performed on that day. You should review the performance of QC of all analysers and compare. If the QC is within range then review the moving average on the analyser. This will give an indication of analyser performance on the day the external QC was processed.

You should consider with your section lead BMS what is the deviation from the mean for the standard samples that you run across all the analysers. A typical laboratory will run the sample through all the analysers within the laboratory three times per week. What is the accuracy of the result obtained in terms of the degree to which the same result is obtained on the same specimen when processed on more than one occasion in the same analyser (reproducibility); when processed in more than one analyser in the same laboratory (consistency); how does the result in your laboratory compare with results in other laboratories?

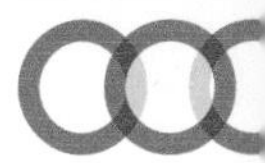

CASE 100

QUESTIONS

The example here illustrates results obtained for a haematomorphology exercise. The distributed slide will typically have been examined by a clinician as well as the laboratory scientists as this would be the normal practice for examination of a strikingly abnormal blood film. Emphasis is on recording observations rather than making a diagnosis, though participants are encouraged to offer a diagnosis.

A 47-year-old female presents with a 4-week history of gradually increasing tiredness

Her blood count shows the following:

Haemoglobin (hb)	94 g/L
White blood cells (WBC)	48 × 10^9/L
Platelets	46 × 10^9/L

Please examine the blood film and record the abnormalities on the attached sheet.

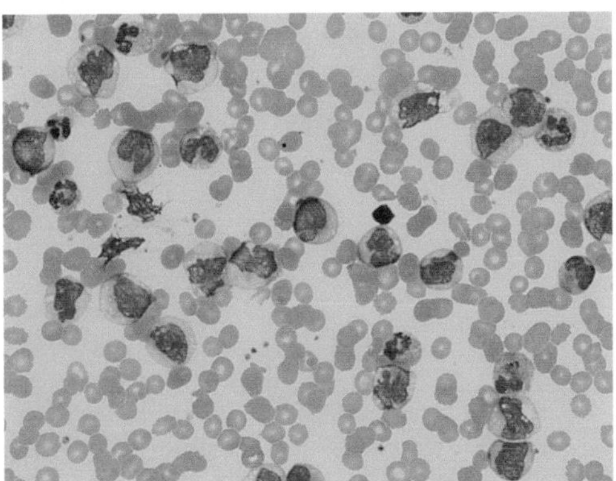

You may offer a diagnosis but you will not be penalised if you do not.

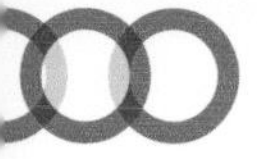

Case 100: QUESTIONS (Continued)

Red cell changes:

002 Microcytes
003 Macrocytes
004 Hypochromic cells
005 Polychromatic cells
006 Mixed cell population (dimorphic)
007 Poikilocytes
008 Crenated cells
009 Fragments
010 Nucleated red blood cells (RBCs)

White cell changes:

201 Agranulocytosis
202 Monocytosis
203 Promyelocytes
204 Myelocytes
205 Blast cells
206 Sezary cells
207 Myelocytes
208 Reactive lymphocytes
209 Basophilia
210 Eosinophilia
211 Lymphocutosis
212 Neutropenia

Other changes:

301 Thrombocytopenia
302 Thrombocytosis
303 Dohle bodies
304 Platelet anisocytosis
305 Macrocytic platelets
307 Megakaryocyte fragments

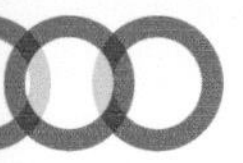

Case 100: ANSWERS

Top 5 Reported Comments	Rank	Number	Your Results	Rank	Number
205 Blast cells	1	480	Blast cells	1	480
301 Thrombocytopenia	2	451	Monocytosis	2	340
212 Neutropenia	3	401	Neutrophilia	3	6
207 Myelocytes	4	387	Myelocytes	4	387
202 Monocytosis	5	340	Nucleated RBCs	5	240

Your suggested diagnosis? Chronic myelomonocytic leukeamia (CMML).

Your performance: within consensus.

The sample was from a female with acute myeloid leukaemia with monocytic differentiation.

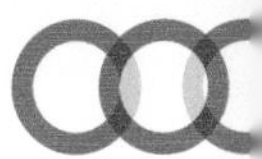

CASE 101

QUESTIONS

Q101.i A 76-year-old male on warfarin. Indication: mechanical aortic valve.

Please perform a prothrombin time (PT) and report the international normalised ratio (INR). Indicate if the patient is underdosed, adequately dosed or overdosed.

Results are shown below.

Test	**INR**
Your result	1.9
Participants in your Group	232
Reagent median international normalised ratio (INR)	1.9
% Deviation	0%
Overall participants	830
Your performance	*Within consensus*
Your previous % deviation	−4.5%
Your dosage interpretation	Adequate
Overall interpretations	
Under dosed	93%
Adequately dosed	5%
Over dosed	2%

Comment on these results.

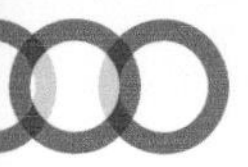

Case 101: ANSWERS

These are standard results from a coagulation exercise. The results of the laboratory tests are assessed alongside the results obtained from laboratories using the same reagents. The laboratory performance for the PT, APTT and the anti-Xa are all within consensus.

A101.i The recommended INR for an individual with an aortic valve replacement is 2.5–3.5. The patient is therefore underdosed, as agreed by the majority of participants in the exercise. The dosage interpretation, which would have been made by the clinician, is out with consensus.

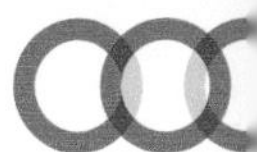

Case 101: QUESTIONS (Continued)

Q101.ii A 27-year-old female has just delivered an infant. She had a deep vein thrombosis at 36 weeks of pregnancy and has been on subcutaneous low-molecular weight heparin.

Please perform an activated partial thromboplastin time (APTT), an anti-Factor Xa assay and indicate if the patient is under dosed, adequately dosed or overdosed.

Results are shown below.

Test	**APTT**
Your result	31.1 s
Your normal range	25–35
Your test/normal ratio	0.97
Participants in your group	301
Reagent specific median	1.05
% Deviation	−7.6%
Overall participants	626
Overall median	1.10
Your performance	*Within consensus*
Test	Heparin assay
Your method	Chromogenic anti-Xa
Your result	0.41
Method n	20
Overall participants	246
Method median	0.44
% Deviation	−6.8
Your performance quantile	a
Your cumulative grades	e / a / a
Your performance	*Within consensus*
Your dosage interpretation	**Adequate**
Overall interpretations	
Adequate	5%
Under dosed	90%
Over dosed	5%

Comment on these results.

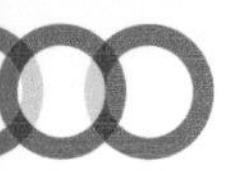

Case 101: ANSWERS (Continued)

A101.ii The laboratory performance with regard to the APTT and the anti-Xa are again within consensus. The clinical interpretation is outwith consensus, as the patient is under dosed. The result of 0.41 is just above the acceptable value of 0.4 which means that the clinical interpretation has correctly been written as 'adequately dosed'. However, the majority of participants reported under dosing and this deviation needs to be explained. Note that only 20/246 participants have used the specific method used by this laboratory. It maybe that the method(s) used by the majority of participants gives a lower overall median which would be below the required level thereby indicating under dosing. This example shows the effect of performing a test using a method that is not widely used.

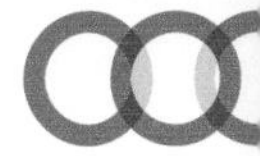

INDEX

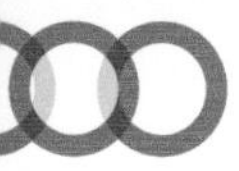

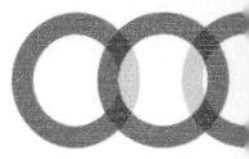

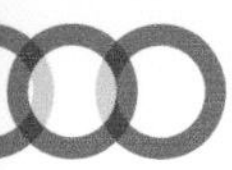

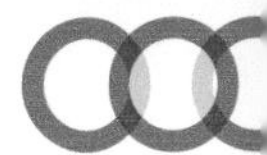

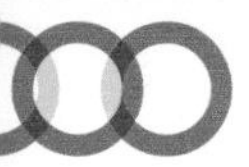

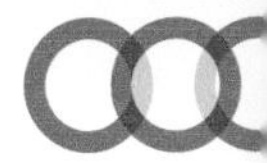